P9-AEX-733

Cystic Fibrosis

FOURTH EDITION

A Guide for Patient and Family

David M. Orenstein, M.D.

Antonio J. and Janet Palumbo Professor of
Cystic Fibrosis
Director, Antonio J. and Janet Palumbo Cystic
Fibrosis Center
Children's Hospital of Pittsburgh of UPMC;
Professor of Pediatrics
School of Medicine
University of Pittsburgh;
Professor of Health, Physical and Recreation
Education (Exercise Physiology)
School of Education
University of Pittsburgh
Pittsburgh, Pennsylvania

Jonathan E. Spahr, M.D.

Director, Pediatric Pulmonology Fellowship
Training Program
Children's Hospital of Pittsburgh of UPMC;
Assistant Professor of Pediatrics
School of Medicine
University of Pittsburgh
Pittsburgh, Pennsylvania

Daniel J. Weiner, M.D.

Co-Director, Antonio J. and Janet Palumbo
Cystic Fibrosis Center
Medical Director, Pulmonary Function &
Exercise Laboratories
Children's Hospital of Pittsburgh of UPMC;
Assistant Professor of Pediatrics
School of Medicine
University of Pittsburgh
Pittsburgh, Pennsylvania

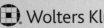 **Wolters Kluwer** | Lippincott Williams & Wilkins
Health

Philadelphia · Baltimore · New York · London
Buenos Aires · Hong Kong · Sydney · Tokyo

Acquisitions Editor: Sonya Seigafuse
Product Manager: Kerry Barrett
Production Manager: Alicia Jackson
Senior Manufacturing Manager: Benjamin Rivera
Marketing Manager: Kim Schonberger
Design Coordinator: Stephen Druding
Production Service: Aptara, Inc.

© 2012 by LIPPINCOTT WILLIAMS & WILKINS, a WOLTERS KLUWER business
Two Commerce Square
2001 Market Street
Philadelphia, PA 19103, USA
LWW.com

Printed in China

Library of Congress Cataloging-in-Publication Data

Orenstein, David M., 1945–
  Cystic fibrosis : a guide for patient and family / David M. Orenstein, Jonathan E. Spahr, Daniel J. Weiner.—4th ed.
    p. ; cm.
  Includes bibliographical references and index.
  ISBN-13: 978-1-60831-753-0 (alk. paper)
  ISBN-10: 1-60831-753-6 (alk. paper)
  1. Cystic fibrosis in children–Popular works. 2. Cystic fibrosis–Popular works.
3. Patient education. I. Spahr, Jonathan E. II. Weiner, Daniel J. III. Title.
  [DNLM: 1. Cystic Fibrosis–Popular Works. WI 820]
  RJ456.C9O74 2012
  616.3′72–dc22

                                                    2011008414

Care has been taken to confirm the accuracy of the information presented and to describe generally accepted practices. However, the authors, editors, and publisher are not responsible for errors or omissions or for any consequences from application of the information in this book and make no warranty, expressed or implied, with respect to the currency, completeness, or accuracy of the contents of the publication. Application of the information in a particular situation remains the professional responsibility of the practitioner.

The authors, editors, and publisher have exerted every effort to ensure that drug selection and dosage set forth in this text are in accordance with current recommendations and practice at the time of publication. However, in view of ongoing research, changes in government regulations, and the constant flow of information relating to drug therapy and drug reactions, the reader is urged to check the package insert for each drug for any change in indications and dosage and for added warnings and precautions. This is particularly important when the recommended agent is a new or infrequently employed drug.

Some drugs and medical devices presented in the publication have Food and Drug Administration (FDA) clearance for limited use in restricted research settings. It is the responsibility of the health care provider to ascertain the FDA status of each drug or device planned for use in their clinical practice.

To purchase additional copies of this book, call our customer service department at (800) 638-3030 or fax orders to (301) 223-2320. International customers should call (301) 223-2300.

Visit Lippincott Williams & Wilkins on the Internet: at LWW.com. Lippincott Williams & Wilkins customer service representatives are available from 8:30 am to 6:00 pm, EST.

10 9 8 7 6 5 4 3 2 1

RRS1105

*To all those patients and families who have so enriched our lives,
and have taught us so well (in the words of Si Kahn),
"it's not just what you're given,
but what you do with what you've got."*

CONTRIBUTING AUTHORS

Louise T. Bauer, R.N.   Nurse Educator and Coordinator, Antonio J. and Janet Palumbo Cystic Fibrosis Center and Pediatric Pulmonology Department, Children's Hospital of Pittsburgh of UPMC, Pittsburgh, Pennsylvania

Robert J. Beall, Ph.D.   President and Chief Executive Officer, Cystic Fibrosis Foundation, Bethesda, Maryland

Garry R. Cutting, M.D.   Professor, Department of Pediatrics, Johns Hopkins University School of Medicine, East Baltimore Campus, Baltimore, Maryland

Elisabeth P. Dellon, M.D., M.P.H.   Assistant Professor of Pediatrics and Medicine, University of North Carolina School of Medicine, Chapel Hill, North Carolina

Raymond A. Frizzell, Ph.D.   Professor, Department of Cell Biology and Physiology, University of Pittsburgh, Pittsburgh, Pennsylvania

Judith A. Fulton, R.D.   Nutritionist, Antonio J. and Janet Palumbo Cystic Fibrosis Center, Children's Hospital of Pittsburgh, Pittsburgh, Pennsylvania

Luigi R. Garibaldi, M.D.   Division of Endocrinology, Children's Hospital of Pittsburgh of UPMC, Professor of Pediatrics, School of Medicine, University of Pittsburgh, Pittsburgh, Pennsylvania

Barbara Karczeski, M.S., M.A.   Senior Genetic Counselor/Program Manager, Johns Hopkins DNA Diagnostic Laboratory, Baltimore, Maryland

Geoffrey Kurland, M.D.   Medical Director, Lung Transplant Program, Children's Hospital of Pittsburgh of UPMC; Professor of Pediatrics, School of Medicine, University of Pittsburgh, Pittsburgh, Pennsylvania

Douglas S. Lindblad, M.D.   Division of Gastroenterology, Children's Hospital of Pittsburgh of UPMC, Pittsburgh, Pennsylvania; Assistant Professor of Pediatrics, School of Medicine, University of Pittsburgh, Pittsburgh, Pennsylvania

Rebecca Mutich, R.R.T.   Respiratory Therapist, Children's Hospital of Pittsburgh of UPMC, Pittsburgh, Pennsylvania

David M. Orenstein, M.D.   Antonio J. and Janet Palumbo Professor of Cystic Fibrosis, Director, Antonio J. and Janet Palumbo Cystic Fibrosis Center, Children's Hospital of Pittsburgh of UPMC; Professor of Pediatrics, School of Medicine, University of Pittsburgh; Professor of Health and Physical Activity, School of Education, University of Pittsburgh, Pittsburgh, Pennsylvania

Christopher Penland, Ph.D.   Director of Research, Cystic Fibrosis Foundation Therapeutics, Bethesda, Maryland

Joseph M. Pilewski, M.D.   Co-Director, Adult Cystic Fibrosis Program, Medical Director, Lung Transplant Program, University of Pittsburgh Medical Center; Associate Professor of Medicine, School of Medicine, University of Pittsburgh, Pittsburgh, Pennsylvania

Jonathan E. Spahr, M.D.   Director, Pediatric Pulmonology Fellowship Training Program, Children's Hospital of Pittsburgh of UPMC; Assistant Professor of Pediatrics, School of Medicine, University of Pittsburgh, Pittsburgh, Pennsylvania

Daniel J. Weiner, M.D.   Co-Director, Antonio J. and Janet Palumbo Cystic Fibrosis Center, Medical Director, Pulmonary Function & Exercise Laboratories, Children's Hospital of Pittsburgh of UPMC; Assistant Professor of Pediatrics, School of Medicine, University of Pittsburgh, Pittsburgh, Pennsylvania

Selma F. Witchel, M.D.   Division of Endocrinology, Children's Hospital of Pittsburgh of UPMC, Associate Professor of Pediatrics, School of Medicine, University of Pittsburgh, Pittsburgh, Pennsylvania

Iris Yann, R.D.   Nutritionist, Antonio J. and Janet Palumbo Cystic Fibrosis Center, Children's Hospital of Pittsburgh of UPMC, Pittsburgh, Pennsylvania

PREFACE

I wrote this book (with a lot of help) for everyone with an interest in cystic fibrosis, whether they be patients, the friends and family of patients, or health professionals who work with patients and their families. It is designed to be of particular use to parents in the initial months that follow their child's diagnosis of cystic fibrosis. It is also written with the intention that it serve as a "refresher" course for people to review areas of treatment and physiology that they may have forgotten. The relatives and friends of a patient may also benefit from this introduction to cystic fibrosis.

An important group for whom this book is written is teenagers who were diagnosed in infancy. While teenagers grow up knowing a lot about cystic fibrosis, they seldom receive the in-depth explanation that their parents received immediately upon diagnosis. I hope that teenagers will use this book to learn more about cystic fibrosis. A final goal of this volume is to provide a foundation for understanding cystic fibrosis that will enable patients and families to understand more fully the advances that are being made so rapidly in this field.

I've tried to stress throughout this book that cystic fibrosis is a serious disease, yet it is one that can be effectively controlled for long periods of time in most patients. It is a life-shortening disease, yet it is also one in which the outlook for patients' length and quality of life has improved dramatically in a relatively short time and continues to do so. It is a disease for which there is currently no cure, yet it is one for which treatment is very effective. It is a disease that creates demands on patients and families for daily treatments; it is also one in which the efforts of patients and families can greatly influence the health and quality of life of the patient. It is a disease that is commonly accepted as inhibiting normal life, yet the reality is that most patients go to school, play sports, and grow up accomplishing all the tasks, and experiencing all the joys and sorrows, of childhood, adolescence, and young adulthood. It is my hope that patients and their families will find this volume to be of help in all these stages of life.

Many patients, families, and health professionals have responded generously to the first three editions of this book and have made suggestions that we've tried to incorporate in this edition to make it more useful. I've been extremely fortunate (and honored) to have been able to convince several of the leaders in the fields of CF research and clinical care to help with this edition. For this edition, it has been my great good fortune to be joined by two of my colleagues, Drs Jonathan E. Spahr and Daniel J. Weiner, with whom I get to work every day. Having their collaboration in producing this fourth edition has made it a true pleasure to work on and, I am convinced, has made the final product that you're holding in your hands even better than it would otherwise have been. It is the hope of all of us that patients, families, and health care workers will find this volume useful.

David M. Orenstein, M.D.

PREFACE

ACKNOWLEDGMENTS

Many wonderful people helped make this book possible. I am indeed fortunate that fate put me in Cleveland from 1969 to 1981 and enabled me to be introduced to cystic fibrosis by five of the most outstanding physicians, teachers, and human beings—LeRoy Matthews, Carl Doershuk, Bob Stern, Tom Boat, and Bob Wood. That they would then accept me as a student, resident, fellow, and finally as a partner is among the most wonderful things that one could imagine. They taught me reams about CF and life; they helped me show the importance of communication and helped me develop my skills in the use of the written word; and they showed me what dedication and compassion are. I am forever grateful to them.

Many patients and their families taught me, too, and have given me so much more than I could ever give them. Quite a few have given generously of their time to make suggestions for the first three editions of this book, and their suggestions have been invaluable.

I am especially grateful to the patients (and colleagues) from across the country and overseas who have been kind enough to let me know that the previous editions have been helpful to them. I hope the same will be true for this edition also.

Colleagues within the Antonio J. and Janet Palumbo Cystic Fibrosis Center at Children's Hospital of Pittsburgh have also continued to make my work rewarding, and even joyful. Louise Bauer, our CF nurse educator for the past 23 years, has taught us more, kept us in line, and made every day fun. Our staff of clinical nurses are amazing in their ability to handle a gazillion phone calls and eight doctors with knowledge, efficiency, understanding, and humor. Drs. Joel Weinberg and Joe Pilewski continue to amaze me with their wisdom and excellence in their care of our adult patients. Liz Hartigan, Sandy Hurban, Adrienne Horn, Judy Fulton, and Caitlin Clark make our CF research projects run without a hitch, but not without fun, for patients, families, and staff. I'm convinced that Beth Lytle, Iris Yann, and Kristen Roberts are the best CF dietitians anywhere. Melisa Kennedy organizes my office life with wonderful efficiency, lollipops, and good cheer; she has perhaps the greatest laugh in all of Pennsylvania. Janet Palumbo's vision and generosity helped make it possible for me to continue to devote my energies—and that of our entire center—to CF; she will be sorely missed.

I've been lucky in my work partners over the years; now I'm delighted that two of the most wonderful CF physicians and colleagues, Drs. Jonathan E. Spahr and Daniel J. Weiner, have not only joined our CF Center in Pittsburgh, but also have joined me in writing this fourth edition. It gives me confidence that if I should stop writing when I hit 100, or even before, this book can continue.

My parents taught me the pleasures of language and humor and showed me their gentle, loving way with people. I was blessed with the best siblings on earth, who have provided me with the best nieces and nephews in the southern (brother) and northern (sister) hemispheres. Then, unexpectedly, Alex came along and brought me—and continues to bring me—profound happiness. She also contributed some pretty terrific siblings, nephews, and nieces, all in the northern hemisphere. Finally, there aren't adequate words to describe the joy and wonder that are ours each day because of Jacob Atticus An Toan Orenstein.

David M. Orenstein

Ditto what he said. We really do have an amazing group of professionals in Pittsburgh doing their best every day to give the most up-to-date and most compassionate care to children and adults with cystic fibrosis. Thank you David O for giving me this opportunity to work with great folks and highlight what I have learned from them.

I would also like to acknowledge my parents, Robert and Diane Spahr and my wife, Laura Spahr. My father is my model for the perfect physician. My mother is my model for the perfect mother. Laura somehow figured out how to be great at the physician *and* mother thing (the complete package).

My kids (Caroline, Dane, and Elyse) are awesome. Jamie Malone, you are an inspiration to people you've never even met. And finally, Garrick Chow, you acknowledged me in your last book, so here's your payback.

Jonathan E. Spahr

My love of children and pediatrics was fostered by my father (Allan Weiner), and my interest in cystic fibrosis was sparked by my mother (Betty Weiner) who performed sweat testing at Children's Hospital of Michigan for many years. I hope that my work does honor to their memories. My mother also introduced me to Dr. Robert Wilmott, who showed me that pediatrics rather than pediatric surgery would fit best with my talents and personality. I am grateful for his mentorship over many years. I am deeply indebted to those who trained me, including Jules Allen and Howard Panitch, from whom I learned to love physiology. On their shoulders have I stood, and, without them, I would not be the doctor I am today. My patients have taught me the rewards of long-term relationships. My fondness for pediatric surgery led me to the love of my life, Dr. Aviva Katz, and together, our lives are greatly enriched by Gabriel, Samuel, Shoshana, and Channah.

Daniel J. Weiner

CONTENTS

Contributing Authors v
Preface vii
Acknowledgments ix
Introduction xiii

1 The Basic Defect 1
Daniel J. Weiner, Raymond A. Frizzell, and David M. Orenstein

2 Making the Diagnosis 13
Jonathan E. Spahr, David M. Orenstein, and Daniel J. Weiner

3 The Respiratory System 21
Daniel J. Weiner and David M. Orenstein

4 The Gastrointestinal Tract 83
Douglas S. Lindblad, Daniel J. Weiner, and David M. Orenstein

5 Other Systems 103
Daniel J. Weiner and David M. Orenstein

6 Nutrition 113
Judith A. Fulton, Iris Yann, Daniel J. Weiner, and David M. Orenstein

7 Hospitalization and Other Special Treatments 135
Jonathan E. Spahr, David M. Orenstein, Daniel J. Weiner,
and Louise T. Bauer

8 Transplantation 153
Geoffrey Kurland, Jonathan E. Spahr, Daniel J. Weiner,
and David M. Orenstein

9 Daily Life 195
Jonathan E. Spahr, David M. Orenstein, and Daniel J. Weiner

10 Exercise 205
David M. Orenstein and Daniel J. Weiner

11 Genetics 221
Barbara Karczeski, Garry R. Cutting, and David M. Orenstein

12 The Family   235
David M. Orenstein and Daniel J. Weiner

13 The Teenage Years   245
Jonathan E. Spahr, David M. Orenstein, and Daniel J. Weiner

14 Cystic Fibrosis and Adulthood   265
Joseph M. Piliewski, David M. Orenstein, Jonathan E. Spahr,
and Daniel J. Weiner

15 Death and Cystic Fibrosis   287
Elisabeth P. Dellon and David M. Orenstein

16 Research and Future Treatments   295
Christopher Penland, David M. Orenstein, and Daniel J. Weiner

17 The Cystic Fibrosis Foundation   311
Robert J. Beall

APPENDICES

A   Glossary of Terms   319

B   Medications   325

C   Airway Clearance Techniques   363

D   Some High Calorie Recipes   375

E   The History of Cystic Fibrosis   385

F   Bibliography and Resources   387

G   Cystic Fibrosis Care Centers in the United States   391

H   Cystic Fibrosis Care Centers Worldwide   411

Index   *445*

INTRODUCTION

David M. Orenstein, Jonathan E. Spahr,
and Daniel J. Weiner

WHAT IS CYSTIC FIBROSIS?

Cystic fibrosis (CF) is a life-shortening, inherited disorder that affects the way in which salt and water move into and out of the body's cells. The most important effects of this problem are in the lungs and the digestive system (especially the pancreas), where thick mucus blocks the small tubes and ducts. The lung problem can lead to progressive blockage, infection, and lung damage, and even death if there is too much damage, while the pancreatic blockage causes poor digestion and poor absorption of food, leading to poor growth and under-nutrition. The sweat glands are also affected, in that they make a much saltier sweat than normal. Anyone reading this book has probably heard about the sweat test used to diagnose CF. Most parts of the body that make mucus are also affected, including the reproductive tract in men and women with CF.

ARE ANY PARTS OF THE BODY *NOT* AFFECTED BY CF?

The list of body parts affected by CF can seem overwhelmingly long. But CF does *not* affect the brain and nervous system (it does *not* cause mental retardation); it does *not* affect the kidneys; it does *not* directly affect the heart; it does *not* affect the muscles; it does *not* affect the blood; and, except in the lungs, it does *not* interfere with the immune system (the body's ability to fight infection).

WHAT CAUSES CYSTIC FIBROSIS?

Cystic fibrosis is an inherited disorder that is present from birth, although signs and symptoms of it may not show up for weeks, months, or even years after birth. Although it is inherited, the parents of a child with CF do not have CF, and most often there is no history of it in the family. We all have two CF genes that determine whether or not we have CF. Both of these CF genes need to be abnormal for us to have CF, and CF is inherited by receiving one abnormal CF gene from each parent. Each parent usually has only one abnormal CF gene, and thus has no sign of CF at all. Cystic fibrosis is very common among white people, and is the most common inherited profoundly life-shortening disease, affecting 1 in every 2500 live babies born. One in 25 people carry a mutation of the CF gene. CF is not caused by anything the parents did—or did not do—during the pregnancy. The only way to get CF is to inherit one abnormal CF gene from each parent. You cannot "catch" CF; it is not contagious.

HOW LONG DO PEOPLE WITH CYSTIC FIBROSIS LIVE?

It is impossible to predict how long a single patient will live. It *is* possible to give some overall statistics. Just a few decades ago, nearly all children with CF died before they reached 2 years of age. By 2010, the average survival had improved to over 37 years, with many people surviving into their 50s and beyond. Some children do still die with CF, but this is much less common than in past years. For one recent year, the death rate among CF patients under 1 year was 0.007 (meaning a rate of 7 babies dying out of every 1000), for children aged 6 to 7 years, it was 0.004 (a rate of 4 children dying out of every 1000), for 14- to 15-year-olds, it was 0.015 (15 of 1000), and for 23-year-olds, it was 0.048.

There are several important factors that explain the tremendous improvement and that explain why the outlook continues to improve almost year by year. First, CF is a newly recognized disease. (It is not a *new* disease, as is related in Appendix E, but a newly *recognized* disease.) It was not until 1938 that Dr. Dorothy Andersen wrote the first medical paper describing a number of children who had died with digestive problems and lung problems. She was the first to recognize that this was not just a coincidence, but represented a single disease, which she called "cystic fibrosis of the pancreas," because the children she examined after they died all had *cysts* (fluid-filled sacs) and scar tissue (*fibrosis*) replacing almost all the normal tissue of their pancreas. The name has been shortened to cystic fibrosis, but her description helped to lay the foundation for recognizing the disease, and therefore treating children who had it. Around this time, antibiotics were becoming available, and lung infections could be treated to a degree. In 1964, Drs. Carl Doershuk and LeRoy Matthews and their colleagues from Cleveland reported the results of 5 years of a comprehensive treatment program. These results were very much improved over previous results, and most modern treatment programs use the same basic principles which these pioneers used.

In the last 50 years, many new antibiotics have become available, making treatment more effective. Further, knowledge of CF has spread widely, so that now most pediatricians and family doctors are able to recognize the signs and symptoms of CF and are able to give children treatment while it can still be helpful, that is, before there is too much irreversible lung damage. Many babies are now diagnosed within the first weeks of life, because of widespread *newborn screening* programs. Very importantly, a nationwide network of CF centers has grown up, where CF experts deliver state-of-the-art care.

The point here is that the medical world has had good comprehensive treatment programs for patients with CF for only a little more than 50 years. This means that there are virtually no patients with CF who are 50 years old *and* were started on a treatment program in the first year of life. There are more and more teenagers and people in their 20s and 30s who were started on treatment programs early in life, before their lungs were in bad shape, and many of these young adults are doing extremely well. Therefore, there is every reason to be very optimistic about the future of a youngster diagnosed and started on treatment today. Certainly, while an average survival to age 37 years reflects a tremendous improvement, it is not something to be satisfied with; but this situation is continually improving. And, for the first time ever, there are now treatments going through clinical trials in patients with CF that are aimed at the very basic cellular defects that underlie all the problems in CF. If these treatments prove their promise, they may well add decades more to patients' lives.

CYSTIC FIBROSIS CARE

Medical care of patients with CF is best carried out at 1 of the 117 CF Centers accredited by the Cystic Fibrosis Foundation, in conjunction with your own pediatrician, family doctor, or internist. Doctors are becoming better informed about CF, but it is important to be in touch with the CF experts who stay up-to-date with the quickly changing field that CF has become. These experts are found in CF Centers, and there are also many specially trained professionals (nutritionists, social workers, nurses, respiratory therapists, physical therapists) at these centers with extensive knowledge and experience taking care of people with CF. The record is fairly clear that CF patients whose care is coordinated by a CF Center live longer than those who do not attend a center. With the health care system changing, it may be more difficult to get a referral to a CF Center, but it is important to insist on it.

It is also important to continue to have care from a general pediatrician, internist, or family doctor, who can be very helpful with the non-CF health issues that arise in everyone's life.

RESEARCH AND THE BASIC DEFECT

When the first edition of this book was published just a little over twenty years ago, the basic defect in CF was not known, and the gene was not yet discovered. Much was understood about the kind of problems people with CF have, how to prevent many of those problems, and how to treat the problems that cannot be prevented. But at a very basic chemical level, no one knew exactly what went wrong within the cells of the body to cause the problems that occurred. What this meant for treatment was that the medications and therapies were all directed at *secondary* problems (problems that are themselves caused by the basic defect) and not at the underlying problem itself. Another way of putting it is that there was no *cure* for CF.

Much has changed in the past few years, and our understanding of what goes wrong within and outside the cells of people with CF has increased tremendously. The gene for CF has been found and cloned (produced in the lab); there is now a

"CF mouse," "CF ferret," and a "CF pig," created through genetic engineering, while previously no non-human animal had CF, and we know infinitely more about the alterations of cell functioning caused by CF (the basic defect is discussed in Chapter 1). There are even some experimental treatments that appear to get around the basic problem with the abnormally functioning cells. However, there is not yet a proven treatment that successfully (and safely) undoes the basic defect, and, therefore, there is still no cure for CF. This may change by the time you read this book.

The situation is similar to that of diabetes. It is known that people get sick with diabetes because they don't have enough insulin to control their blood sugar. These people can lead normal lives by taking daily insulin shots, but they still have diabetes and will have it until scientists discover and eliminate the cause of inadequate insulin production.

When the second edition of this book was published just 15 years ago, there was no national network to coordinate clinical research on new CF treatments. Such a network was not really needed then, because the increased knowledge about the basic defect in CF cells had not yet led to possible treatments. How different the story is now! The Therapeutics Development Network of the CF Foundation was established in 1997, and enables the testing of new treatments that have been developed as a result of the explosion of our knowledge of the basic defect. Tremendous progress has been made in the search for the ways to undo or get around the basic defect in CF. This is a very exciting time in CF research, because nearly every month an important piece of the puzzle is discovered and new experimental treatments come to light and enter into collaborative clinical studies. The prospects for ever better treatment in the upcoming years are very bright.

A WORD TO NEWLY DIAGNOSED PATIENTS AND FAMILIES

If you are reading this book because you (or, more likely, your child) have (has) just been diagnosed with cystic fibrosis, this is a hard time for you. Many people in your situation feel panicked, numb, or "spacey." You may be angry, frightened, disbelieving. For some of you, along with the bad feelings, there may also be a sense of relief at having a diagnosis, particularly if you've known something was wrong but couldn't get your fears taken seriously, or couldn't get your questions answered. Or, as is becoming increasingly common, you may have been "blindsided" by the news with a call from your doctor's office, telling you about the abnormal results of a newborn screening test. This may be a time when you don't want to hear any more information, or it may be a time when you want to learn absolutely everything there is to know about CF. However you are feeling, it may be a little hard to take in a lot of new information. However you are feeling, you can be certain that there have been many, many people who have experienced these same feelings. It may be helpful to talk about how you're feeling with people in the CF

Center, and in some cases with other families who have been through what you're going through now. The people in the Center can help you find such people if you're interested. As you learn more about CF, and get used to the idea that you (your child) have (has) it, and as you see that in most cases people can live quite a normal childhood, adolescence, and beyond, your emotions will become less raw and times will be less hard.

HOW CAN PEOPLE LEARN ABOUT CYSTIC FIBROSIS?

The purpose of this book is to help you learn about all aspects of CF, including how it is inherited, the problems it causes, how it is treated, and current research. Cystic fibrosis centers and the Cystic Fibrosis Foundation can provide information also. Some of you will want to plow through the book cover-to-cover now, while others may not be able to face even the first chapter just yet. But the book will be here when you're ready for it and can certainly be referred back to when a new question comes up, or if you find you've forgotten something. Encyclopedias and many general medical books are *not* a good source of information, since they are likely to be outdated. Newspapers, especially the tabloids we all see in the checkout line in the grocery store, are also not good sources, for they are likely to announce the discovery of a cure that bears little relation to medical truth. Even if you hear something that sounds encouraging on a national TV news show, be sure to check it out with your CF Center or someone who is knowledgeable and up-to-date on research developments.

There have been several instances of incorrect information—even dangerous information—being reported as medical truth on supposedly reputable news shows. In one of these instances, it was announced that CF was caused by a deficiency of *selenium* (a mineral we all need and one that most of us—with or without CF—get plenty of in the diet), and that a cure existed in taking huge doses of selenium. Several babies died as a result of that report, after being given massive overdoses of selenium. Usually, information about CF that appears in the news is not harmful and is even fairly accurate. But it is wise to be cautious about "dramatic breakthroughs" that are announced. Most often, medical progress is made not by dramatic breakthroughs but rather by tiny steps, with one group of scientists building upon the work of previous researchers. Your CF Center and the CF Foundation are informed of all the reputable work in the field worldwide and will be happy to provide you with this information.

The Internet has many sites related to CF, some of them excellent. But anyone who has had any experience "surfing the net" knows that alongside superb sources of information, there can be not-so-reliable (and sometimes even "wacko") sources. This rule holds true for CF-related sites as well. In Appendix F, you can find a number of web sites that should be reliable. As with any other information source, be sure to check any new information you're not sure about (and maybe some that you *are* sure about) with CF Center staff.

ORGANIZATION OF THE BOOK

The goal of this book is to cover all the important topics that concern people with CF and their families. The opening chapter discusses the basic defect in the cells of people with CF, going over some amazing discoveries that have been made just within the past few years. (Our co-author on this chapter, Dr. Ray Frizzell, is responsible for a lot of the exciting research that is unlocking the secrets of the cellular abnormalities in CF.) Next comes a short chapter summarizing how the diagnosis of CF is made. The respiratory system (lungs), how it normally works, the changes brought about by CF, and the treatment of the lung problems are the subject of Chapter 3. Chapter 4, on the digestive and gastrointestinal system, also reviews both normal functioning and that affected by cystic fibrosis. After these sections, there is a brief chapter on the other body systems affected by cystic fibrosis. Then follows a chapter on nutrition.

Chapter 7 discusses hospitalization and other types of elaborate treatments and is followed by a chapter on organ transplantation for CF (mostly about lung transplantation and a bit about liver transplantation), and then a chapter dealing with various aspects of daily life including day care, school, sports, home responsibilities, and travel. Exercise is considered separately in the following chapter. Next is a chapter on the genetics of CF, which describes the manner in which CF is inherited and a lot of the very new information about molecular genetics, how they determine the abnormalities seen in CF, and even prospects for gene therapy. (One of our co-authors on this chapter, Dr. Garry Cutting, is one of the most prominent experts in CF genetics.)

We then switch gears for a chapter that deals with emotional and psychological issues (growing up with CF, effects on the family of a child with CF, etc.). Teenagers get their own chapter—Chapter 13. The special problems of the adult with cystic fibrosis are discussed in Chapter 14, where we're joined by Dr. Joe Pilewski, one of our colleagues here in Pittsburgh, and the co-director of our own adult CF program. The next chapter discusses the difficult issues surrounding dying with CF. For this chapter, we've been joined by Dr. Elisabeth Dellon from the University of North Carolina, who is recognized for her work with dying patients as well as with patients doing well.

Research—past, present, and future—and some speculation about future treatments are the subjects of the next chapter (co-authored by Dr. Christopher Penland, the Director of Research Programs for the CF Foundation). The national Cystic Fibrosis Foundation is discussed by its President and Chief Executive Officer, Dr. Robert Beall, in the final chapter.

The volume includes several appendices: a glossary of technical terms; a listing of commonly used medications, giving brand names and generic names, uses, and side effects; diagrams illustrating the proper techniques for performing chest physical therapy, and discussions of other airway clearance techniques; a short but chubby group of high-calorie recipes; a brief appendix on major historic landmarks in CF; a list of CF Centers in the United States; and a list of CF Centers worldwide.

Finally, the last appendix is a brief bibliography of outstanding readings (mostly technical) on CF and listing of web sites on the Internet dealing directly or indirectly with CF.

A FINAL NOTE ON THE ORGANIZATION AND CONTENT OF THIS BOOK

Each of the chapters starts with a section labeled The Basics, which includes a few of the most important points of that chapter. Some chapters are very long and have much more detail than you'll need or want at any one time. Some of the science presented—particularly in Chapter 1 (*The Basic Defect*) and in parts of Chapter 11 (*Genetics*)—is *very* difficult to understand, and can be daunting, especially the first time 'round. Try not to be intimidated by it, but keep in mind that it's been hard even for most physicians to keep up with the torrid pace of CF research, and it's taken some of us months or years to become comfortable with these concepts.

For each chapter, The Basics may give you an idea of what's there, and you can skim the chapter for what you want to get out of it. The details will be there when you want them.

The Basic Defect

1

Daniel J. Weiner, Raymond A. Frizzell, and
David M. Orenstein

THE BASICS

1. The main problem with the cells that make up the lungs, pancreas, and sweat glands in people with cystic fibrosis (CF) is that chloride and bicarbonate (part of what makes up common table salt and baking soda, respectively) cannot pass through the cells normally.

2. Another problem is that too much sodium (the other part of salt) is transported through the cells, at least in the lung.

3. Both of these problems cause lung and pancreatic fluid to be reduced so that mucus builds up and blocks the airways and ducts. Also, sweat is saltier than normal.

4. Cell function is affected to different degrees in people with CF, depending on which CF gene mutation they have.

5. New treatments are being designed which target these basic cell abnormalities.

Until recently, it was not known what caused the various problems that people with cystic fibrosis (CF) have. One fact almost explained all these problems: Extra thick and sticky mucus seemed to be secreted by most of the organs of the body affected by CF: Thick mucus clogged bronchial tubes in the lung, blocked ducts and tubes leading from the pancreas or liver to the intestines, and sometimes blocked the intestines. One of the most noticeable abnormalities in patients with CF is their salty sweat. The salty sweat is the reason the sweat test is still considered the best test to diagnose CF, even though it has been around for 50 years. (In the sweat test, as most people reading this book probably already know, sweat is collected from a patient and is then analyzed for its salt (sodium and chloride) concentration: A "positive" sweat test is one in which the saltiness of sweat is more than three times higher than normal.) Mucus—thick or thin—has nothing to do with sweat glands, and so it can't be blamed for the salty sweat seen in patients with CF. When CF doctors used to try to explain CF, there was always that little stumbling block: "All the problems are caused by thick mucus—the lung problem, the pancreas and digestive problem, the intestine problems, and so on . . . Oh, and by the way (we'd say softly), there's the little matter of the sweat glands that seems different."

ELECTRICAL CHARGES IN THE NOSE!

In the 1980s, researchers in North Carolina made important discoveries that, for the first time, seemed to tie together all the abnormalities in CF. These researchers happened to be interested in measuring the electrical charge in people's noses. They measured what we now refer to as the nasal potential difference (PD) or, simply the electrical charge, across the mucous membrane in the nose. As it turns out, everyone has a negative electrical charge across these mucous membranes. In almost everyone, this is a small charge [−5 to −30 millivolt (mV)], but virtually everyone with CF has a much larger PD (−40 to −80 mV). The measurement of nasal PD is somewhat difficult to do correctly, but if experienced people perform the measurements, the PD result distinguishes people with CF from those who do not have CF at least as well as—and maybe even better than—the sweat test.

At the same time as the discovery of different PD in the nose of people with CF, other researchers in California found changes in the electrical charge across the cells lining the sweat glands of people with CF. Not long afterward, the cells making up the lining (the epithelial surface) of the intestines and pancreas were also found to have changes in their electrical properties that were similar to those found in the nasal mucosa. For the first time, all the organs that are affected by CF were found to have a single abnormality: The electrical charge across the cells making up the epithelial surfaces in people with CF was different from the electrical charge seen in the epithelia in people without CF.

One of the things that made these discoveries, taken together, even more exciting than they might have been individually was that they occurred around the same time as molecular biologists discovered the CF gene (more about this in Chapter 11, *Genetics*). The scientists who discovered the CF gene predicted that the protein produced by this gene was like a number of previously discovered proteins that direct the traffic of various chemicals across cell membranes. The electrical charge across membranes depends on the speed of sodium (positive charge) and chloride (negative charge) movements across these membranes. Sodium and chloride make up salt, thus we're back to the salty sweat. In the next section, we give a few more details about what we've now learned about salt traffic across cell membranes in the organs affected by CF.

MOVEMENT OF SALT AND WATER ACROSS CELL MEMBRANES

The protein whose production is directed by the *CF* gene is called CFTR (for cystic fibrosis transmembrane conductance regulator), and, as you might guess by its name, this protein is extremely important in regulating how much salt (sodium and chloride) gets across cell membranes.

Here's what seems to happen: For the proper functioning and cleansing of the lungs, there needs to be a certain amount of fluid and mucus lining the airways. This fluid comes from within the cells that line the smallest bronchi, far out in lungs, and the mucus comes from the specialized mucus-secreting cells that lie along the airways. The cells lining the smallest bronchi secrete fluid; that is, they push fluid out onto the airway surface. Although each of these airways is very small and does not hold much fluid, the total amount of fluid in all the thousands of small airways is tremendous, and is as much as 4,000 times greater than the volume of the larger airways. (This is because there are fewer of the large airways.) Since the fluid is constantly moving upward toward the trachea, eventually reaching the back of the throat, this means that the cells in the larger bronchi are required to absorb the fluid in order to keep the layer of fluid roughly the same depth all along the airway. If the fluid layer becomes too thin, the fluid cannot be moved properly (cleared) out of the airways, and, therefore, mucus builds up.

The way healthy bronchial cells secrete fluid (Figure 1.1) is that they allow chloride and bicarbonate (since the same thing happens to both of these ions, we will talk only about chloride in the rest of this chapter) to pass out through the luminal membrane of the cells (the part of the cell's membrane that lies on the airway surface, where the air flows). There are several different channels in the cell's luminal membrane through which the chloride can flow. One is opened by increased calcium in the cell and is called the *calcium-dependent chloride channel*; it may provide an alternative pathway for chloride flow to the one that is missing in CF. But the main one for chloride flow onto the airway surface is CFTR itself. Remember its name ends with "transmembrane conductance regulator," meaning that it is responsible for regulating salt and water movement across the membrane. Every

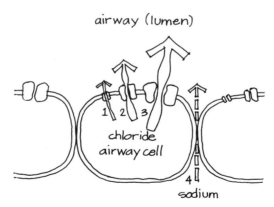

FIGURE 1.1 Non-CF cell chloride secretion. Chloride is secreted out of the cell into the airway lumen through several channels. The main chloride channel is CFTR (*3*). Another channel shown is the *calcium-dependent channel* (*2*). Yet another channel (*1*), called the outwardly rectifying chloride channel, is also present. When chloride leaves the cells, sodium passively follows, in this case probably between cells (*4*), in order to keep the positive and negative charges equal, and (not pictured), where sodium and chloride go, water is pulled, so chloride secretion results in fluid being added to the airway surface.

little chloride ion carries a negative charge, and since (as in many aspects of life) opposites attract, the negative charge of chloride pulls a positively charged ion with it, namely, sodium. There is a law here—the law of electrical neutrality—that says the number of positive charges in a solution must be same as the number of negative charges. So, whenever a negative charge (chloride) leaves, a positive charge (sodium) is pulled along with it, and vice versa. Therefore, chloride and sodium are transported *onto* the airway surface when the fluid layer is too shallow and *off* the airway surface when the fluid becomes too deep. No matter, it gets to where it's supposed to go, to maintain a very thin fluid layer, which is needed for moving out the mucus and bacteria. Fluid (water) goes onto or off the airway surface following the sodium chloride. In summary, secreting cells open channels, such as CFTR, to allow chloride into the lumen; the chloride pulls the oppositely charged sodium with it (opposites attract), and the combination of sodium and chloride pulls in water, by osmosis, to form the airway lining fluid. The opposite happens when fluid is removed from the airway surface (see below).

As the fluid moves up the tracheobronchial tree from the small bronchi (see Chapter 3 , *The Respiratory System*), the depth of the airway lining fluid is adjusted by salt secretion (see Figure 1.1) or salt absorption (Figure 1.2). Because a lot of fluid is produced in the small airways, salt absorption tends to be very important in controlling the volume of the airway lung fluid. As you can see in Figure 1.2, fluid absorption starts with sodium ions being pumped out of the airway fluid across the epithelial cells. As the positively charged sodium ion leaves, it pulls the negatively charged chloride ion, and water, with it. Sodium absorption is a two-step process, where sodium enters the airway cell through a channel (a channel that can be blocked by

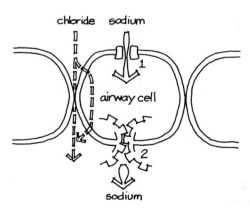

FIGURE 1.2 Non-CF cell sodium absorption. Sodium enters the cell from the airway through a sodium channel (*1*). The driving force for sodium entering the cell from the airway lumen is that sodium is actively pumped out the other side of the cell (*2*). Where sodium goes, chloride follows (not pictured). In this case, it is not yet known if chloride passes through the cell membranes or between cells. Once again (not pictured), where sodium and chloride go, water is pulled, so sodium absorption results in fluid being removed from the airway.

the drug amiloride) and is pushed out of the other side of the cell into the bloodstream by a protein that functions like a pump. In most circumstances, there's only a small force pulling on chloride to go with the sodium, and because chloride normally moves easily, the electrical charge difference across these membranes is normally small.

Changes in CF and the CFTR Protein as a Chloride Channel and Regulator of Sodium Transport

This system of airway fluid regulation does not work well in people with CF. As you can see in Figure 1.3, there are problems in both secretion and absorption of salt and water. Both problems lead to less fluid in the airway lumen and drier,

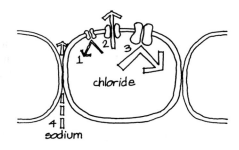

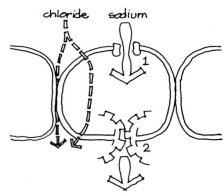

FIGURE 1.3 CF cell secretion and absorption. **A:** Chloride secretion abnormality. With CF cells, the CFTR channel (*3*) is blocked or nonexistent, so chloride cannot exit. A small amount of chloride probably can exit through the calcium-dependent chloride channel (*2*). With limited chloride secretion, there's also limited sodium (*4*) and fluid (not pictured) entering the airway lumen. **B:** Sodium absorption abnormality. With CF cells, the sodium channel (*2*) is overactive, leading to excessive sodium being absorbed across the luminal membrane (*1*), which also leads to excessive fluid absorption (not shown).

stickier mucus contents of the airway fluid layer, making it harder to move and more hospitable to bacteria:

1. The secretion problem is that the main channel to let chloride out of the cell is the CFTR protein. *In someone with an altered or missing CFTR protein* (because of having two abnormal *CFTR* genes, as everyone with CF has), *this channel is absent or doesn't function correctly: Chloride cannot easily exit from the cell.*
2. Then, the absorption problem is that the sodium channel, which is open to allow sodium to get into the cell and out of the lumen (fluid absorption), is *over*active, so more sodium (and more positive charge) than normal enters the cells and gets absorbed. This makes the electrical charge (PD) across the airway larger in CF and is the basis of the test for the nasal PD (see the preceding section). This overactivity of the sodium absorption system seems to be determined by the absence of functional CFTR protein at the cell surface.

Together, these problems mean that there is an imbalance in salt and water transport. More fluid is removed from the airway luminal surface, and the secretion that would normally replenish that fluid is blocked by absent or defective CFTR. The airway surface is too dry and mucus secreted onto the surface accumulates.

WHAT ABOUT THE PANCREAS AND SWEAT GLANDS?

The lungs are not the only organs affected by the abnormal CFTR protein. The pancreatic ducts are also affected in a very similar manner. The CFTR chloride channel is absent or abnormal there, too, and this leads to plugging of the ducts (because fluid secretion is depressed) and to eventual destruction of the pancreas. In the sweat glands, chloride (and therefore sodium) cannot be absorbed out of the gland fluid (see Chapter 5) as that fluid retains a high concentration of chloride and sodium, resulting in salty sweat—a hallmark of the disease.

WHAT CAUSES CF AIRWAYS TO BECOME INFECTED?

We have long thought that people with CF got frequent bronchial infections because their airway secretions were drier, stickier, and harder to remove (clear) than normal secretions. This explanation is supported by more recent findings related to salt movement across bronchial epithelial cells. The idea that there is not enough salt and water on airway surfaces means that the thin film of fluid that is normally there becomes dehydrated. This impairs the major defense mechanism that protects the airways from infection, namely, the ability of the beating cilia that project from the luminal membranes of airway cells to move mucus up and out of the airways to the throat where it is swallowed. (See Chapter 3, *The Respiratory System,* for more about cilia.) Each time we clear our throat, we are clearing a bit of these secretions from the airway surface. If there is too little surface fluid, which depends on the salt transport function of CFTR, then the cilia are bent over like a wheat field after a hurricane. They cannot beat effectively to clear the mucus out, and eventually it sticks to the airway surface. Normally, the bacteria we inhale stick to the mucus, but when its clearance is impaired, then bacteria build up as well, leading to chronic airway infection that is characteristic of CF disease. In addition to chloride, bicarbonate secretion also depends on a functional CFTR, and the lack of bicarbonate may make the mucus more dense and sticky. This makes it easier for *Pseudomonas* bacteria (see "Lung Infections," in Chapter 3) to set up housekeeping in the airways, and they eventually form organized colonies called "biofilms" that are very difficult to penetrate with antibiotics.

Another concept is that normal, healthy lung cells respond in a very localized way to inhaled particles, including bacteria. In ways that we don't fully understand as yet, the cells can detect when a foreign invader has landed, and they open their chloride channels to let chloride out of the cell; sodium and water quickly follow, in tiny amounts, but enough to wash away the bacteria or dust particle from this small area. If the chloride channels cannot open, the bacteria stay there long enough for the next line of defense, namely white blood cells, to be called in to fight them off. Unfortunately, as you'll see in Chapter 3, these white blood cells secrete agents that can damage lung tissue along with the bacteria they attack. Thus, when the airway cells can't wash away bacteria at sites where they have landed, the airways become damaged and filled with thick mucus and debris from dead bacteria, exhausted white blood cells, and also damaged airway cells.

There are many more details, but it is clear at this point that the lung problems are related to the abnormal CFTR and the abnormal movement of salt and water across bronchial cells. This new knowledge has set the stage for treatments designed to correct these basic defects in airway hydration.

ARE THERE DIFFERENCES AMONG THE DIFFERENT CF MUTATIONS?

Chapter 11 (*Genetics*) discusses the different ways in which the *CFTR* gene (and the protein it makes) can be abnormal. You will see in that chapter that geneticists think that there are over 1,800 different ways in which this one gene can be abnormal! You will also see that there's a lot of interest in trying to find out how (or if) these different changes (mutations) cause different problems for patients. In this section, we will briefly discuss what is known about whether different mutations in the *CFTR* gene and protein produce differences in the basic defect, that is, in how the cells work.

The way the CFTR protein seems to work in healthy cells is shown in Figure 1.4. There are four steps involved: (a) the protein is made within the cell (*production*), then (b) it has to fold in a particular way, that is, it has to adopt a shape that allows it to be transported to the cell's surface membrane (*folding*),

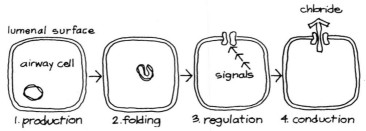

FIGURE 1.4 The four steps needed for proper functioning of the CFTR protein in healthy cells. (*1*) The protein is made within the cell (*production*), then (*2*) it has to fold in a particular way so that its shape allows it to be transported to the cell membrane (*folding*), where (*3*) it responds to certain chemical signals that activate it (*regulation*), and it does its job, (*4*) including opening for brief periods to let chloride out (*conduction*).

where (c) it responds to certain chemical signals from the cell that activate it (*regulation*), and it does its primary job, (d) opening to let chloride and bicarbonate out onto the luminal surface (*conduction*).

Different mutations in the *CFTR* gene can cause it to get "hung up" on its way to the cell membrane or not work correctly, and usually a mutation interferes with one of these four steps. Geneticists and other scientists have grouped the different CFTR mutations into different "classes," depending on which of these steps is primarily affected. For example:

1. There are quite a few CF gene abnormalities that are known (or suspected) to prevent the CFTR protein from being made at all (defective *production*). These include mutations called *W1282X, G542X, 3905 insT,* and *R553X* that are sometimes called as STOP mutations since they stop protein production. (Class I)
2. The most common CF mutation (Δ*F508*, pronounced "delta-F 508") results in the second kind of problem (abnormal *folding*): CFTR protein is made, but it folds into an abnormal shape, and therefore it is not transported to the cell membrane to do its work. In the laboratory, when researchers have moved the abnormal ΔF508 CFTR protein into the cell membrane, it has worked somewhat, but not as well as the normal CFTR. Several other mutations seem to have a similar folding problem that prevents their delivery to the surface membrane, including Δ*I507, N1303K,* and *S549R.* (Class II)
3. There are several CFTR mutations that have abnormal *regulation:* The CFTR protein is delivered to the membrane, but it is not able to respond normally to the usual chemical signals that should tell it to be active as a chloride channel (this means it doesn't open normally to let chloride pass through the membrane). These mutations include *G551D* and several others that are very rare. (Class III)
4. There are a few mutations with abnormal chloride *conduction:* These altered CFTR proteins seem to be made and transported to the cell membrane correctly, and under experimental conditions they respond normally to the chemical-activating signals. Yet, under usual circumstances, they let a less-than-normal

amount of chloride pass through the cell membrane (they open, but either not wide enough or not for a long enough time). The three most common of these mutations are *R117H, R334W,* and *R347P.* For the R117H CFTR protein, there's an explanation of its subnormal chloride current: Although this protein channel opens normally in response to the appropriate signals, it remains open for a much shorter time than normal. (Class IV)

5. For another group of *CFTR* gene mutations, for example, *A455E,* and one with the unwieldy name *3849 + 10kb C→T,* some CFTR protein is made, but less than normal. Basically, the *production* of CFTR is inefficient. (Class V)

We know less about how different CFTR mutations affect the overactive sodium-reabsorbing channel. It is possible that the changes in sodium transport will be different for each kind of CFTR mutation, but related to the level of function of CFTR for that mutation.

SO WHAT?

Only some of the CFTR mutations make much difference in how the patient is affected: Patients with most CFTR mutations have similar CF diseases. Some exceptions include the patients with CF with the last two types of problem (i.e., conduction or limited production), caused by *R117H, R334W,* and *R347P,* or *3849 + 10kb C→T* and *A455E,* who are likely to have relatively normal pancreatic function (see Chapters 4 and 11) and less severe lung disease.

What is becoming more important, especially as therapies are developed to treat the basic CFTR defect, is that if we know how someone's abnormal CFTR is handled by his or her cells, then there may be specific ways to treat patients depending on the type of *CFTR* gene mutation they have, a strategy known as personalized medicine. One example that may be useful in helping us to understand the situation is the most common mutation, which produces ΔF508 CFTR. Remember from a few paragraphs ago that this CFTR protein does not escape from the inner portion of the cell where membrane proteins are made, and it is not effectively delivered to the surface membrane. However, if a scientist can use an experimental trick to put it into the surface membrane, then it functions about one-quarter as well as the normal CFTR. What if there were a way to free the ΔF508 CFTR from the cell interior so it could get to the surface of the cell? In the laboratory, there are a couple of ways:

1. In cells growing at normal body temperature (37°C, 98.6°F), the ΔF508 CFTR protein is trapped inside the cell, but if the cells are grown at a cooler temperature (26° to 30°C; 80° to 86°F), some of the protein escapes and makes it to the cell membrane, where it partially functions. Now, it is not possible to lower everyone's body temperature by 12° or 16°F, but it is helpful and encouraging to know that there's something that can make the protein behave closer to normal.

2. There's also evidence that chemicals such as glycerol, which are protein stabilizers, can have effects similar to low temperature: The ΔF508 cells grown in the laboratory in the presence of lots of glycerol have some CFTR protein that makes it to the cell membrane. From a more practical standpoint, scientists are developing drugs that can move CFTR with mutations that impair its folding to the cell surface. These drugs are called "correctors," and they are currently being tested in patients (in clinical trials).

Drugs that target the defects in other CFTR mutations are also being devised. The regulation mutant, *G551D* (Class III, see above), cannot open to let chloride out of the cell in response to signals that should turn it on. Drugs that improve the opening of CFTR are called "potentiators," and extremely encouraging results have emerged from clinical trials in patients having this mutation who have been treated with a potentiator. It is also possible that potentiators will be useful for other CFTR mutations in which some protein channel gets to the surface membrane (e.g., Class IV or V, above) or even in combination with correctors of protein folding to increase the amount of CFTR activity. Also, other drugs in clinical trials may help some patients who cannot make the CFTR protein. These different and specialized drugs reflect the need for personalized medicine to treat a disease like CF in which so many different kinds of problems arise with different mutations in CFTR. In addition to drugs that target CFTR itself, it should be possible to slow down the overactive sodium channel, and there are also clinical trials underway with this aim in mind. A more complete listing of the drugs that are being developed to treat CF can be found in Chapter 16 (*Research and Future Treatments*) and at the CF Foundation website (look for "Drug Development Pipeline"). For example, amiloride is a drug that has been around for a long time and has been used as a diuretic (it makes you lose certain salts in the urine). Amiloride works by blocking the sodium channel. Better versions of amiloride are being developed to specifically treat the increased absorption of sodium in the airways that we see in patients with CF. Other drugs, such as uridine triphosphate, are being developed to increase chloride flow through the calcium-activated chloride channel in the surface membrane (not the CFTR channel—see Figure 1.1). The molecular basis of these channels has been recently identified, which should make the development of activators (or potentiators) of these channels easier. Thus, it is evident that there are a number of promising agents in the pipeline that target CFTR or related ion channels to improve airway surface hydration, and this is expected to produce a substantial change, from primarily treating the symptoms of disease to treating the core defect of the disease.

DOES THE BASIC DEFECT EXPLAIN WHY THE *CF* GENE HAS SURVIVED FOR SO LONG?

Scientists always wonder how an abnormal gene sticks around, over centuries, instead of dying out. That question is especially puzzling for an abnormal gene that ends up with people dying before they are old enough to reproduce (as was true of CF until just the past decade or two, compared to the thousands of years that CF has been around). In a number of different genetic diseases, there has been something good found out about the mutation in the gene to offset its bad effects. That "good" is usually something that gives an advantage to the people who carry one copy of the abnormal gene. A well-known example is the case of sickle cell disease, a terrible problem afflicting some 1 in 300 African Americans. Like CF, sickle cell disease is a recessive disorder (more about this in Chapter 11), meaning that to have the disease, someone has to have two copies of an abnormal gene, inheriting one from each parent. The parents almost always have one abnormal gene and one normal gene (as do 10% of African Americans). Having one normal and one abnormal gene for sickle cell disease is called having the "sickle trait," and people with sickle trait are quite healthy. As it turns out, not only are they healthy, but having sickle trait *protects* them from the ravages of malaria. So, if whole villages were being wiped out by malaria, someone with sickle trait would have a survival advantage and would have been more likely to live through the malaria epidemics and *continue to pass on the abnormal gene.*

For CF, a number of different advantages for carriers (parents of patients with CF and others who carry only one abnormal *CFTR* gene) have been guessed at over the years. Recently, researchers working with CF mice found that carrier mice (those with one normal and one abnormal *CFTR* gene) were protected from having the terrible diarrhea that comes with being infected with cholera. Cholera causes severe illness and death in many places around the world. The damage is done by a chemical made by the cholera bacteria ("cholera toxin"), which makes the intestines secrete chloride in huge amounts. As we have seen above, when cells secrete chloride, sodium and water will follow. Airway cells secrete into the lumen of the lungs' airways; intestinal cells do the same thing into the lumen of the intestine. A large amount of chloride, sodium, and water pouring into the intestinal lumen creates a watery diarrhea. So people with cholera become dangerously—often fatally—dehydrated. It now appears that the intestinal cells of CF carrier mice do not secrete as much salt and water after they've been exposed to cholera toxin. We know that having two abnormal *CFTR* genes makes chloride secretion very much below normal. It appears that having one normal and one abnormal *CFTR* gene may allow healthy levels of chloride secretion under usual conditions. But under unusual conditions (e.g., infection with cholera), perhaps the cells cannot increase their chloride secretion much above the usual level; that is, they can't increase their chloride secretion to the point where these people become dangerously dehydrated because of too much fluid lost in diarrhea. Since this is different from the noncarriers (who increase chloride and water secretion dangerously), it is not "normal," but since it protects against fatal dehydration, it certainly is an advantage for the CF carrier. This is an attractive hypothesis: If carriers of the abnormal *CFTR* gene have been protected from cholera or other similar intestinal infections over the centuries, while people with no "CF trait" were being wiped out, that would explain the persistence of the abnormal *CFTR* gene that causes so much trouble. (It is not a *perfect* explanation, though, since the worldwide distribution of cholera is not the same as the distribution of CF. However, the intestinal protection probably extends to other infectious diarrheas, with a geographic distribution more similar to that of CF.)

In summary, the basic defect in CF is becoming better understood. It involves abnormal transport of salt and water across and through the epithelial cells that line the airways, pancreas, intestinal tract, and sweat glands, which affects the level of hydration in the lumens of these organs. As we have seen in the airways, this determines whether mucus and bacteria are being effectively removed; in other organs, it determines whether there is blockage. The different ways in which the salt and water transport are abnormal in people with different CFTR mutations are leading to new and personalized treatments of their disease, many of which are showing promise for improving the quality of life of CF patients.

Making the Diagnosis

Jonathan E. Spahr, David M. Orenstein, and
Daniel J. Weiner

2

THE BASICS

1. The sweat test is the best test for cystic fibrosis (CF) *if* it is done in a laboratory that has a lot of sweat testing experience.

2. Genetic testing can help to tell whether a patient has CF.

3. With genetic testing, a "positive" test means the person probably has CF, but a "negative" test does not completely rule out CF.

4. If there is any question about the possibility of a person's having CF, then that person needs to be tested.

Making the diagnosis of cystic fibrosis (CF) is one of the most important things that can be done for the health of people with CF. It can clear the way for starting extremely effective treatment that will have a tremendous influence on how healthy they will be and how long they will live. The earlier the diagnosis is made, the sooner treatment can begin, and the better the outlook for the patient. Making the diagnosis will also have a big impact on the patient's family, in several ways. It will have a big emotional impact, perhaps overwhelming at first. For some families, it will actually be a relief or a vindication, since they might have known for a long time that something was wrong, yet they had not been able to discover what. (See Chapter 12, *The Family*, which has more discussion on the emotional impact of CF on patients and families.) It will certainly influence the family's time, finances, insurance, and perhaps even employment (since having good insurance will become a very important part of job considerations).

For these and many other reasons, making the correct diagnosis and making it early are extremely important. Yet in CF centers, many patients are seen who have received an incorrect diagnosis of CF. Some have had negative test results, and their families were told they did not have CF (or CF was never mentioned), when they really did have CF. Alternatively, others had positive test results and were told they had CF, when they really did not have it.

In this chapter, we'll discuss the various ways of making the diagnosis of CF, including sweat tests, newborn screening, and DNA analysis (sometimes called "genetic testing"). We won't discuss prenatal testing and carrier testing because these are covered in Chapter 11, *Genetics*.

Before a CF test can be done, someone has to think about ordering one (there must be a suspicion of CF), so we will begin with a brief consideration of who should be tested.

WHO SHOULD BE TESTED?

Not everyone needs to be tested for CF. Anyone with any of the signs or symptoms that are part of CF should be tested for it. The most important of these signs and symptoms are listed in Table 2.1 and are discussed throughout the book.

In order to make the diagnosis of CF, there must be a suspicion of disease plus a confirmatory test. The clinical suspicion is triggered by the sign or symptom that brings the patient to the doctor in the first place. In the case of newborn screening (discussed below), we will see that the diagnosis can be made even before there are signs or symptoms that would make someone suspicious for CF.

WHAT CONFIRMS A DIAGNOSIS OF CF?

To make the diagnosis of CF, most experts require a positive sweat test (discussed below) from a reliable, experienced laboratory, and one or more of the following: (a) pulmonary symptoms, (b) gastrointestinal symptoms, and (c) family history of CF.

In some cases, genetic testing that shows two abnormal CF genes can substitute for any of the items on the above list. In most cases, CF experts will be willing to say that someone has CF if the person has two abnormal CF genes.

In the case of newborn screening, most experts will make the diagnosis on the basis of a "positive" newborn screen and a "positive" sweat test or a "positive" newborn screen and genetic testing positive for two abnormal CF genes.

Let's now consider the different tests.

Sweat Tests

The sweat test has been the "gold standard" for diagnosing CF for over 50 years, and when it is done in an experienced, reliable laboratory, it is still the best test for CF. It is a superb test. It is painless, relatively inexpensive, and gives definitive answers within a few hours. There are almost no false positives (people who test positive for CF, but don't really have it) or false negatives (people whose tests say they don't have CF, but really do have it). Furthermore, in almost every case, the result of the test is positive or negative: There are almost no people who have test

TABLE 2.1

Reasons to Test for Cystic Fibrosis

Abnormal Newborn Screening Result
  Abnormal IRT result with only one or no gene mutations identified
  Abnormal IRT and gene analysis, but one or both genes are "novel" or very rare
Family History of CF
  Every sibling of a patient with CF should be tested; cousins should be tested if
    there are signs, symptoms, or worry of CF
Respiratory System
  Upper respiratory system
    Nasal polyps
    Sinus disease with radiographic findings showing "pansinusitis" (all the sinuses
      abnormal)
  Lower respiratory system
    Recurrent or severe bronchiolitis
    Severe or nontypical "asthma"
    Frequent productive cough
    Persistent cough, especially with hard coughing spells
    Coughing up blood
    Recurrent pneumonia
    Throat or sputum culture positive for *Pseudomonas* organisms
    Collapsed lung or partially collapsed lung
Gastrointestinal System
  Meconium ileus (bowel obstruction in the newborn)
  Frequent bulky, loose, oily, foul-smelling stools that float in the toilet
  Failure to gain weight, especially with a big appetite
  Rectal prolapse (see Figure 4.3)
  Liver disease
  Pancreatitis (inflammation of pancreas)
Miscellaneous
  Tastes salty when kissed
  Finger clubbing (see Figure 3.15)
  Male infertility

CF, cystic fibrosis; IRT, immunoreactive trypsinogen.

results in an "in-between" range (or "gray zone" or "intermediate range"). The test can be performed—with accurate results—on patients of any age. Many physicians mistakenly believe that sweat tests are not reliable in young infants. Some young babies may not make enough sweat for the laboratory to analyze, but most will produce enough. If a baby doesn't produce enough sweat on a sweat test, it should be repeated, either the same day or, at most, a week later.

Details on how the sweat test is performed and interpreted can be found in Chapter 5, *Other Systems*. Sweat is collected from the arm or leg of the patient and is then analyzed for its salt (sodium chloride) content. To do this, the laboratory measures the concentration of chloride (and sometimes sodium). A positive test is one in which the concentration of chloride (or sodium) is 60 milliequivalents per liter (mEq/L) or higher. Almost everyone with CF has values between 60 and 110 mEq/L. A negative test is one in which the concentration of chloride (or sodium) is 40 mEq/L or lower. Very few people have values between 40 and 60 mEq/L. (Later in the chapter, we'll talk about what to do with these few difficult cases.) There are very few cases of positive sweat tests caused by rare diseases other than CF. These diseases are readily distinguished from CF. Lists of these diseases can be found in any pediatric textbook.

Recently, CF experts have decided that the values of sweat chloride concentrations should be a little different for young babies. That is, in a baby younger than 6 months, sweat chloride values less than 30 mEq/L are considered to be normal. If a baby with a suspicion for CF has sweat chloride values greater than 30 mEq/L, then it is recommended that the sweat test be repeated or other testing, such as genetic testing for CF, be performed. The reason for this is that some young babies with CF can have lower sweat chloride values.

Once a test result is positive, it is always positive, with very few exceptions. Sweat test values do not change significantly as a patient grows older. And sweat test values do not vary when the patients have colds or other temporary illnesses. There is no point in saying: "It is positive now, but the baby is sick; let's repeat it when she feels better." Two rare exceptions to this rule are the child who is undernourished because of psychological deprivation and the adolescent who is suffering from anorexia nervosa. These children may test positive until they are treated for their emotional or environmental causes of malnutrition, at which time their tests turn negative.

Another exception with regard to the sweat test results has to do with recent, and very exciting, medications that have been developed to treat CF. It appears that new medications that treat the underlying cause of CF (cystic fibrosis transmembrane conductance regulator [CFTR]—the protein responsible for CF) have the ability to decrease sweat chloride values (nearly to normal levels). This is, to put it mildly, earth-shattering, since it suggests that these medications work to replace or repair the defective CFTR protein wherever it is in the body.

We need to stress again the importance of the experience of the laboratory doing the tests. Most CF centers find that CF has been misdiagnosed in about half of all the patients they see who have been tested by inexperienced laboratory personnel. The mistakes happen in both directions: People who do not have CF are told they do and vice versa. Sweat test laboratories associated with an approved CF center have passed accreditation by the national Cystic Fibrosis Foundation, and can be trusted. Many other laboratories are also good, but it is harder to know about those that are not associated with CF centers, as they have not had to pass an accreditation process.

Newborn Screening

Nearly all babies born in the United States are tested for CF at birth. Since early diagnosis is so helpful to the long-term health of patients with CF, all 50 states plus the District of Columbia have newborn screening. The test used for newborn screening is called the IRT. The initials stand for **i**mmuno**r**eactive **t**rypsinogen, and the test is discussed in Chapter 4, *The Gastrointestinal Tract*. For our purposes here, it will suffice to say that the test is done on a spot of blood that is taken from the baby's heel within the first few days of life. Almost every baby with CF has a high level of IRT. Different screening programs use this information in different ways: Some programs get the results of the initial IRT in a week or two, and if it's elevated, they notify the baby's doctor, who calls the family to bring the baby for a repeat test. The repeat test is needed because many babies (not just those with CF) have high IRT levels on the first test. By the time the test is repeated, the IRT levels for most babies without CF will have fallen to normal, whereas most babies with CF will still have high IRT levels. If the level is still high on the second test, sweat testing is needed. In other programs, genetic testing is done on blood spots with elevated IRT levels (more about this in the next section).

Newborn screening has its good and bad features: The good is that very few babies with CF are missed by this test; the bad is that lots of babies who don't have CF have to come back for the second test, and some who don't have CF have to get a sweat test. This means that many families have days or weeks of worrying that their little ones have CF, when it will turn out that they do not. Most families and CF experts now think that the good of getting babies diagnosed and getting started on treatment early outweighs the bad of some temporary worry for the families whose babies end up getting a clean bill of health.

Gene Testing

Gene testing is discussed further in Chapter 11, *Genetics*.

We all have two CF genes, one from our mother and one from our father, that determine whether we have CF. Both of these genes must be abnormal (have mutations) for us to get CF. If one is abnormal, we are said to be a "carrier," meaning we don't have the disease, but we carry the gene and can pass it along to our children. (Then, if we do pass on the abnormal CF gene to our children, whether our children get CF depends on whether they also get an abnormal CF gene from our spouse.)

The CF gene is very large, and there are many sites along the gene that can have changes ("mutations") that cause problems. To date, scientists have discovered more than 1,800 different ways in which the CF gene can be abnormal! A few of these mutations are common and are found in different combinations in most patients with CF; many of the CF gene mutations are uncommon. There are even some that are found in only one family. There are some patients with CF whose mutations have not yet been discovered. We can analyze blood or other tissues and see whether people have CF gene mutations of a type that has already been described. Most patients with CF have two common CF gene mutations that are identifiable on genetic testing. However, some patients have abnormal CF genes that standard genetic testing cannot find because they are rare, and the standard tests look only for the most common mutations. Since the normal structure of the CF gene is known, it is possible to analyze the entire CF gene to see if it is abnormal in any way, including ways that have not previously been recognized. Testing of the entire CF gene for *any* mutation is automated, making it much easier to identify all patients with CF from a blood test or cheek brushing.

With the testing now available for CF mutations, if we consider the diagnosis of CF and do genetic testing, finding two known abnormal CF genes pretty much tells us the person has CF. But finding one or no known CF mutation doesn't give a definite answer. It may say the chances are better that the person doesn't have CF, since most people with CF have two of the abnormal genes we've been looking for, but it doesn't tell us for sure. Also, the gene mutations that are found cannot be used to determine a prognosis or the severity of CF. While we know that certain gene mutations are likely to cause certain problems (like whether the pancreas works or not), the genes do not tell the whole story. This is evident when siblings with CF who have the same gene mutations have different manifestations of disease (one may be healthier than the other).

Some newborn screening programs automatically test all blood spots or all samples with elevated IRT for the most common CF gene mutations. Throughout most of the world, the most common gene mutation is called Δ*F508*, pronounced "delta-F 508." (Some geneticists are now calling this mutation "F508del," but for now we'll stick with Δ*F508*.) Finding two of this particular CF mutation (as happens in about 50% of people with CF in North America) pretty much confirms the diagnosis. All states test for Δ*F508*. But since different populations have different groups of gene mutations (more about this in Chapter 11, *Genetics*), each state or country may have a slightly different newborn screening program from the next, where they look for different sets of mutations.

There are some unusual situations in which genetic testing might be done instead of sweat testing. These situations might include a patient who does not make enough sweat for analysis or who lives far removed from a reliable sweat testing laboratory. In these cases, it would probably make sense to send a blood sample (or a simple painless cotton-tipped swab rubbed on your inner cheek) for genetic analysis. If the test comes back with two CF mutations identified, the diagnosis is almost certain. If the test comes back with one or no abnormal CF genes found, you won't know whether there's CF or not, and you'll have to go to a good sweat testing laboratory after all, but nothing's been lost.

Other Testing: "Nasal Potential Difference"

A very few specialized laboratories can perform a test called "nasal potential difference." This test is discussed a little more in Chapter 1, *The Basic Defect*. The test measures the electrical charge (also called the potential difference) inside a person's nose. People with CF have a large electric charge, while people without CF have much lower values. This test is probably even better than the sweat test in separating those with CF from those without. The problem is that it is very difficult and time consuming to do correctly, and very few centers are set up to do this testing.

What About the Unusual Cases?

In some cases, it might be difficult or impossible to make the diagnosis in the usual way. Examples might include a patient who doesn't make enough sweat to analyze or one of the rare individuals whose sweat test results are in the "gray zone"—neither clearly positive nor clearly negative—and genetic testing has been inconclusive. We'll assume that testing of nasal potential difference is not available. In these cases, the physician has to consider the whole picture: What are the patient's lungs like? What germs grow on throat cultures? Does he or she have abnormal sinuses on radiographs (x-ray films)? Are the stools abnormal? Is there finger clubbing? (All these signs and symptoms are discussed in Chapter 3, *The Respiratory System*, and Chapter 4, *The Gastrointestinal Tract*.) Occasionally, the physician and family will decide that the wisest course of action is (a) to accept the fact that for the time being a definite diagnosis cannot be made, and (b) to decide to treat the child *as if he or she has* CF. This makes sense because the treatment is not harmful for someone who does not have CF, but not getting the treatment could be very harmful for someone who does have CF.

Sometimes, even when you think you have made the diagnosis, it may still not be clear what to expect or what you are dealing with. Remember earlier when we were talking about certain genes that may make CF less severe? There are some genes we know of that can cause a range of symptoms from typical CF lung disease to no apparent disease at all. One of the best known ones is the *R117H* gene mutation. Paired with another usual gene mutation for CF (like Δ*F508*), *R117H* can cause lung and sinus diseases or apparently no problems. There are other gene mutations that act in a similar fashion to *R117H*, but *R117H* is the most common (and probably even more common than we know).

This *R117H* situation can be a little tricky, especially early on. The severity of the disease with *R117H* tends to depend also on other gene alterations. We label these other alterations as 5T, 7T, and 9T. The "T" stands for thymidine, which is one of the very basic building blocks of DNA. If you have fewer thymidines (5T), it is likely that the pancreas will work and sweat chloride values may be low (that's good in CF), but there still may be significant lung disease. If you have more thymidines (7T or 9T), it is likely that the pancreas will work, sweat chlorides may be *normal* and there may be no signs of lung disease. This, as you may imagine, can be very confusing. It is so confusing that even the experts haven't really figured out what to do in this situation. That is because with normal sweat test results and two gene mutations for CF, we have conflicting data about the diagnosis of CF. This is why, especially in the past, some CF doctors believe that patients with *R117H* (7T or 9T) *have* CF and others believe that they *don't have* CF.

Fortunately, we are getting a little smarter about this situation, and the CF scientific community has recognized that this "nonclassic" CF can occur. We know that the amount of functioning CFTR protein available in the body can be important for how significant the disease is (see Chapter 1, *The Basic Defect*). That is, with mild gene mutations (like *R117H* with 7T or 9T), there tends to be more functioning CFTR protein available, or at least the defective CFTR protein is "good enough" to do some of the work that CFTR needs to do (conduct chloride). This makes CF lung disease less severe. That is not the whole story, but a large part of it. Because of this, we have realized that there can be diseases related to CFTR function, and so a new category has arisen: "CFTR-related disease" or the even-bulkier "CFTR-related metabolic syndrome." Now that we have found that some people can have enough functioning CFTR to avoid having classic CF, but not enough to avoid having recurrent bronchitis and pneumonia, sinusitis, or asthma, we can begin to learn more about how to monitor and treat these people. Learning more about CFTR-related disease also helps us know more about CF in general because if we know why some people have mild disease we may be able to figure out why and how to make severe disease mild or no disease at all.

So what does this mean for people with "nonclassic" or CFTR-related disease or those who have *R117H* with 7T or 9T? What we generally recommend is that patients and their parents and doctors take a close look at what symptoms or problems might be occurring and treat the patient, and not the laboratory test. In other words, if someone is having frequent bouts of pneumonia, it really doesn't matter if they have "mild" genes. Take the stance that we will make sure that we do all that we need to do to keep the lungs healthy. For some, that may mean just checking in with the CF clinic every 6 months or so. For others, it may mean coming to the CF clinic every couple of months, monitoring growth, doing airway clearance, and aggressively treating infection (usual CF care).

The Respiratory System

3

Daniel J. Weiner and David M. Orenstein

THE BASICS

1. The lungs are the most important part of the body in people with cystic fibrosis (CF), and they cause most of the sickness and more than 95% of the deaths from CF.

2. Thick mucus blocks the bronchial tubes in people with CF, causing infection and inflammation.

3. The lung problem is progressive, meaning it keeps getting worse as time goes by.

4. With very good treatment, the progression of the lung disease can be slowed dramatically, and the lungs can be kept relatively healthy for long periods.

5. Regular treatment to keep the airways clear of mucus and infection is extremely important.

6. New or increased cough is usually the first sign of worsened infection and inflammation. If cough increases, you should call your CF doctor for treatment.

The respiratory system is usually the most affected organ system for patients with cystic fibrosis (CF). Problems with this system account for more than 95% of the sickness from CF and also for more than 95% of the deaths from this disease. In the years since CF was first recognized, treatment of lung disease has improved considerably, resulting in the tremendous improvement in longevity and quality of life that CF patients can now expect.

The three sections of this chapter are devoted to: (a) a discussion of the normal anatomy and functioning of the respiratory system, (b) an explanation of how CF changes the functioning of this system, and (c) a review of the treatments that are aimed at preventing, correcting, or minimizing the changes that CF brings about in the respiratory system.

ANATOMY AND FUNCTION OF THE RESPIRATORY SYSTEM

All tissues in the body, especially the brain and the exercising muscles, need oxygen to function. It is the task of the respiratory system to bring in oxygen from the air that surrounds us and transfer it to the bloodstream. Once oxygen is in the bloodstream, the cardiovascular system (heart and blood vessels) delivers it to all the parts of the body that need it. It is a further responsibility of the lungs to dispose of excess carbon dioxide, which is made in the process of normal metabolism. These tasks are essential to life, since all body tissues need oxygen to survive, and if too much carbon dioxide builds up in the bloodstream and the brain, it can put someone so deeply to sleep that he or she will not breathe.

The Airways

The actual transfer of oxygen from the air we breathe to the bloodstream (and carbon dioxide from the blood to the air we exhale) takes place deep in the lungs, in the alveoli (air sacs), which are located at the end of a long series of tubes. At the beginning of these air-carrying tubes, or "airways," are the nose and the mouth, followed by the throat, then the larynx (or "voice box," another name given to this area, which includes the vocal cords), and the trachea (also called the "windpipe"). As the trachea enters the chest, it divides into two branches, and each branch leads into a lung. These branches are referred to as the bronchial tubes, or simply, bronchi (Figure 3.1). Each bronchus reaches into its lung where it divides again, and yet again, forming a network of bronchi that extend into the various lobes, or sections, of the lung, the segments of each lobe, the subsegments of each segment, and so forth. Each time the bronchi branch, they become smaller and are thus able to distribute air to the smallest and farthest reaches of the lungs. (The word "branch" is frequently used to describe the bronchial system, for it does look very treelike.)

The bronchi divide, or branch, approximately 23 times before they reach the alveoli. It is in these air sacs that oxygen finally leaves the inhaled air and enters the bloodstream. Throughout most of this branching network, the bronchial tubes are referred to as "bronchi," or, for the smaller ones, "small bronchi." Toward the very end of this network, the bronchi become quite small and are referred to as "bronchioles." Bronchioles are the last segment of tubes through which air passes before it reaches the alveoli.

The difference between bronchi and bronchioles, aside from their size, is that bronchi have cartilage in their walls and bronchioles don't. Both bronchi and bronchioles need something to stiffen their walls so that they maintain their shape and, particularly, so that they stay open. In healthy lungs, there is a tendency for the bronchi and bronchioles to enlarge slightly as the chest expands with each breath inhaled, and to narrow with each breath exhaled. If breathing is particularly

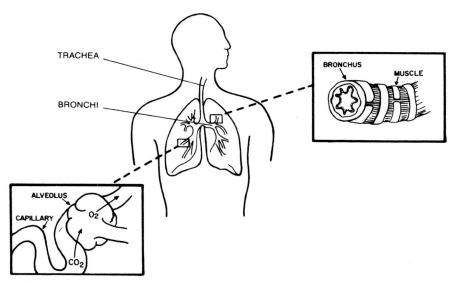

FIGURE 3.1 The lungs, including bronchi and alveoli. Note the muscles in the bronchial wall. Oxygen enters the bloodstream by passing from the inhaled air through the wall of the alveoli and into the blood cells in the capillaries.

strenuous, or if the support of the bronchial walls is not very strong, the bronchi and bronchioles can collapse during exhalation, making it difficult for the proper amount of air to leave the lungs.

In addition to cartilage, other tissues help support the bronchi. One of the most important is muscle: the bronchi and bronchioles have bands of muscle running around their walls. If a dangerous substance threatens to enter the lungs (such as a chemical with toxic fumes), these muscles can contract, squeezing down and making the bronchial opening much smaller than normal. With the bronchial passage blocked in this way, it is difficult for anything to get deep into the bronchial tree. This action protects the lungs only if it happens briefly, and only if it happens when there is a true danger. However, this "protective" mechanism can actually be harmful if the bronchial muscles squeeze down at inappropriate times.

Gas Transfer and Delivery

The transfer of oxygen from the inhaled air to the bloodstream takes place at the alveoli. Running past each alveolus is a tiny blood vessel called a "pulmonary capillary." The walls of the alveoli and the capillaries are membranes so thin that oxygen and carbon dioxide can pass directly through them. It is through these walls that oxygen passes from the alveoli to the bloodstream, and that carbon dioxide passes from the bloodstream to the alveoli. There are 20 million of these tiny air sacs in a newborn infant's lungs and 300 million in an adult. The enormous extent of these figures can be better grasped by imagining that, if you were to lay out the working surfaces between the alveoli and capillaries side by side, they would span an area of the size of a tennis court.

After oxygen has been supplied to the blood, the task remains of getting the blood to the tissues that need oxygen (brain, exercising muscles, etc.). Fortunately, there is an excellent system that accomplishes the task of pumping the blood to where it is needed. The pump, of course, is the heart.

Actually, the heart is a muscular double pump. The right side of the heart pumps blood through the lungs, where the blood becomes oxygenated through the process just described (and where the carbon dioxide is dumped out of the blood). After the hemoglobin molecules, which are the oxygen-carrying elements in the blood, are loaded with as much oxygen as possible (that is, they are fully saturated with oxygen), the blood flows back to the heart. It then enters the left side of the heart, where it is pumped to the rest of the body. Oxygen is removed from the blood by the tissues that need it. The deoxygenated blood then returns to the heart through the veins and enters the right side of the heart. The heart then pumps the blood back to the lungs, where it is loaded with oxygen once again. At rest, an adult's heart will pump 4 to 5 liters of blood per minute (1 liter is approximately equal to a quart). During heavy exercise, that amount can increase to 25 or even 30 liters per minute.

The condition can arise in which the oxygen levels are too low and the carbon dioxide levels are too high. This is called "respiratory failure" and can result from several circumstances. If someone with normal lungs is paralyzed in a car accident, for example, the breathing muscles (see the section "The Respiratory Muscles" later) could also become paralyzed and thus be unable to accomplish the work of breathing. Brain injury or brain disease, or drug overdoses, may also result in respiratory failure by damaging the brain's ability to direct the muscles to move the chest, in which case breathing will not occur. Serious lung disease can also cause respiratory failure if oxygen cannot be brought into, or carbon dioxide removed from, the bloodstream.

Control of Breathing

Among the many amazing things our body can do without our awareness is regulating how much we breathe. The main job of the lungs is to bring in the right amount of oxygen and eliminate the right amount of carbon dioxide that has been produced. This is a balancing act that is controlled with astounding precision.

In general, the more we breathe, the more oxygen we bring into the body and the more carbon dioxide we breathe out. When we exercise, our muscles use as much as 10 to 20 times as much oxygen as when we're resting, and even more carbon dioxide is formed, which needs to be eliminated. During strenuous exercise, we breathe 5 to 10 times as much air as when we're resting, and our heart pumps five or six times as much blood each minute, yet all the while the levels of oxygen and carbon dioxide in the bloodstream remain almost exactly the same! You'd think that a little extra oxygen would come in, or not quite enough, or that a bit too much carbon dioxide would be breathed out, or not quite enough, but this doesn't happen. In healthy people as well as in most people with lung disease (including those with CF), the blood levels of oxygen and carbon dioxide remain steady, regardless of what the person is doing.

This tight control is achieved by the brain's response to the two gases that the lungs manage—oxygen and carbon dioxide. Carbon dioxide is usually the more important regulator. If the breathing slows down (as it does in all of us now and then), less carbon dioxide will be breathed out and it will begin to build up in the body. As soon as this happens, the brain senses the buildup and sends the signal to the breathing muscles to breathe more, until the carbon dioxide level is back down to normal. The opposite occurs also: if the carbon dioxide level gets too low, the brain sends out the signal to slow down the breathing. Most of the time this is very fine tuning, requiring such small changes in breathing effort that we are unaware of the adjustments that are being made.

If the lungs are severely affected by disease and are not able to eliminate carbon dioxide effectively, the carbon dioxide level will build up and the brain will "instruct" the body to increase the rate and depth of breathing. After a while, however, the brain acts as though it has "gotten tired" of the message that the carbon dioxide level is too high, and it ignores the message. In its place, the brain will respond to another signal that regulates breathing—the oxygen level. It notices that the oxygen level is too low and continues sending the message to the breathing muscles to increase breathing more. It is in this way that severe lung disease (from whatever cause) may alter the way the brain controls breathing patterns. Various drugs may also affect breathing patterns, either by making us breathe more or by making us less sensitive to breathing commands, and therefore breathe less.

The Respiratory Muscles

Once the message to breathe is sent from the brain, it must be carried out. The work of breathing is done by the respiratory (or ventilatory) muscles. The most important ventilatory muscle is the diaphragm, which separates the inside of the chest from the abdomen. Since the chest wall (ribs, chest muscles, skin, etc.) is relatively firm, when the diaphragm contracts and moves downward, it leaves more space inside the chest for the lungs to expand. This action creates a vacuum inside the chest, and air rushes into the trachea and bronchi (through the nose and/or mouth) and fills that extra space. When it is time to breathe out, most of the force comes as the lungs and the chest wall just naturally spring back into their usual resting size. With hard breathing, exhalation gets a boost from the expiratory muscles, which include the abdominal muscles, the muscles between the ribs, and some muscles in the neck. During very hard breathing, inhalation gets extra help, too (even the tiny muscles that widen the nostrils contribute to inhalation). All of these muscles are called the "accessory muscles of respiration," since they are helpful, but are not absolutely necessary for normal quiet breathing. It is possible to see these muscles at work during hard breathing: when the muscles between the ribs (the intercostal muscles) are used, the skin seems to sink in between the ribs (this is called "retracting"), and when the neck or abdominal muscles are used, they stick out prominently. If the nose muscles are pitching in, you can see the nostrils widening, a sign called "nasal flaring," or simply "flaring."

Lung Defenses

The air we breathe has an abundance of potentially harmful elements in it (in addition to the good), such as cigarette smoke, pollution, dust, bacteria, viruses, and other germs. And yet, in most people, the lungs stay fairly clean, remaining unclogged by these substances and free from infection. This is the result of a very efficient lung protection system at work.

The Nose and the Mouth

The defense of the lungs begins in the nose and the mouth. Many of the largest particles breathed in get trapped here, especially in the hairs of the nose.

However, some of the smaller particles do make it past the air conditioning and filtering system of the nose and mouth and reach the trachea or bronchi. When they reach the bronchi, they get stuck in the mucus that lines the airways. Fortunately, the lung defenses are very active in these lower airways and can remove small particles through coughing, and through the action of the mucociliary escalator (see later).

Cough

A cough is an explosive release of air from the lungs. It is something we can do voluntarily, but it can also happen without our conscious control. The steps to producing a cough begin with the stimulation of nerves in the nose, throat, trachea, bronchi, or diaphragm. Some of these nerves can be triggered by pressure, others by noxious chemicals, and others by being touched by inhaled particles. Once the cough signal is sent out, there is a deep breath in, followed by a sudden forcible attempt to breathe out at a time when the upper portion of the airway (around the vocal cords) is tightly shut. Since air cannot get out through this closed door, pressure builds up within the lung. Then, after about one-fifth second, the upper airway suddenly opens and the air bursts out at a speed reaching 600 miles per hour! This burst of air is very effective in carrying mucus (with its trapped particles of dirt or bacteria) to at least as far as the back of the throat, where it can be spit out or swallowed into the stomach. This tremendous air force is effective only in the largest bronchi and trachea, for the air moves much more slowly in the smaller bronchi farther out in the lungs. Coughing is therefore not an effective method for mucus clearance in the smaller bronchi, and another action is used, which involves the mucociliary escalator.

The Mucociliary Escalator

Many of the cells lining the trachea and bronchi have tiny hairlike projections, called "cilia." A thin layer of fluid bathes these cilia and reaches partway up their length but not to their tips (Figure 3.2). Resting atop the cilia—and atop the fluid layer—is a blanket of mucus, which has been produced by special glands within the bronchi and bronchioles. This layer of mucus protects the airways by trapping substances that might be harmful to the lungs and removing them through the action of the cilia. The cilia beat approximately 1,200 times per minute in a coordinated action that sweeps the mucus (and everything trapped in the mucus) toward the largest bronchi. When the mucus reaches the large central bronchi, it is carried up the trachea in a movement that is similar to that of an escalator. Hence, this system is sometimes referred to as the mucociliary escalator. When the mucus reaches the top of the trachea (the back of the throat) it is swallowed, usually without our being aware of it. This amazing escalator clears about two teaspoons of mucus each day. Cigarette smokers and others with extra mucus are often aware of the mucus that has been carried to the back of the throat. If there is an especially large amount, or if it is particularly thick, it may be coughed up once it gets to the large central bronchi. Once it is coughed up, it can be spit out, or it can be swallowed down into the stomach, sending it on its way through the digestive tract, where it will do no harm. The functioning of this wonderful airway-cleaning

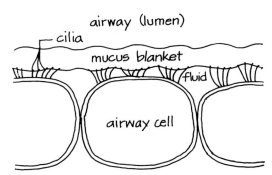

FIGURE 3.2 Cilia project into the airway from atop airway cells. The cilia are bathed in airway fluid almost—but not quite—to their tips. Above the fluid, and just at the tips of the cilia, is a blanket of mucus and trapped inhaled particles.

escalator depends in part on the composition of the mucus, in part on the composition of the fluid layer, and in part on other factors. If the mucus is too thick and dry and sticky, it may be hard for the delicate cilia to move. If the fluid layer is too shallow, the cilia may not stand up straight enough to be effective. As you've seen in Chapter 1, the composition of the fluid lining the airway is controlled in part by the protein (CFTR) made under the direction of the CF gene. This protein helps regulate both secretion of fluid and salt from the airway cells into the airway and absorption of fluid and salt from the airway back into the cells. Abnormal CF genes—as everyone with CF has—make for defects in this CFTR protein, which in turn makes for abnormal secretion and absorption of salt and water by these cells, almost certainly leading to abnormal fluid, and very likely interfering with the functioning of the mucociliary escalator.

Other Protection Against Lung Infection

It is thought that airway cells may be able to sense when they are touched by inhaled particles (including bacteria). The theory goes that when they sense an "invader," they suddenly secrete a burst of fluid that attacks or washes away the invader. If this doesn't happen (e.g., if there is a defect in the ability of the cells to secrete fluid—as seems to be true of CF airway cells), then bacteria may not be removed immediately, or not completely, by the mucociliary route. When this happens, further steps are taken to protect the lungs. One such step is the delivery of **white blood cells** to the area where there are foreign substances and bacteria. These blood cells work in two ways: they can completely surround the bacteria and other particles, capturing them within the blood cells. Then, when the blood cell is removed from the lung, the bacteria or other particles are removed also. They can also release chemicals that attack and destroy the bacteria. These are potent chemicals, some of which degrade structural proteins of the bacteria, and are called "proteases" (the -ase ending means "breaks down"). A particular one of these proteases is called elastase, and its main target is elastin, an important structural protein. It is unfortunate but true that these proteases can also attack proteins that make up airway cells—not just bacterial proteins. The lungs have a finely tuned system that produces antiproteases to keep the proteases in check and to prevent degradation of proteins that are important for the structure of the airways.

There are certain proteins in the blood that also protect the lungs against infection. Immunoglobulins, also known as antibodies, are part of a system that recognizes and attacks materials that are foreign invaders in all parts of the body. Other proteins that can fight infections include the "defensins," named for their role in defending the body against infection, and "cathelicidins."

Another factor that influences infection in the airways is how tightly bacteria stick to airway cells. The stickiness of these cells seems to be related in part to the electrical charge on the surface of the cells.

THE RESPIRATORY TRACT IN CYSTIC FIBROSIS

The Upper Respiratory Tract

There are two major differences between the normal upper respiratory tract and that in people with CF. The first difference is in the condition of the sinuses and has relatively little to do with the person's health or day-to-day comfort. The second difference is the presence of nasal polyps, which affects only about 20% of people with CF.

The Sinuses

The sinuses of people with CF almost always look abnormal in x-rays. In the x-rays, the sinuses appear as though they are badly diseased, indicating a condition called "pansinusitis" (-itis meaning "inflamed," pan- meaning "all"; thus, "all the sinuses are inflamed"). It is useful to understand the meaning of the appearance of pansinusitis on sinus x-rays for several reasons. First, because it is very unusual to find in children, except in children with CF, the appearance of pansinusitis on the sinus x-rays may help make the diagnosis of CF. Second, the appearance of the x-ray will suggest that problems such as headaches may be due to sinus inflammation. However, in children with CF, this is rarely the case. There may be some sinus infection, but this, too, is relatively uncommon. (Sinus infections are discussed in more detail later: "Infections of the Upper Respiratory Tract.")

At some point a child may have skull x-rays or a head computed tomographic (CT) scan taken, and if the child has CF, the x-rays will most likely show abnormal sinuses. It is important for parents to know that the appearance of sinus abnormality is primarily a problem with the x-ray, that (in the absence of symptoms) it is not something that bothers the child, and that nothing needs to be done about it.

Typically, treatment is not needed for the sinuses in people with CF. Some patients—particularly adults—with CF may have sinus infections that actually cause discomfort. In these cases, antibiotics might be helpful, but this is relatively uncommon. In rare cases, CF patients with repeated or persistent sinus problems may benefit from surgery to help the sinuses drain better. However, there is little evidence that sinus surgery is of any use to the majority of patients with CF. If a specialist who is not very experienced with CF suggests surgery for the sinuses, a second opinion should be sought.

The Nose

About 20% of patients with CF at one time or another will have nasal polyps. Polyps are growths of extra tissue that form in various parts of the body. The formation of polyps in the nose occurs much more commonly in patients with CF than in people who don't have CF. In fact, this can be another diagnostic clue: if a child has a nasal polyp, this is a strong indication that she or he has CF. Nasal polyps are also found in people who don't have CF, especially in those who have many allergies. In children, however, it is very uncommon to find nasal polyps, except in those with CF.

Generally, having a nasal polyp is not a major problem. It is never life-threatening, and it never becomes cancerous the way other polyps can in people without CF. What it may do is block up one side of the nose. When there is one polyp, there are often others, and both sides of the nose may become blocked. Rarely, they become so large that they can protrude from the nostril. In either of these cases (when the polyp blocks the nose or sticks out of the nostril), it is a nuisance but not a threat to the person's health. Since it is usually a significant nuisance at this point, it is advisable to have the polyps removed. One other instance in which it is wise to remove polyps is when, after some time, the bridge of the nose grows wider in response to the increasing size of the polyps inside the nose.

It is not yet known why 20% of patients with CF do get polyps, why most people without CF don't get polyps, or why some patients with CF get a polyp once, whereas others get them often.

Treatment of Nasal Polyps

Polyps are strange growths that have a mysterious course of development. They frequently get larger or smaller without treatment, making it difficult to tell whether medications are effective. If a polyp gets smaller after medication, one can't be sure that it wouldn't have gotten smaller on its own. Nonetheless, some medications, such as nasal steroid sprays (see Appendix B), may help shrink polyps.

If the medicines don't work, and if the polyp is completely blocking one or both nostrils, or protruding from the nostril, or is widening the outside of the nasal bridge, then surgery to remove the polyp or polyps (polypectomy) is advisable. This surgery is best done by an ear, nose, and throat surgeon familiar with CF, in the hospital, and under general anesthesia. Simple polypectomy (just removing the polyps the surgeon sees in the nose) or a more extensive procedure called "functional endoscopic sinus surgery" (FESS) can be done. With the FESS, the surgeon uses an endoscope [a tube for looking (-scope) into (endo) things] to enable him or her to see further into the sinuses to get to the roots of some of the polyps. It is not clear yet whether the more extensive procedure actually gives better results. In most cases, a very short (overnight) hospital stay is all that is needed for either procedure. After the surgery, the nose is packed with gauze for several hours to make sure any bleeding has stopped, and once the gauze is removed, the patient can go home. In older patients, the simple polypectomy procedure may even be done in the surgeon's office, with local anesthetic. Most often, CF physicians, surgeons, patients, and families feel more comfortable if the surgery is done in the hospital, while the patient is asleep under a general anesthetic.

Surgery is very effective in removing the polyps, and once they are gone, they may never reappear. In some people, though, they may come back, once, twice, or many times.

The Lower Respiratory Tract (the Lungs)

More than any other factor, the lungs determine the health and life span of the large majority of patients with CF. In little more than one generation, the greatly improved treatment of the lungs has transformed the outlook for infants with CF from one consisting of a few difficult months to one entailing many bright years. Infants with CF are born with lungs that appear normal, but, at varying times after birth, they begin to develop problems. In some, these problems may become noticeable within the first weeks, whereas in others, it may take years or even decades before any problems become apparent. Without treatment, lung problems will eventually appear in everyone with CF and the problems will progress. With treatment, this progression can be slowed, in some, almost to a halt.

The problems in the lungs can almost certainly be blamed on the abnormal movement of salt and fluid through the airway cell membranes. This abnormal traffic of salt and fluid and the abnormal electric charge associated with it (see Chapter 1) are caused by the abnormal CFTR protein whose production was dictated by the two abnormal CF genes that everyone with CF has. The salt and fluid problem leads to dry, sticky mucus clogging the smallest airways (the bronchioles). In turn, the mucus plugging leads to infection and inflammation. Infection and inflammation of those bronchioles is called "bronchiolitis." The inflammation then readily spreads to the larger airways, the bronchi (bronchitis). If the mucus is too dry and sticky (or the cilia too bent over) then the normal mechanisms, such as the mucociliary escalator, may not clear that mucus, and it becomes very easy for germs (viruses and bacteria) to take hold, making it hard for the lungs and body defenses to combat them. (In addition, it may be that other factors related to the abnormal electrical environment make it easier for certain bacteria to take hold in the CF airway.)

The more inflammation there is within the bronchi and bronchioles, the more swelling there is (Figure 3.3), and the narrower the opening becomes to these airways, or, said another way, the greater the bronchial (and bronchiolar) obstruction. With increasing obstruction it becomes more difficult for air to move in and out, which forces the respiratory muscles to work harder. Also, when the airways become obstructed, it is difficult to clear them of mucus. Other mucus-clearing mechanisms, especially cough, are then used more frequently to force the mucus up and out of the bronchioles and bronchi. ***Increased cough is often the first sign that the bronchial infection and inflammation are getting out of control.***

If the bronchial and bronchiolar infection and inflammation remain out of control for too long, they can damage the bronchioles and bronchi. Bacteria can cause direct damage to the bronchial walls, and the body's response to the bacteria can cause even more damage: you've seen earlier ("Other Protection Against Lung Infection") that white blood cells are sent to kill bacteria. These white blood cells release chemicals that cause inflammation to attack and destroy the bacteria. Unfortunately, these chemicals (sometimes called "mediators of inflammation," including proteases like elastase—see earlier) cannot distinguish between

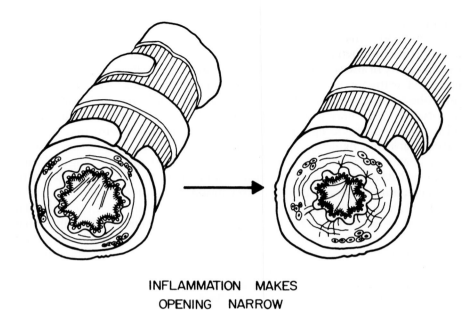

INFLAMMATION MAKES
OPENING NARROW

FIGURE 3.3 Inflammation within the bronchi makes the bronchial opening ("lumen") smaller.

bacteria and airway tissue, and they can also damage the cells lining the airways. In recent years, we've come to understand that this damage from inflammation from our own white blood cells is just as harmful as—or even more harmful than—the harm from the bacteria (which also release chemicals that cause inflammation). If the damage to the airways continues, it can weaken their walls so that they become floppy, and the airways enlarge (dilate)—this is referred to as *bronchiectasis* (abnormal dilatation in the airways). If the lung damage progresses, it can lead to permanent changes such as infected cysts and scar tissue (*fibrosis*), which are indicated by the name of this disease.

The progression of lung damage is most often very slow and subtle but it can be relentless. This is why the lung disease of CF is often referred to as "progressive"— if left on its own (and even in the majority of cases with treatment), it gets worse and worse. If this progression of infection, inflammation, and lung destruction continues uninterrupted for too long, it will eventually reach a point where there is no longer enough healthy lung to bring oxygen into the body or to eliminate carbon dioxide.

As a particular episode of increased infection and inflammation develops, or as the lung disease increases over the years, the following progression occurs: first, there is more cough. Someone who usually doesn't cough at all may develop a mild cough for a few minutes in the morning, or someone who coughed only in the morning may now cough during the day or through the night. Morning is a common time for people with CF to cough, since they have been in one position for many hours, making it easier for the lung mucus to stay down in the lungs. During the day, when people are active and breathing harder, mucus is more easily shaken loose and sent on its way out of the lungs.

Along with increased cough (and part of its cause) there is often an increase in lung mucus production and an increase in *sputum* (mucus that is coughed up and spit out of the lungs): the patient is more likely to feel "crud" in the lungs that feels like it needs to come up. The airways now contain mucus made by the bronchial glands and increasingly large amounts of other material. This other material includes DNA (genetic material contained in all cells) that has been released from white blood cells (*neutrophils*) that have died fighting the bronchial infection. There is also a stringy substance called actin. The neutrophil DNA and the actin account for a lot of the thickness of CF sputum. There are also numerous dead bacteria and old airway cells that contribute to the thickness and stickiness of CF airway secretions.

With the progression of the lung disease, patients often have decreased exercise tolerance, with quicker tiring and even some shortness of breath (difficulty breathing).

As the particular episode of infection and inflammation subsides—on its own or with treatment—the symptoms also subside, either fully or partly, depending on whether any new lung damage has been caused. The goal of treatment is to get back to the baseline (the condition prior to the onset of the problem) after each episode of worsening (*exacerbation*) of lung infection. This is often, but not always, possible.

Asthma

Asthma affects people with or without CF and is a condition in which the muscles that surround the bronchi squeeze down readily. This ability of the muscles to tighten and make the opening of the bronchi smaller is basically a protective mechanism (see earlier, "The Airways"), since it can prevent dangerous substances that have been breathed in (*aspirated*) from getting deep into the lungs. But if bronchial wall muscles go into spasm (*bronchospasm*) when there isn't a real threat to the lungs, the end result is that this "protective" mechanism does more harm than good. The bronchi become partly squeezed shut, making it difficult to move mucus out and to breathe air in and out. The airways also become inflamed in people with asthma. When the bronchi are narrowed from bronchospasm and inflammation, there is often a characteristic whistling sound to the breathing. This sound is called *wheezing* and is heard especially when someone breathes out.

Asthma episodes can be related to allergies, infections, exercise, cold air, or to breathing irritating substances such as cigarette smoke or air pollution. In some babies, a condition known as *gastroesophageal reflux* ("GE reflux," simply "reflux," or "GER") can also cause bronchospasm (see Chapter 4, *The Gastrointestinal Tract*). Between 10% and 40% of patients with CF also have asthma.

Infections of the Respiratory Tract

This subject can be confusing since there are many different kinds of respiratory infections (which may or may not present serious problems for people with CF), and it is not always clear which are the potentially dangerous ones and which are merely a nuisance.

Infections of the Upper Respiratory Tract

Sinusitis

Sinusitis is an inflammation of the sinuses, usually caused by infection. This is not often a problem for children with CF, even though sinus x-rays always look as though there is an active sinus infection. Many people attribute their cough (or their child's cough) to sinus problems ("mucus drips down my throat and makes me cough"), and this may be, but much more of the cough in people with CF is caused by lung (bronchial) infection. Some patients—mostly adults—do have bothersome sinus problems. Symptoms of sinusitis may include nasal drainage, headache (especially from the frontal sinuses), facial pain, low-grade fever, and cough. Sinusitis symptoms can usually be controlled with antibiotics. In a very few patients, sinus surgery may be able to allow the sinuses to drain better and prevent recurrent sinus infections.

Colds

Colds are often referred to as "URIs," for *upper respiratory infections*. Everyone gets colds and has experienced firsthand what they are: They are infections of the nose and throat that may produce mucus in the nose, sneezing, and a sore throat. The person with a cold feels generally bad. There may or may not be a fever. Fairly often there is some cough, and scientists don't agree about the cause of the cough. Some say that the cough means that there is inflammation in the trachea and bronchi, as well as in the nose and throat, whereas others say that it results from nose (or sinus) mucus dripping down the back of the throat and tickling the nerves that activate the cough.

Colds are caused by viruses. The main source of cold viruses is other people. People catch colds from other people who have the cold viruses in their noses and throats. The closer the contact with the infected secretions, the easier it is to catch cold. Sneezing on someone is probably one way to give that person your cold, but the most common way the cold virus is passed around is from one person's respiratory secretions to his or her hand, to the next person's hand, and to that person's mucous membranes in the nose or the eyes. Despite what everyone's grandmother has said, *you do not get colds from going out without your galoshes* or from playing in the snow, or from being outside in cold weather! In fact, it's probably safer to be outside during cold weather than inside, where there is less ventilation and closer contact with people who might have cold viruses in their noses and on their hands. During the fall and winter seasons, children in day care or school are almost constantly in contact with cold viruses and are likely to carry those viruses home with them to share with the whole family.

AVOIDING COLDS

Unfortunately, there is little that can be done to avoid catching colds. It is possible to try to avoid colds by staying away from all public places, such as shopping malls, church or synagogue, and school. However, even this will not be effective in avoiding all contact with the cold viruses. While it is probably sensible to avoid snuggling with someone who has a terrible cold, this also won't do the trick completely, since people can have the cold viruses—and pass them on—*before* they feel sick with a cold themselves. If you have a cold, you can help prevent passing it on to others by washing your hands regularly (especially with an alcohol-based hand gel) and coughing into your sleeve or elbow rather than into your hands.

Most colds for people with CF are no worse than colds for other people: You feel miserable, but they do not damage the lungs and they have no long-lasting consequences. Some colds definitely can lead to bronchial infection and can be serious, especially in infants, whose bronchi are tiny and therefore harder to clear of infection. Bronchial infections can be more serious than an infection that stays in the nose and the throat, but most often bronchial infections can be successfully treated. In some cases, it may actually be helpful to get a cold: when we are exposed to viruses, our body's immune system produces antibodies that will prevent infections with these same viruses when we are exposed to them at another time. Many infections are more severe later in life, so it's good to get them early and get them over with. Mumps and chickenpox are viral infections that are more severe in adults than in children, but fortunately, almost nobody has to get these infections now in childhood or adulthood because we have such good vaccines to prevent them. Unfortunately, we don't yet have a cold virus vaccine. This doesn't mean that people with CF should try to get as many colds as possible. It just means that it's not worth losing sleep worrying about colds, and no one should disrupt the patient's or family's life in attempting to avoid all colds.

Infections of the Lower Respiratory Tract

Colonization and Infection

Most patients with CF have some bacteria in their lungs most of the time (people without CF do not). Whether the bacteria are merely colonizing the lungs (i.e., the bacteria are there and have set up colonies but aren't causing any inflammation or destruction) or whether there is actual infection (i.e., bacteria are present and the body has set up an inflammatory reaction to those bacteria, possibly with tissue damage) may be hard to say at any one time. Recent studies have shown that some patients with CF may have bronchial inflammation even without any bacteria or viruses present, and most CF scientists believe that there is actual infection in the airways of most patients with CF most of the time, but the infection is kept fairly well controlled by the body's own defenses most of the time.

Bronchiolitis

Bronchiolitis (infection and inflammation of the bronchioles) is most commonly seen during the winter months in babies, with or without CF, and is most often caused by viruses. The most common cause of bronchiolitis in infants is respiratory syncytial virus (RSV). As many as 25 babies in 100 without CF will get bronchiolitis in the first 2 years of life. Babies with bronchiolitis may cough and wheeze, become very sick, and need extra oxygen. They may tire to the point of being unable to breathe independently and require assisted ventilation, also called "mechanical ventilation." Both of these terms mean that a machine is used to do the work of breathing for the baby by blowing air and oxygen into the baby's lungs. Of course, like most other infections, bronchiolitis can also be a mild disease and can cause just a little cough and wheezing. Many infants with CF have bronchiolitis as the first sign of a lung problem.

Bronchitis

"Bronchitis" (infection and inflammation of the bronchi) is a term that is often used incorrectly to refer to a cough that has no obvious cause. Many children and adults with CF have true bronchitis, which is caused by bacteria or viruses. As was mentioned above, bronchiolitis and bronchitis are the main types of infection that affect the lungs of people with CF. It is these infections that, if not controlled, can lead to lung damage and scarring (fibrosis). Therefore, controlling the episodes of increased infection and inflammation in the bronchi is the most important part of the treatment of someone with CF. The more the lung damage can be prevented or delayed in someone with CF, the better and longer that person's life is likely to be.

Pneumonia

Pneumonia occurs when bacteria, or the blood cells sent to fight bacteria, get into the air sacs (alveoli) or in the lung tissue between the sets of airways. Bacteria and white blood cells are frequently found in these areas in people with CF, but since the infection starts and is mostly confined to the airways, CF lung infections are most accurately thought of as bronchiolitis and bronchitis and not as pneumonia. Even if someone with CF is diagnosed as having "pneumonia," it is almost never the dreaded kind of pneumonia that kills elderly patients.

Causes of Lung Infection in Cystic Fibrosis

Often it is not clear why a particular lung infection occurs, or why it gets out of control when it does. In some instances it is clear, as, for example, when someone has a cold, and a slight cough that develops into a worse cough remains long after the runny nose has disappeared. In a case such as this, the virus infection that caused this cold has thrown off the balance of the lung defenses enough for some of the hardier bacteria in the lung to multiply and cause problems. In someone who has asthma, the asthma may become worse because of pollution, allergies, cigarette smoke, and so forth, and lead to a serious infection (it may be difficult in this case to tell how much of the problem is asthma and how much is infection, and which came first). In some cases, there is no explanation of why a lung infection has gotten worse.

Bacteria, Viruses, and Fungi

Bacteria and viruses are the most important types of germs that cause infection in people with CF; fungi can occasionally cause problems as well.

Bacteria

Bacteria are probably the major cause of bronchial infection (and lung damage) in people with CF. Bacteria are larger than viruses and can usually be killed by antibiotics. Normally, the number of bacteria in the lungs of someone with CF is relatively small, and the body's defenses (immune system) are able to keep these bacteria under control. But when something happens to offset this balance, the bacteria can multiply and cause inflammation. In this situation, there is bronchial infection and not just colonization.

There are several different bacteria (which seem to change their names as often as some people change their socks) that most often colonize and infect the lungs of people with CF: For example, *Haemophilus influenzae*, sometimes called H. flu (not to be confused with the influenza virus); *Staphylococcus*, or "staph"; and *Pseudomonas aeruginosa*. Other bacteria that can be found include *Klebsiella*, *Escherichia coli*, *Serratia*, *Stenotrophomonas maltophilia* (formerly called "*Xanthomonas maltophilia*" and before that *P. maltophilia*—!), *Alcaligenes xylosoxidans* (now most often called "*Achromobacter xylosoxidans*") and *Burkholderia cepacia* (formerly called "*P. cepacia*"). *Streptococcus pyogenes*, which causes strep throat, and *S. pneumoniae* ("*Pneumococcus*," sometimes called the "pneumonia germ" because it is the most common cause of pneumonia in people with normal lungs) are not especially common in people with CF.

The most prevalent bacteria affecting people with CF are staph and the various types of *Pseudomonas*. More than 80% of people with CF eventually have *Pseudomonas* in their throat or sputum cultures. The *Pseudomonas* family has a reputation, which is only partially deserved, of being particularly dangerous bacteria. Though most *Pseudomonas* are harder to kill than other bacteria—especially with antibiotics that are taken by mouth—it is not true that *Pseudomonas* (or any other particular bacteria) are the kiss of death. The important factor is not *what bacteria* are in the lung but rather *what harm* they are causing. Although it is probably true that—*as a group*—the few patients who never have *Pseudomonas* in their cultures survive longer than patients who do have *Pseudomonas* in cultures, the generalities that apply to groups are not useful in considering individual patients. Many people with CF have *Pseudomonas* colonization of the bronchi for many years and experience little or no trouble. If someone has no cough, no problems exercising, and no trouble breathing, it doesn't much matter if a throat or mucus culture has shown *Pseudomonas*. On the other hand, if someone does have all those problems and the culture grows only staph, the person is still sick.

Some years ago, it appeared that *B. cepacia* was an especially dangerous form of bacteria, causing death shortly after colonization, and it does appear that some forms of these bacteria are very bad. It is now clear, however, that this is not always the case: there are multiple bacteria in the *B. cepacia* complex, and that some types of *Burkholderia* are no worse than other CF bronchial bacteria, like *Pseudomonas*. Others, such as *B. cenocepacia*, may be worse. The major issue is how much damage they cause, and how readily they are killed by antibiotics.

Viruses

Viruses are smaller than bacteria and generally cannot be killed by medicines. Antibiotics have no effect on viruses. Viruses are the most common cause of upper respiratory infections (colds) and may affect the bronchi as well. Not only can viruses cause infection but infection with viruses makes it easier for bacteria to take hold in the bronchial tree, perhaps because the viruses interfere with mucociliary clearance. Some 20% of episodes of increased bronchial infection in patients with CF are associated with virus infections (either viruses alone or together with bacteria). Some of the common respiratory viruses are RSV, parainfluenza virus, rhinovirus, and influenza virus. This last virus, influenza ("flu"), causes epidemics in the winter, afflicting many people with miserable cold-like symptoms. Influenza can cause a very serious pneumonia, which can even be fatal. Some of the common childhood illnesses, such as chickenpox, measles, mumps, and rubella (German measles), are caused by viruses. On rare occasions, measles can cause a very serious pneumonia. This is true of chickenpox (varicella) as well, although chickenpox pneumonia is extremely rare in people with CF. Prevention of these infections, with vaccinations, is an important way to stay healthy (see later).

Fungi

Fungi, especially the fungus *Aspergillus fumigatus*, are sometimes found in the bronchi of patients with CF. They can cause trouble, but not usually in the same way as viruses or bacteria. The problem with *Aspergillus* is not usually infection with tissue damage but rather an allergic reaction (*allergic bronchopulmonary aspergillosis, or ABPA*), which induces swelling within the bronchi. In many patients with CF, *Aspergillus* may be present and cause no problems at all. As many as 80% to 90% of patients with CF have *Aspergillus* in their airways at one time or another.

Treatment of the Lungs in Cystic Fibrosis

Since the main problems in the lungs are obstruction of bronchioles and bronchi and the resulting infection and inflammation, treatment is aimed at relieving bronchial blockage and fighting infection and inflammation. There are also some general principles to be observed.

General

CF is unusual in how much of the outcome (how healthy someone is, indeed, how long people live) can be influenced by what the patient and family do for care of the patient's lungs. Being careful not to miss treatments (or to miss as few as possible), getting adequate rest and exercise, paying attention to good nutrition, avoiding cigarette smoke, and getting regular CF clinic visits all have been associated with better outcomes.

Cigarette Smoke

Everyone knows that smoking is not good for the smoker. More and more people are beginning to realize that it's also harmful for "innocent bystanders," who breathe the smoke coming from the end of the cigarette or the smoker's exhaled smoke (*second-hand smoke*). This has been shown very clearly for patients with CF: those who are exposed to smoke in the home have worse lungs than those who aren't. So, at a minimum, parents who smoke should not smoke in the house (even from another room the smoke can get to where it can do harm) or in the car. Parents who have thought about quitting for their own health but haven't been able to are often able to stop for their children's health and life. In many cases, the drive to protect our children is even stronger than the drive to protect ourselves. Certainly, teenagers and adults with CF who feel peer pressure to take up smoking should resist that pressure.

Medical Care

Regular check-ups with your CF physician are extremely important to be able to detect small signs of lung infection and inflammation, before these problems have caused irreversible damage. When someone appears to be doing well it is very tempting to put off a time-consuming (and perhaps expensive and anxiety-producing) visit to the CF center, but these visits are important. One study showed a clear difference in actual patient survival between centers that saw their patients frequently (best survival) and those that saw their patients less frequently (worst survival). Visits to your regular pediatrician or family doctor are also important for good health maintenance.

Relieving and Preventing Obstruction: Airway Clearance Techniques

Chest Physical Therapy

A major portion of most treatment programs is aimed at keeping the airways as free of mucus as possible. The methods seem crude but are quite effective. There are many different techniques, and they all can be considered "airway clearance techniques," often abbreviated "ACT." The most common method is based on a principle taken from everyday life, namely, the "Ketchup Bottle Principle": If you want to get a thick substance out of a container with a narrow opening, you turn the container upside down so that its opening is pointing downward, and then you clap it, shake it, and vibrate it. If the thick substance is mucus, and the container is the various segments of the lungs, the procedure is the same and may be equally effective: you turn the child (or yourself) in various positions, with each position allowing one of the major portions of the lungs to have its opening pointing downward, and then you clap firmly on the back or chest over that part of the lung and actually shake the mucus loose (for details on positioning for these treatments, see Appendix C). Once it's shaken loose, the mucus can fall into the large central airways and then be coughed out. This form of treatment goes by many different names, a few of which are *postural drainage* (PD), *chest physical therapy* (chest PT, or just CPT), and *percussion and drainage*. Often, children and families invent their own pet names like "exercises," "clapping," "boom-booms."

CPT treatments are not painful; in fact, they can be very soothing and relaxing in the way that a massage is. Babies who may be crying at the beginning of their CPT are often asleep halfway through the procedure. The treatment can be time-consuming, however (from 1 to 2 minutes for each of 10 or 12 positions), and can be a bother to children, adolescents, and adults alike, since it interferes with the day's agenda. It may also keep an older child or adult tied to home, since it is awkward to perform on oneself and may require accommodating to someone else's (usually a parent's) schedule.

There are several pieces of equipment that make these treatments easier to perform at home. The first is the high-frequency chest compression vibrating vest (Figure 3.4).

This looks a bit like a life-vest, and it is hooked to high-pressure air hosing that rapidly inflates and deflates the vest, causing a vibration that seems to help shake loose airway mucus. Although it cannot be used in the youngest infants and children, it seems to have been helpful in many adults and children older than 3 years or so. There are now at least three vendors of these devices, but they remain very expensive (about $16,000). It has the advantage of freeing an adult or adolescent patient from dependence on someone else (parent, most often; perhaps a spouse) for treatments and the corresponding advantage of freeing

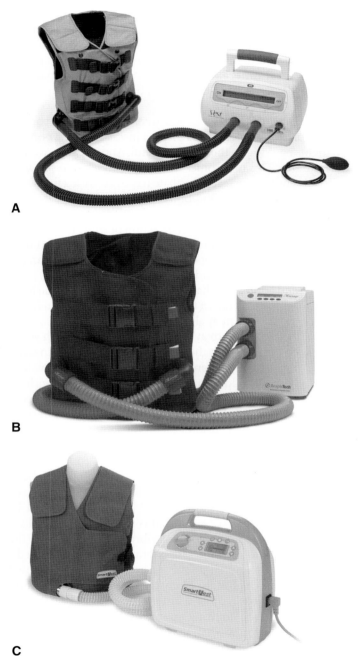

FIGURE 3.4 A: Hill-Rom model 105a vest. **B:** Respirtech InCourage vest system. **C:** Electromed SmartVest.

that parent or spouse from the time-consuming and sometimes physically challenging job of manual CPT. The devices can be adjusted in terms of how fast (frequency) and hard (pressure) they compress the chest. There is some ongoing research to determine how to determine "best" settings, but most patients should probably utilize several different frequencies. In addition, patients need to remember that the devices loosen the mucus, but coughing is required to clear it from the airways.

Another in the category of devices-you-wear is a percussor pack, which you slip on like a backpack. This device has pistons inside the pack pounding on the back. Some patients have found these packs useful. Another device is the mechanical percussor/vibrator. This tool comes in various models, the simplest of which is like an electric jigsaw that instead of a blade has a rod with a firm cushion on it. The cushion is held on the chest and bounces firmly and repeatedly where it is aimed. Most models have variable force and speed; some models are driven by electricity and others by compressed air. The action of some models is a pounding motion, whereas others vibrate; some models can do both, depending on the setting selected. Treatments with the good mechanical percussors can probably be just as effective as those done by hand.

Some children (and adults, too) have a strong preference for the hand, whereas others prefer the machines. Clearly, a treatment by either method is considerably more effective than no treatment at all.

Another device that simplifies treatment is a PD table. Although vest treatments are done entirely with the patient in the seated position, manual chest PT requires the patient to be turned in many different positions, which can be awkward. Treatments for infants and small children are done most comfortably with the child on a parent's lap, but when the child outgrows the parent's lap (either because of size or not wanting to be treated "like a baby"), the table becomes very useful. The person receiving the treatment can sit or lie on the table, which can be set at different angles, thereby making proper positioning easier to achieve. Tables and percussors can be bought from commercial suppliers.

There are several airway clearance techniques that do not involve hitting the chest but seem to be very effective for adults, adolescents, and children old enough to cooperate: The first of these uses the Flutter® valve. This is a hand-held device (Figure 3.5), small enough to carry around in your pocket, that looks a little like a kazoo. It has a stainless steel ball in it that vibrates up and down (flutters, you might say) as you blow into the tube. The vibrations are transmitted backward down through the patient's mouth into the trachea and bronchi, where they shake mucus free from the bronchial walls. Many teenagers and adults who had done traditional CPT for years have become "Flutter® converts," saying that the Flutter® is more effective in helping them bring up mucus, letting them feel when there's excess mucus there, and to know when they've cleared their airways. Like some of the mechanical devices, the Flutter® has the advantage of enabling patients to work on airway clearance without help (except perhaps the reminder from a parent that so many children seem to need to do any job).

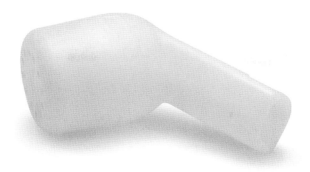

FIGURE 3.5 Flutter (Scandipharm). Oscillating positive-pressure device.

The Acapella® (Figure 3.6) is a newer device that works similarly to the Flutter, but is less dependent on proper positioning, and in addition, also provides an adjustable positive expiratory pressure (PEP). This positive pressure in the airway can help prop open collapsible airways, allowing better clearance of the mucus. The Quake® (Figure 3.7) also provides oscillating PEP that is generated by the patient cranking a handle and provides oscillation during inspiration and exhalation. These handheld devices are quite portable and relatively inexpensive (approximately $50 wholesale for an Acapella®).

Other PEP techniques have had more use in Europe or Canada than in the United States. These techniques include one called a "PEP mask." The patient breathes through a special mask that has an exhale valve that requires some air pressure to open. It is thought that this expiratory pressure is transmitted back

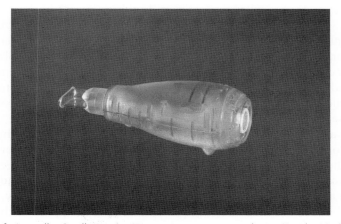

FIGURE 3.6 Acapella. Oscillating positive expiratory pressure device (Smiths-Medical).

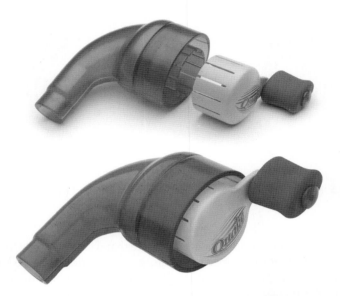

FIGURE 3.7 The Quake (Thayer Medical) provides oscillating positive expiratory pressure. The oscillating frequency is determined by the patient's cranking of the handle.

down the airways and helps to prop them open during the exhalation, allowing mucus to be pushed out along with the air (remember that usually during exhalation, the airways tend to narrow a little bit, so this keeps them wider open than they'd normally be). The TheraPEP (Figure 3.8) or PARI-PEP devices have the patient exhale against resistance into a mouthpiece, and generating positive pressure in the airways. The latter can be used with a nebulizer.

Another method is called the "active cycle of breathing technique." This technique has three phases: breathing control (quiet breathing), thoracic expansion (deep breaths in), and forced expiration or huffs (quick, strong—but never violent—breaths out, with the mouth and throat open). Autogenic drainage involves a series of breaths controlled so that some are done with very little air in the lungs, some with a medium amount, and some done with the lungs filled almost to capacity. This technique requires instruction by someone very skilled in its use before it can be effective in mobilizing mucus.

There are some other mechanical devices that have been used by patients with CF for airway clearance, although there is very little research evidence to support their use. The Intrapulmonary Percussive Ventilator (IPV, Percussionaire®) uses very fast minibursts of pressure through a mask or mouthpiece to shake the airway walls and can deliver an aerosol at the same time. The Frequencer™ uses sound waves through handheld speakers applied to the chest to mobilize mucus.

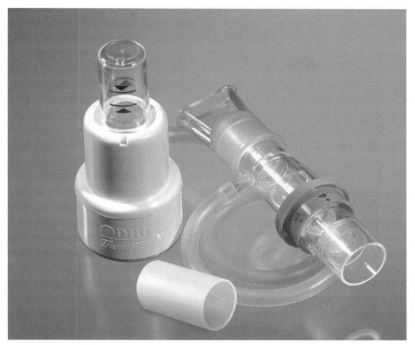

FIGURE 3.8 TheraPEP positive expiratory pressure device (Smiths-Medical).

Exercise

Many people believe that vigorous exercise may be helpful to loosen mucus and to keep bronchi clear. Certainly, hard exercise, or laughing or crying, often results in a coughing spell that brings up mucus, even in people who do not raise mucus during the traditional CPT treatments. Since there is not yet any scientific evidence that exercise can successfully replace the time-honored CPT treatments, it is best to encourage patients to be very active *and* to do their treatments. Several studies have shown that exercise *plus* ACT treatments clear more mucus than ACT treatments alone. (Exercise is discussed at greater length in Chapter 10.)

An Important Note on Airway Clearance Treatments

One important point to keep in mind is that a method may be helpful even if it does not result in the immediate expectoration of large amounts of mucus. Mucus might be shaken loose from the smallest bronchioles and started on its way to the central bronchi, but it will not cause a cough until it actually reaches the large, central bronchi. There is good evidence that regular airway clearance treatments are helpful, even though a single treatment makes little or no apparent difference. In one study, a number of children stopped their CPT for 3 weeks and had a significant deterioration in their lung function (even though they didn't *feel* any different); when they resumed their treatments after the 3-week experimental period, their lung function returned to its previous level. This can be a problem for patients with CF and their families: the treatments are time-consuming, and it is not uncommon to see or feel no obvious results right after the treatments. That means it's easy to convince yourself that skipping the treatments won't hurt. But it will! Often, people have realized too late that they have harmed their lungs by not keeping up with their treatments. Of course, for many patients with CF, the benefit of the treatments is very obvious even during the individual treatment sessions.

Breaking up Mucus

For decades, the idea of somehow breaking up, thinning, or watering down the thick CF airway secretions has been appealing, and numerous attempts have been made to accomplish this and, most of them not very successful. For many years, patients with CF slept all night in *mist tents*, which surrounded them with a dense fog of water. It turned out that this didn't really help. The next approach—still used by a very few patients—was a medication called "acetylcysteine" (Mucomyst®), which is inhaled as an aerosol. When Mucomyst® is mixed with CF mucus in a test tube, it does make the mucus thinner and easier to move. However, human bronchi and tracheas are different from glass test tubes and may react with inflammation when Mucomyst® is inhaled. Some people have developed increasing bronchial obstruction because of inflammation, or even bronchospasm, after inhaling Mucomyst®. While some people do improve with this treatment, most are neither helped nor hurt by it.

A new era in thinning bronchial mucus began in the 1990s on the basis of our better understanding of what makes CF mucus thick. Remember that DNA that's been released from white blood cells is an important component of CF mucus; it happens to account for some 40% of the stickiness of CF mucus. There is now a genetically engineered medication that breaks down this DNA: DNase (the ending -ase refers to enzymes that break down other substances). DNase (*Pulmozyme®*) is extremely effective in liquefying CF mucus in the test tube (as was true of Mucomyst®). Taken by aerosol, it also seems to be very safe for most patients with CF (with the possible exception of those with very severe lung disease and huge amounts of mucus in their airways—these patients do better if all that mucus is not mobilized all at once). Studies in large numbers of patients have suggested that breathing in DNase once a day does seem to bring about a small (5%) improvement in lung function as compared to the gradual deterioration that might be expected. Perhaps surprisingly, this benefit is not restricted to patients with a lot of trouble bringing up thick mucus but seems to help improve lung function even in some patients with mild lung disease. An additional benefit is that it decreases the number of "pulmonary exacerbations," or times when there are more symptoms or need for antibiotics. However, not everyone does benefit, and the drug is extraordinarily expensive: about $24,000 a year. The approach many CF doctors (especially in Europe) have taken is to have patients try DNase for 1 to 3 months, comparing pulmonary function before and after. If the patient feels better and/or the pulmonary function tests (PFTs) have shown an improvement, then it makes sense to use it. There are some patients who do feel better, without any measurable improvement, and we don't know how to explain this.

Another medication that thins the mucus was discovered recently by surfers with CF in Australia. These surfers recognized that their cough was more productive after a day at the beach, and their doctors determined that this effect was due to breathing air containing salty water! The higher salt concentration pulls water into the airway tubes, loosening the mucus and making airway clearance treatments more effective. Hypertonic saline (HyperSal®, containing 7% saline, or about seven times as much salt as is in the salt water used intravenously) when inhaled twice daily has been shown to decrease pulmonary exacerbations and improve lung function. The medication can cause increased cough or bronchospasm, but for most patients this can be prevented by taking their bronchodilator medication (see next section, *Treating Asthma*) first. It is attractive because it is quite inexpensive ($900 per year) and is directed at the underlying cause of CF airway disease (not enough moisture in the airways). Studies of hypertonic saline in infants and young children with CF are now under way.

It is possible that even better mucus-thinning medications—or combinations of medications—will be developed.

Treating Asthma

When asthma is present in addition to CF, there is increased bronchial obstruction with which to contend. Bronchospasm makes the opening of the bronchi smaller than normal, making it much more difficult to get the mucus out. Several very effective bronchodilator medications that dilate (open) the bronchi are available. These medications are most effective when taken by inhalation (they are available for oral use, but are less effective and more likely to give side effects when taken orally). The aerosols are delivered by an aerosol machine, which is composed of an air compressor, a length of tubing, and a nebulizer (Figure 3.9). The compressor sends air through the tube to the nebulizer, which holds the liquid medicine. As the air rushes by, it lifts the medicine, breaks it into a mist, and blows it out through the mouthpiece or mask to be inhaled. Some medications are available in handheld metered-dose inhalers. These devices deliver a measured amount of medicated mist with each puff. Valved holding chambers (Figure 3.10A and 3.10B) are available with a mouthpiece (for older children or adults) or a mask (for younger children) that attach to the opening of the inhaler and temporarily trap the medication until the next breath, improving the delivery of the medication. Some bronchodilator medications are albuterol (Ventolin®, Proventil, ProAir®), levalbuterol (Xopenex®), metaproterenol (Alupent®, Metaprel®), and ipratropium (Atrovent®) (see Appendix B). Most people with asthma benefit from medications that prevent airway inflammation, particularly inhaled steroid preparations. These

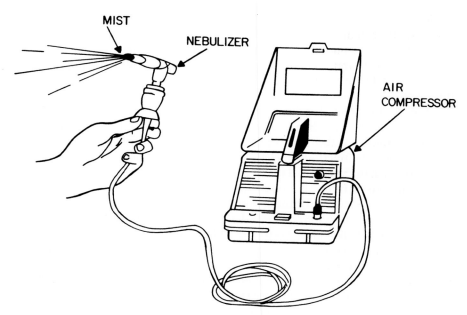

FIGURE 3.9 Aerosol machine. The machine blows compressed air through the tubing, over the liquid medication that is held in the cup of the nebulizer, creating a mist from the liquid medication. The patient then breathes the medicine.

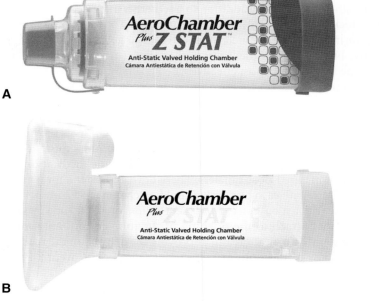

FIGURE 3.10 A: Valved holding chamber (Aerochamber, Monoghan Medical) with mouthpiece. **B:** Valved holding chamber (Aerochamber, Monoghan Medical) with face mask for toddlers.

steroids (mostly) do not get absorbed into the bloodstream and therefore do not cause side effects that can be seen with oral or injected steroid medications. Some inhaled steroids are budesonide (Pulmicort®) and fluticasone (Flovent®). There are also some preparations that combine a longer-acting bronchodilator with a steroid (e.g., Advair® and Symbicort®).

Reducing Airway Inflammation

Airway inflammation often accompanies infection and/or asthma (see earlier, "The Lower Respiratory Tract"), making the airway opening that much smaller and possibly damaging the cells that line the airway. Although inflammation is a normal part of fighting infection (see earlier, "Other Protection Against Lung Infection"), if it gets out of control it can do more harm than good. Excessive inflammation appears to be a very important cause of the progressive damage to CF airways, and therefore prevention and treatment of airway inflammation has become an important focus of CF research. Some medications, most notably a group of drugs called *steroids*, can reduce inflammation wherever it occurs, including in the bronchial tree. Prednisone (one of the steroids) has been studied in a number of people with CF and has appeared to be effective in improving their lung function.

Prednisone, however, is a very potent drug that has many possible side effects (see Appendix B). One of the most serious of these side effects is oversuppression of the immune response, which makes the body unable to fight infection. Prednisone can also bring out a tendency to develop diabetes and can interfere with growth. Although the chances of dangerous side effects are much lower if prednisone is given on alternate days (Monday–Wednesday–Friday, etc.), instead of every day, there are still some risks. In fact, in the largest study done to date in patients with CF, prednisone was given on alternate days, and improved pulmonary function, but (after a couple of years) did cause side effects in some patients, so if prednisone is to be used, patients need to be checked fairly frequently.

Steroids have been developed in a form for inhalation, and these drugs have been very helpful in preventing airway inflammation in people with asthma. Although they are commonly used for people with CF (because some CF symptoms overlap with symptoms of asthma), it is not yet known which patients are helped by these medications. As the inhaled steroids are not absorbed into the bloodstream (or are absorbed in only tiny amounts), side effects from inhaled steroids are much less a concern than from oral or injected steroids.

There are other drugs that reduce inflammation without interfering with the body's ability to fight infection. These drugs include aspirin, ibuprofen, and related drugs, which are used for people with arthritis. A small study with ibuprofen in patients with CF gave promising results: the drug seemed to slow the rate of decline of pulmonary function over a 4-year period. However, ibuprofen has its own problems, as well. Many (non-CF) patients taking the high doses of ibuprofen needed for the beneficial effects have had bleeding ulcers, whereas others have had kidney failure. Although these worrisome side effects have not been seen commonly in patients with CF, worry about them has kept many CF doctors from prescribing ibuprofen for their patients. The antibiotic azithromycin has been shown to have some anti-inflammatory effects, apart from its bacteria-killing effects, and a fairly large study showed improved pulmonary function and fewer pulmonary exacerbations in patients with CF with positive cultures for *Pseudomonas* who took azithromycin each Monday, Wednesday, and Friday for 6 months. Some experts think that improvement can be attributed to reduced inflammation. Studies are currently under way to see whether other medications might have anti-inflammatory effects without side effects and whether azithromycin has the same benefit in patients with CF whose cultures do not grow *Pseudomonas*.

Reducing Bronchial Infection
Antibacterial Drugs (Antibiotics)

Antibiotics are probably the most important single factor responsible for the tremendous improvement in the outlook for people with CF, both in terms of length of life and quality of life. Antibiotics are very effective in reducing airways infection and therefore in preserving lung health. (See Appendix B for a more complete discussion of antibiotics.) Most CF physicians agree that antibiotics should be used when there is evidence of increased airways infection (such as increased cough and mucus production and decreased exercise tolerance). There is no agreement, however, on whether it is helpful to give antibiotics on a regular basis to prevent infection. One large multicenter study suggested that the preventive ("prophylactic") use of continuous antibiotics was not helpful for young patients with CF.

Oral antibiotics are usually taken when the infection is caused by *Staphylococcus* (Staph) or *Haemophilus*. (See Appendix B for a review of these antibiotics.) Oral antibiotics may also be helpful for *Pseudomonas* infections, but often throat and sputum culture results will say that they will not work, and in fact, in many cases they will not bring these infections under control. Sometimes oral antibiotics will work fine, even when the culture reports suggest that they will not. But if they do not, someone may need treatment with aerosolized or intravenous (IV) antibiotics. Compared with oral antibiotics, the aerosolized and IV antibiotics are more powerful, more likely to get to the site of infection within the bronchial tubes, or both. IV antibiotics most often require a hospital stay (see Chapter 7, *Hospitalization and other Special Treatments*).

Preventing Bacterial Infection: "Infection Control"

There is no proven effective method for preventing bacterial bronchial infections. However, in recent years, people have devoted a *lot* of attention and energy to ways of reducing the risks of developing and maintaining bacterial infection in CF airways. Two of the areas that have received the most attention (and that have caused the most emotional upset among patients with CF, families, and caretakers) are (a) *patient-to-patient transmission of bacteria* and (b) the first positive culture for *Pseudomonas*.

Patient-to-Patient Transmission of Bacteria: Contact with Other Patients with Cystic Fibrosis and Their Bacteria

The sources of bronchial infection in patients with CF are not completely understood. Some of the bacteria and viruses that cause these infections are all around us—in the air, in soil, and so on. But we have found out that some of the bacteria can be passed directly from one patient with CF to another. A prime example of this "person-to-person transmission" of CF airway bacteria is *B. cepacia*. As you've seen above, these particular bacteria have in some cases been associated with an especially bad sickness. Because of dangers from *cepacia* for some people, and other bacteria (including antibiotic-resistant *Pseudomonas*), and because of the possibility of person-to-person spread of these bacteria, most experts are now recommending that patients with CF limit their contact with other patients with CF. These recommendations have been carried out in different ways by different individuals, and different CF centers and organizations have all set up different guidelines (or none at all). Nationally and internationally, there has been a lot of attention paid recently to "*infection control.*"

Some typical recommendations for infection control include:

- No direct or physical contact (like kissing, or perhaps even hand-shaking) between patients with CF; keeping a 3-foot distance between patients with CF
- No prolonged close contact between patients with CF (no playing together for young children, no long car rides together, etc.)
- No holiday parties for groups of CF families
- No patients allowed to attend the traditional "Family Education Days" that many CF centers have had
- Careful hygiene: thorough hand-washing (especially with alcohol-based products like Purell™) for patients with CF and their caretakers; cover your mouth and nose during coughing spells, carefully dispose of tissue that has sputum in it, etc.
- *Changes in procedures in clinic and during hospitalization:*
  - Clinic: attempts to prevent prolonged waiting times in crowded waiting rooms—some clinics have instituted a beeper system similar to what you find in some restaurants: check in, get a beeper, then go wander around until your beeper goes off, letting you know that your clinic room is ready.
  - Hospital: patients can't room together, can't be in the same room during aerosols or chest PT; must wear masks outside their rooms; caretakers wear some protective gear (gowns, gloves, masks, or some combination) when they are in contact with patients in their rooms.

One of the things that makes these new recommendations difficult is that they are not all based on solid scientific proof. Take masks, for example: it seems to make sense that wearing a mask should keep a patient from spreading his own germs to others or breathing in someone else's germs, but we don't know for certain that this works with all bacteria. Masks are different from each other and some are probably better than others; they probably work better right when they're put on and less well as they get wetter from exhaled humid air; bacteria are different, and some likely are blocked more effectively by masks than others, and so forth.

Another challenge in this area is that different experts recommend different guidelines, and (as is true of experts in any field) some of these experts put forth their views—which might conflict with other experts' views—as the *only* right ones. Meanwhile, the nonexperts (patients, families, nurses, doctors) have to try to figure out what to do.

This is a very difficult issue to deal with. Patients with CF and families have always received information, friendship, and a sense of shared experiences from contact with each other, and those patients who have had to spend any time in the hospital have been able to enjoy a fairly free fun time with access to computers, playrooms, classrooms (OK, so that's not always *fun*), and other patients. It would be a shame to lose all that. It would also be a shame for someone who is relatively well to get dreadfully ill if that could have been avoided. Many patients have taken advantage of the Internet and e-mail to try to get around some of these problems— they can "talk" with other patients without fear of getting a new infection. Discuss these issues with your own CF physician. It should be possible to find a safe and humane approach that's right for you and your family.

Treating the First Pseudomonas Culture

This is a relatively new concern for patients and CF physicians. For decades, the approach in good CF centers was to use the results of throat and sputum cultures *to help guide treatment, if treatment was warranted by the patient's symptoms or test results* (e.g., PFTs—see later in this chapter). Cultures were not used to decide whether treatment was needed or not. Recently, however, there has been a lot of talk about aggressive antibiotic treatment of patients the first time (or times) *Pseudomonas* shows up on a throat or sputum culture. The reasons for this are that (a) it's probably better not to have *Pseudomonas* than to have it and (b) it *might* be possible to get rid of *Pseudomonas* if it's treated soon after it first appears in the lungs. This possibility has come mostly from the experience of patients with CF in Denmark, where CF physicians report that *Pseudomonas* can be eliminated with early antibiotic treatment. Denmark is a country where in general antibiotics are used *very* aggressively in CF care. For example, in Denmark, patients are admitted to the hospital for 2 weeks of IV antibiotics every 3 months, even if they are feeling well! What is not yet known is whether the Danish experience can work elsewhere and whether there might be more drawbacks than benefits to using antibiotics in patients with no symptoms. The possible benefit is clear: elimination of *Pseudomonas*. The possible drawbacks include (a) *Pseudomonas* organisms developing resistance to antibiotics, thus making treatment more difficult when it's needed when a patient develops symptoms, (b) side effects from the antibiotics, and (c) expense. At the time this book goes to press, there are several multicenter studies (one called EPIC, one called ELITE) being completed to try answer these important questions; preliminary results suggest benefit from using an inhaled anti-*Pseudomonas* antibiotic the first time *Pseudomonas* is found on culture. Until we have definitive results, patients and their physicians will have to act on the basis of their best beliefs and the latest information available.

Fighting Viral Infections

There are very few safe drugs that kill viruses, and, therefore, no safe, effective drug treatment for viral bronchiolitis or bronchitis.

One exception is the influenza virus, which can be treated with various medications, including amantadine, rimantadine, and oseltamivir. These medications are taken by mouth and are used primarily by people who become infected with influenza during an epidemic. People who are at risk for influenza infection, such as patients with CF who have not had the flu vaccine, may also take these drugs as a preventive measure, during a community outbreak of influenza.

Preventing Viral Infections

See also Avoiding Colds, above.

The most common type of viral infection, namely, the common cold, cannot be effectively prevented (see earlier, "Infections of the Upper Respiratory Tract"). There are other viral infections that can be prevented, though, including measles and influenza ("flu"). All children should be immunized against measles, and all children with CF (or other abnormal lung conditions) should receive a flu shot each year. These vaccines are effective and are safe except in people with very severe egg allergy. Sometimes a new strain of influenza may crop up (recently the H1N1 influenza, so-called "swine flu"), requiring an extra flu shot.

There is a medication available that can decrease the severity of infection with RSV (see earlier). Palivizumab (Synagis®) is a "monoclonal antibody" (see Appendix B) fairly widely used now for sick and tiny infants. This has to be given by injection once a month during the winter viral season. Although its effectiveness has not been studied in babies with CF, it is recommended by some CF centers.

There is a varicella (chickenpox) vaccine available, and the American Academy of Pediatrics recommends it for all children. It is safe for children with CF. Another chickenpox-related medication is **varicella-zoster immune globulin**, or VZIG. It is not a vaccine but rather a gamma-globulin-like shot that is given to prevent chickenpox. Most CF physicians feel, however, that this is unnecessary for people with CF, since the chances that someone with CF would have lung complications from chickenpox are very small. In addition, a major drawback to VZIG is that once it is given, it has to be repeated every time there is an exposure to chickenpox. Nonetheless, some CF physicians recommend VZIG for nonimmunized patients who have been exposed to chickenpox.

Steps in Treating Worsened Lungs

In CF, the lungs get worse from time to time. These periods of worsening, called *"pulmonary exacerbations,"* are most often caused by increased airways infection and can usually be brought under control if proper steps are taken.

In order for pulmonary exacerbations to be treated, they must first be recognized, which is not always easy. The signs that the lungs are worse may be very subtle and may at first escape attention. These signs include more cough than usual, more mucus, decreased energy, poor appetite, difficulty exercising, and shortness of breath. In most people, the amount of cough is the single most important clue. Many people will not have lessened activity or shortness of breath, nor will they have fever, so the absence of these clues should not be taken as proof that there's not a problem. It is important to recognize when there are more signs of infection than are usual for you, since everyone is different. For example, if your usual pattern is to cough only a little bit in the morning, but you begin to cough after laughing or crying and find that the cough lasts just a bit longer, then you will know that your condition is not quite as good as it usually is. On occasion, someone else, such as your doctor or a relative who doesn't see you everyday, may point a difference out to you that you haven't noticed. Sometimes, however, it may take an x-ray or PFT to show that a change has occurred. For this reason, it is quite important to make fairly frequent clinic visits. It's very tempting to say, "I [or my child] am doing so well that there's no need to go for a checkup." There are far too many patients with CF (usually teenagers) and parents of patients who have used this reasoning, only to return to regular care after irreversible lung damage has been done. Regular visits, which would include physical examinations, throat or sputum cultures, and periodic chest x-rays and PFTs, can often spot a problem while it is still reversible. Since the progression of lung disease in CF is usually very gradual and subtle—and is *not* characterized by sudden dramatic deterioration—it is easy for patients and families to miss signs of deterioration. Sometimes your family doctor or pediatrician may listen to you and say "the lungs are clear, so we don't have to treat you." This is a common misunderstanding. Most CF specialists recognize that someone with CF can have clinically important airways infection, and still sound wonderful by stethoscope. Your physician may be able to recognize these signs, because a change in the weeks or months since your last visit is easier to detect than small day-to-day changes and because sensitive laboratory tests (PFTs and x-rays) help clarify your condition.

Once you have recognized that there is a problem, it is important not to wait until you're terribly ill to do something about it. That wait can give the infection and inflammation an opportunity to destroy a small portion of lung, leaving a little scar tissue behind. A little scar tissue with each inadequately treated infection adds up over the years. Scar tissue can never become normal lung tissue, so it's important to prevent its formation. It is impossible to tell at any one time whether bronchial obstruction is because these tubes are filled with mucus and bacteria and white blood cells—that could be gotten rid of, or because of permanent irreversible scarring.

Oral Antibiotics

During a period of worsening, your physician will probably prescribe an oral antibiotic or change the antibiotic if you are already taking one. The choice of antibiotics is based on several factors, including how the individual patient has responded in the past, how sick the person is at the time, and what recent throat or sputum cultures have shown (what bacteria are there and which antibiotics kill those bacteria in the laboratory). The physician may also recommend increasing the number of airway clearance treatments you're doing to clear out the extra mucus that builds up with infections.

If an infection does not improve quickly, and certainly if it becomes worse, it is advisable to take the next step: changing antibiotics. This change will be to a more powerful antibiotic or to one that is better at killing the particular bacteria a culture has shown to be in your system. If a more powerful or appropriate oral antibiotic is not available, or if the physician feels that an oral antibiotic would work too slowly, then he or she may recommend an aerosol antibiotic or even IV antibiotics. Most often, symptoms will improve nicely with oral antibiotic treatment. In fact, patients are often back to their baseline (usual state of health) even before the antibiotic prescription has run out. In these cases, it's tempting to stop the medicines as soon as you feel better, but this is usually not a good idea. Infectious disease experts tell us that one of the surest ways to make bacteria become resistant to an antibiotic (not be killed by it) is to give antibiotics for too short a time. So if your doctor has prescribed 2 weeks of antibiotics and your cough is gone (or back to your usual) in 1 week, you should take the second week of antibiotics anyway.

Aerosol (Nebulized) Antibiotics

Several different kinds of antibiotics can be breathed directly into the lungs as aerosols, using the same kind of machine that we use for bronchodilator aerosols (see Figure 3.9). For decades, CF physicians have prescribed nebulized antibiotics for patients with CF, usually using the form of the antibiotic that was designed for use in IVs. The most commonly used nebulized antibiotics were gentamicin and tobramycin, but quite a few others were also used successfully. Then, beginning in 1997, pharmaceutical companies, often along with the CF Foundation's Therapeutics Development Network (see Chapter 16) began to develop antibiotics specifically designed for nebulization into the lungs. TOBI® (the nebulized form of tobramycin) was the first such drug, followed by aztreonam (Cayston®) in 2010. As this book goes to press, there are a number of other nebulized antibiotics in the final stages of clinical trials, almost ready for prime time. CF physicians continue to prescribe a wide array of IV antibiotics for use in the nebulizer. Despite the fact that they are not specifically formulated for the airways, many CF physicians have felt that they have been beneficial for specific patients. There are widely varying doses of these medications, and you should be sure that you know how much your doctor wants you to take.

Intravenous Antibiotics

If these steps do not work, or do not work fast enough, it may be time for IV antibiotics. In almost every case, putting antibiotics into a vein is the most effective way of treating infection, especially if the infection is caused by *Pseudomonas.* Typically, the administration of IV antibiotics requires a hospital stay. In some cases, it is possible to get IVs at home. (For more information about IVs and hospitalization, see Chapter 7.)

The length of time to give IV antibiotics should be determined by how the patient is responding to treatment. Patients seldom improve (and may perhaps even worsen) in the first 4 or 5 days on IVs. Thereafter, most people improve for several weeks, returning to their usual condition or even to an improved condition. On occasion, someone may stop improving without having returned to his or her previous baseline. Studies have shown that the level of lung function achieved after in-hospital IV treatment of a pulmonary exacerbation can be maintained for at least several weeks but usually does not continue to improve after discharge from the hospital. Therefore, it makes sense to get the most mileage possible from the IV and hospital treatment and not to stop after a predetermined number of days have gone by. Some people will have gotten the maximum benefit from the intensive treatment in as short a time as 10 days, but most people take about 2 weeks and quite a few people take even longer. Keep in mind that this investment of time can pay off in the long run if it keeps even a small portion of lung from becoming scarred. Figure 3.11 shows a time curve for when someone should enter the hospital and when he or she should leave.

Other Treatments

In some cases, other treatments may be used with IV antibiotics or tried before them. One example is trying medications to decrease bronchial inflammation, like prednisone. Another example is altering anti-asthma medications by increasing their dosage or by adding different ones. The best steps to take will differ under different conditions.

General Questions About Using Antibiotics

HOW DO WE KNOW WHETHER TO GIVE ANTIBIOTICS OR NOT?

For individual episodes of increased cough, we will often have the question, is this a cold that does not involve the lungs, and therefore shouldn't need antibiotics, or is it a bronchial infection, which definitely should be treated with antibiotics? And we can't always tell. Given that we can't tell for sure, we have to base treatment decisions on an educated guess and keep in mind the possible consequences of a wrong guess. If we guess that this is bronchial infection and it's really only a cold, we would have given unneeded antibiotics. The consequences of that mistaken decision would be: (a) financial (had to pay for antibiotics that weren't needed), (b) small risk of allergic or other reaction to the antibiotic, and (c) small theoretical risk of encouraging

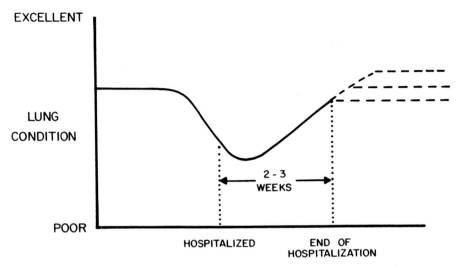

FIGURE 3.11 Timing of hospitalization. When it is recognized that the patient is not doing well out of the hospital, she or he is admitted to the hospital for treatment. Improvement begins within 4 or 5 days. Hospital treatment then continues until the patient is not longer improving. This is usually when she or he has returned to his or her usual state of health, but in some cases the patient might be better than she or he has been in some time. Unfortunately, in a few patients, they may not quite make it back to their pre-IV state of health.

the bacteria to become resistant to the antibiotic. If, on the other hand, we guess that this is a simple cold with no bronchial infection, and we don't give antibiotics, and we've guessed wrong (there really was infection), then the consequences are much worse: possible lung damage, some of which could be irreversible. Given those choices, we'll almost always take the chance of giving antibiotics when they might not have been needed rather than not give them when they might have been needed.

What's "Too Much" Antibiotics? Will I Become "Immune" to the Effects of the Antibiotic?

People often worry that they or their bacteria will "become immune" to the antibiotics (or as physicians say, the bacteria become resistant to the antibiotics). This can happen over time but not nearly as easily as many people fear. Furthermore, if the choice is between treating an infection that we know can cause lung damage—even irreversible damage—or not treating it because of the remotely possible development of resistance to a single antibiotic, most experts would go with the treatment every time. In fact, the history of CF has shown this to be the correct approach: we use a lot more antibiotics now than a few decades ago, and there are more resistant bacteria now, but patients live well into adulthood instead of dying before school age. One important study showed that the survival of patients was much better in centers that use a lot of antibiotics than in those that are stingy with their antibiotics.

WHAT IF WE "RUN OUT" OF ANTIBIOTICS THAT ARE EFFECTIVE?

On occasion, a patient's cultures (see the end of this chapter) may show that one or more of the bacteria in the lungs have become "resistant" to some, many, or even all of the available antibiotics. When this happens, it can be frightening to a patient or parent, for it may signal to them the end of effective treatment for lung infections. While it is undeniably better if the bacteria are all sensitive to readily available antibiotics, the problem of resistance is not completely straightforward and therefore not always as bad as a culture report may make it seem. We have known for decades that patients often respond well to antibiotics that "shouldn't" work, for example, when a patient's respiratory tract bacteria are "resistant" to the particular antibiotics. Why should this be so? There are several possible explanations: One (as you'll see at the end of this chapter) is that "resistant" is not an absolute term, that is, although it may sound as though it means that the antibiotic in question has no effect on the particular bacteria, this is not the case. Often it means that the antibiotic doesn't kill all the bacteria, or that you need a lot of the antibiotic to kill the bacteria. So, some killing may be possible. Another important part of the explanation is that the testing for bacterial sensitivity or resistance takes place in a test tube or culture plate—not in the body. The body has its own defenses, including white blood cells, antibodies, and so on that help to kill invading bacteria, and these aren't measured in the bacteriology laboratory. Finally, it has come to light in recent years that antibiotics have important effects other than their ability to kill bacteria. Erythromycin, for example, has usually been shown in the laboratory to be good for killing staph, but not *Pseudomonas*, yet has seemed to be effective in improving the lungs of patients with CF whose only cultured bacteria are *Pseudomonas*. Why? Well, we now know that erythromycin has powerful anti-inflammatory effects separate from its ability to kill bacteria. Since *Pseudomonas* causes damage largely through inflammation—from the chemicals it itself releases or those released by white blood cells that have come to fight it—lessening the inflammatory response to *Pseudomonas* may do just as much good as killing it.

WHAT IF THE CULTURE REPORTS ARE RIGHT, AND THE ANTIBIOTICS REALLY DON'T WORK ANY MORE?

This happens occasionally and is very serious. In these cases, when the antibiotics really seem unable to make any dent in a patient's symptoms of lung infection, the physician may try other means to fight inflammation (for example, steroids). In some unusual situations, physicians have been able to stop antibiotics for a while and let the bacteria become sensitive to the antibiotics again, so that when the antibiotics are resumed, they are effective once again. This is a risky business, and you should definitely not try it without your doctor's direction, for there is a strong chance that it won't work, and stopping the antibiotics will allow the infection to worsen, without changing the sensitivity pattern of the bacteria.

Finally, there is the helpful fact that the pharmaceutical industry is well aware of the problem of emerging resistance and is continually at work developing new antibiotics. As with so many other aspects of CF care, there is almost always hope even when things might appear bleak. If you're worried about your (or your child's) culture results and their implications for the future, be sure to let your doctor know.

Complications

There are several problems that can be an indirect result of CF. These problems are often referred to as complications of CF. The most important complications related to the lung disease of CF are hemoptysis, atelectasis, pneumothorax, respiratory failure, heart failure, and chest pain. Other complications that relate to the lung disease of CF affect the bones and/or the joints.

Hemoptysis

The literal translation of this term is to "cough up blood" (*heme* is the Greek word for "blood," and *ptyein* translates as "to spit"). Hemoptysis is very uncommon in young children with CF, but as many as 50% of adults with CF will on occasion have some streaks of blood in the mucus they cough up and spit out. A relatively small proportion of patients (3% to 5% of those older than 15 years) will cough out large (more than 10 oz) amounts of blood at a time. This problem, called "massive hemoptysis," can be fatal, although it rarely is, even in people who bring up very large amounts of blood. In most cases, the significance of hemoptysis is the same as that of an increased cough, namely, both are signs of increased infection. A major difference, however, between having a bit more cough than usual and bringing up bright red blood is that it is very frightening to see the blood, especially the first time it happens. One's first reaction is to panic and to assume that all of one's lungs must be bleeding. This is not the case: It's extremely important to know that hemoptysis is a fairly common problem that is almost always simple to treat.

What is happening is that the increased infection in one small area has irritated a capillary or small artery and made a small hole in its wall, causing blood to leak out into the airway. Remember that the size of the working surface of the lungs is about the same as a tennis court; the problem area in someone with hemoptysis is about the size of a little pebble on that tennis court. It helps to keep this in mind if you should see some blood mixed in with mucus sometime. If you see pure blood, you should notify your doctor, because you do need treatment, but there's no need to panic.

In unusual cases, hemoptysis can mean something other than just increased infection. It can indicate a more general bleeding problem. Bleeding problems can be caused by inadequate vitamin K (this would be uncommon in someone with

CF who is getting a good diet and taking the prescribed enzymes), by advanced liver disease, or rarely by a drug side effect. In some unusual situations it may be difficult to tell where spit-up blood has come from. Bleeding in the stomach or esophagus can be confused with bleeding in the lungs. Fortunately, bleeding in the stomach or the esophagus is not common in people with CF.

Treating Hemoptysis

The treatment required for someone who coughs up bloody mucus, or pure blood, depends on the cause of the bleeding. In most cases, the cause is an increase in bronchial infection that has irritated a blood vessel, and the treatment therefore is the same as the treatment for any increased infection, namely, antibiotics and airway clearance treatments. There is little or no controversy about the need for antibiotics (or for stronger antibiotics in someone who is already taking antibiotics). Not all CF specialists agree on the usefulness of ACT, and, in fact, some experts recommend stopping ACT in someone who has brought up a large amount of blood. However, in most cases, the clapping and vibrating are very unlikely to cause any bleeding and should be continued.

In some people who bring up blood, a gurgling sensation is felt in the chest (they can sometimes even tell which part of the lung it's coming from) just before the blood comes up. If someone feels a gurgling every time he or she goes into a particular position, the head-down position, for example, then that position should be avoided. In general, though, the treatments should be continued as much as possible, for three reasons: (a) blood is not good for cilia; (b) blood can make an infection worse by providing a hospitable environment for bacteria; and (c) even if the blood itself is not a problem, one of the underlying principles of treating bronchial infection in someone with CF is to lessen bronchial mucous obstruction as much as possible.

In most cases in which a person has brought up a large amount (more than a cup) of pure blood, hospitalization is recommended. In the hospital, IV antibiotics can be given easily, and patients can be watched carefully to make sure that the bleeding is under control. If the bleeding is very severe and much blood has been lost, blood transfusions may be necessary, just as they would be if the bleeding were caused by a car accident, for example. It is quite uncommon, however, for a transfusion to be required.

Extra vitamin K is usually given to someone with CF who has hemoptysis, since a lack of that vitamin can cause bleeding problems. If the bleeding is not controlled fairly quickly, it may be necessary to do various tests. These tests would check for a generalized bleeding problem (as might occur in someone with severe liver disease) or examine the possibility that the bleeding is a side effect of a drug or drug combination.

In a few cases of massive hemoptysis that can't be controlled by the above means, more difficult methods may be needed. The most effective procedure is called "bronchial artery embolization." An embolus is a clot or other plug in a blood vessel that blocks the circulation in that vessel (*embolos* is the Greek word for "plug"). Emboli are usually bad, but they can also be helpful when a bronchial artery is leaking. In this case, a radiologist may be able to thread a catheter (a thin, flexible tube) into the artery and inject a plug (typically made of a synthetic substance called Gelfoam®) through the catheter that will then seal the leak and stop the bleeding.

There are several problems that make this procedure less than perfect. The first is that it is not always possible to find the artery that is leaking, even with the sophisticated radiologic technology that is available. Second, a fair proportion of people whose bleeding has been stopped with bronchial artery embolization will bleed again from that spot in the future.

In a very few cases—when there is massive bleeding and bronchial artery embolization cannot be performed or is not successful—surgery may be necessary to remove the lobe of the lung that is the source of bleeding. There are numerous problems with this approach, a major one being that, although the person will obviously not bleed again from the removed lobe, he or she will also not have the use of that lobe for breathing. In addition, general anesthesia and chest surgery carry their own risks, especially in someone with severe lung disease. Finally, even with the chest open, it may not be possible to identify the lobe that is the source of bleeding with absolute certainty. There are too many cases of patients with CF who have had a lobe removed in a hospital inexperienced in CF care, only to be transferred to a CF center because the bleeding didn't stop. Nonetheless, there are some cases in which surgery is necessary and very successful.

Because of the problems and uncertainties with the invasive means of dealing with hemoptysis, many CF experts prefer to treat patients—even those with massive hemoptysis—as conservatively as possible, with antibiotics, ACT, vitamin K, transfusions if necessary, and careful observation.

Pneumothorax

This complication is also called "collapsed lung." The term actually means "air inside the chest," which doesn't sound all that abnormal, since that's where air is supposed to be. But it actually refers to air that's within the chest but outside the lung (Figure 3.12). That is very abnormal and can be dangerous, since once air gets outside the lung, it can press in on it and cause it to collapse. If there is enough air under enough pressure or tension, it can even squeeze the blood vessels (venae cavae) that bring the blood back to the heart. This will mean that there won't be enough blood to pump out to the body to keep it functioning normally. This does not usually happen with a pneumothorax in someone with CF. It is unusual for pneumothorax to occur in someone younger than 10 years, and after age 10, between 10% and 25% of patients with CF will develop a pneumothorax. Pneumothorax is much more likely to happen in someone with CF if there is relatively severe lung involvement than if the lungs are in very good shape.

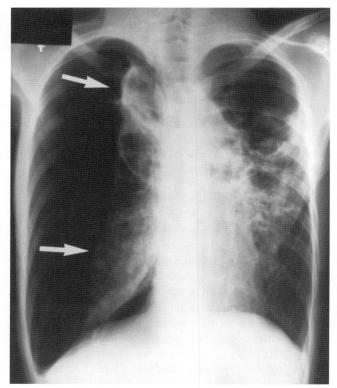

FIGURE 3.12 X-ray appearance of pneumothorax. The air outside the lungs appears black, while the lungs are lighter in color. Arrows show edge of collapsed lung.

Pneumothorax develops when mucus partially blocks a bronchus or bronchiole and functions as a one-way valve or "ball-valve" (Figure 3.13). This kind of blockage allows air to go in only one direction past the blockage. Bronchi enlarge with inhaling and get smaller with exhaling (see The Airways). When mucus fills up a portion of a bronchiole, the bronchiole will enlarge enough with each breath so that some air can get beyond the mucous plug. But while exhaling, the bronchus may collapse to the same size as the plug, so no air will escape. When this happens, the alveoli beyond the blockage will get bigger with each breath in, until, like an overfilled balloon, they finally burst. If these overfilled alveoli are at the edge of the lung (especially at the apex, or top, of the lung), when they burst, the air leaks out of the lung.

A pneumothorax almost always causes sudden, sharp pain in the chest, side, or back, and difficulty breathing (shortness of breath). The only way to tell for certain whether someone has a pneumothorax is with a chest x-ray (see Figure 3.12). The x-ray will show an area inside the chest that is completely black, rather than

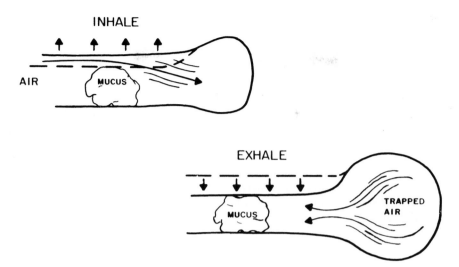

FIGURE 3.13 Partial obstruction of bronchi may cause progressive overinflation of a portion of lung, leading to pneumothorax. The bronchi enlarge slightly when one inhales, allowing air to get into the lungs past mucus. When one exhales, the bronchi get smaller, trapping the air behind the blockage. With each breath, more and more air can become trapped, leading to progressive overinflation and eventual tearing of the tissue, allowing air to escape from the lung.

the usual combination of white and gray; there will also be a clear outline to the edge of the collapsed lung. Some doctors "score" pneumothoraces on the basis of how much of the lung is collapsed on the x-ray. A "25% pneumothorax" means that air outside the lung takes up 25% of the space that the lung normally occupies, and that the lung itself has collapsed to 75% of its normal size. If someone with relatively healthy lungs develops a pneumothorax, this can be a useful description. But when a pneumothorax occurs in someone with CF, it's less helpful, since the lungs tend to be stiff in people with CF and therefore may not collapse readily, even with quite a bit of air outside, under quite a bit of tension. So, what looks like a small amount of air may actually be a lot.

Since pneumothoraces need to be treated, you should let your doctor know if you ever develop sudden chest pain and shortness of breath.

Treatment of Pneumothorax

The treatment for pneumothorax usually requires hospitalization and is directed toward accomplishing three goals: (a) relieving the pressure on the lung by evacuating the air from around the lung, (b) sealing over the hole through which the air has escaped, and (c) ideally, preventing recurrence. There are rare instances in which there is a tiny pneumothorax—just the smallest bit of air outside the lung, with the leak already sealed off by itself—and no treatment is needed. Much more commonly, if there is a pneumothorax, all three treatment goals should be met.

The pressure is usually relieved by a chest tube. This is a tube that goes through the skin, between the ribs, and into the pleural space, which is the space between the chest wall and the outside of the lung. This is the space where air accumulates if it leaks out of the lung. The tube is hooked up to a vacuum that sucks the air out continuously and allows the lung to expand to its normal size. The system of tubing used to evacuate the air from the pleural space must have a good valving system (most often provided by having the tubes pass through a series of vacuum jars or a water seal) so that air can pass only out of the chest and not back into it. The physician makes a small skin incision to place the chest tube and then pushes the tube into place and hooks up the vacuum. Placement of the tube can be painful, and having a tube in place is also uncomfortable. If the treatment chosen is only chest tube placement, the treatment is often successful in the short run but unsuccessful in the long run. Since most air leaks will seal themselves eventually, a chest tube can evacuate the air, and sooner or later the air will stop accumulating, and the tube can be pulled out. Unfortunately, it may take many days for this self-sealing to occur, and during this time, the painful chest tube will interfere with the deep breathing and coughing needed to keep the lungs clear. Even when the leak does seal itself, between 50% and 100% of these pneumothoraces will recur within months or years unless further steps are taken to prevent this from happening.

There are two main approaches to sealing the leak and preventing recurrences of pneumothorax. Both approaches purposely cause inflammation of the pleural surface (the covering of the lung), almost like a burn, so that when the irritated, inflamed surfaces heal, the healing scar tissue will cover over any weak, leaky area. The first approach is called *chemical sclerosing or chemical pleurodesis*. For this method, it is necessary to have a chest tube in the pleural space (the space between the lung and the chest wall). An irritating chemical (such as tetracycline, talc, or quinacrine) is sent through the tube once a day for 3 days in a row. When the chemical is pushed through the tube, the patient rotates through different positions, holding each one for several minutes in order to distribute the chemical to all surfaces of the lungs. The head-down position is particularly important, since the weakest spots are usually at the apex (top) of the lung. If the treatment is successful, it causes intense inflammation and therefore is often very painful. Pain medication prior to the daily procedure is essential.

Another method of stopping the leak at the surface of the lung is with a surgical operation, during which the patient is asleep under general anesthesia. The surgeon either makes an incision between the ribs and spreads the ribs (a "thoracotomy") or inserts a camera through an incision (a "thoracoscopy") and examines the lung for weak spots (blebs). These areas are then cut out and the remaining hole is sewn closed. In some cases, the pleura is stripped off the upper part of the lung, which leaves the lung surface raw and irritated. In other cases, the surgeon will take a piece of gauze and rub the surface roughly to set up the same kind of irritation and inflammation. The surgeon can also instill chemicals to irritate the surface of the lung. These maneuvers are all designed to have the reinflated lung "stick" to the inside of the chest wall and prevent a future pneumothorax.

When the chest is closed, a chest tube must be left in to drain the extra air outside the lung. Usually that tube can come out when the air has been fully evacuated and when it is clear that the leaks have been sealed. Although this procedure sounds brutal, the patient is asleep and feels no pain. After the surgery, the main discomfort is from the chest tube, which is usually removed within a few days. It is surprising, but true, that most people have less discomfort with the surgical treatment than with the chemical sclerosing. This treatment by an experienced surgeon is nearly 100% successful in preventing recurrences of pneumothorax in the involved lung.

Atelectasis

This term is derived from two Greek words (ateles + ektasis), meaning "incomplete" and "expansion" and refers to different kinds of incomplete expansion of the lung or part of the lung. Like pneumothorax, atelectasis is a kind of collapsed lung, but is very different from a pneumothorax. In someone with CF, atelectasis is almost always caused by mucus that completely blocks a bronchus leading to one of the lobes or segments of a lung (much more often in the right lung than the left and more often in the upper lobe than in other lobes). If the opening to a lobe or segment is blocked, air cannot get into that portion of the lung. Eventually all the air that was in that lobe or segment gets absorbed, leaving the lobe or segment airless. On an x-ray it will appear white (solid) instead of the usual combination of white and gray (Figure 3.14). About 1 of every 20 people with CF will develop atelectasis at some point. This problem is more common in infants than older people, probably because their bronchi are smaller and therefore more readily blocked. Usually, atelectasis does not cause any specific signs or symptoms but is likely to occur during a period of worsened lung infection.

Treating Atelectasis

Since atelectasis occurs when mucus totally blocks the opening of the bronchi in a segment or lobe of a lung, the treatment is similar to the maintenance care designed to keep the bronchi clear on a regular basis. The mainstay of the treatment is airway clearance techniques, especially CPT and percussion. Once atelectasis is identified, the physician will recommend increasing the frequency of CPT treatments, perhaps to as often as four times a day. Most physicians will also recommend antibiotics, since infection may have caused the bronchial obstruction (by generating more mucus) and may also result from the obstruction. Physicians who don't usually advise their patients to inhale mucus-cutting drugs such as DNase (see Appendix B) may make an exception in treating atelectasis. There is little or no information to support its use in this particular circumstance, however.

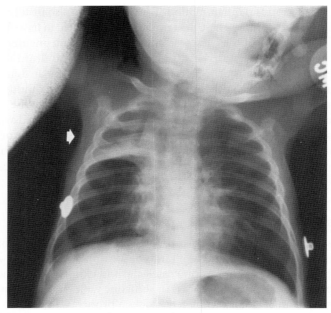

FIGURE 3.14 X-ray appearance of atelectasis of right upper lobe (arrow, x-ray taken as though we are looking at the front of the child, so his right side is on our left). The portion of the lung with more mucus and less air (the atelectatic portion) appears white, whereas the rest of the lung is darker.

Bronchoscopy (looking into the lung with a flexible tube that is passed through the nose or the mouth) with lavage (washing out mucus from the bronchi) is sometimes employed in treating atelectasis. This is an appealing kind of treatment based on the logic that if mucus is blocking the bronchi, why not just go in and wash it out? Although it is logical, this treatment, unfortunately, is rarely successful because only the first several branches of the airway tree can be seen with the bronchoscope, and the mucus is not usually confined to a single location that is visible.

The most inclusive study to examine the results of treating atelectasis with many different methods has shown that the traditional methods of CPT and antibiotics are just as successful as invasive methods such as bronchoscopy. Successful treatment of atelectasis, regardless of the method chosen, may be slow, and it may take weeks or even months before the condition resolves.

Low Oxygen Level

Most people with CF who have any more than the mildest amount of lung disease will have a lower-than-normal blood oxygen level (called "hypoxemia"). In most cases, this causes no problems. If someone lives at sea level, extra oxygen is needed only when the lung disease is very severe. At higher altitudes, the air pressure is so low that it's harder to move oxygen from the air in the alveoli into the bloodstream. At the top of Mount Everest, the air pressure is less than half of what it is at sea level; up there, everyone needs to breathe extra oxygen. In Denver (and in the passenger cabins of commercial airliners), the pressure is about four-fifths of the sea-level pressure. For people with normal lungs, this presents no problems; however, for someone with lung disease, it is likely to mean that extra oxygen will be needed. This can be determined with special testing in the pulmonary function lab.

With the appropriate treatment, which is simply getting extra oxygen to breathe, it's remarkable how better a person can feel. The various ways to obtain oxygen are outlined in Appendix B.

Respiratory Failure

As its name implies, respiratory failure is the condition in which the job of the respiratory system is not being accomplished, which is usually defined by the blood oxygen level being too low (hypoxemia), and the blood carbon dioxide level being too high (hypercapnia). This problem can occur in different people for different reasons (see Gas Transfer and Delivery). Most often, respiratory failure occurs at least partly because of lung disease. If the lungs are very severely affected by CF, it may be difficult for oxygen to be absorbed into the bloodstream at the alveoli; there will also be airway obstruction which can be so great that the work of breathing becomes too difficult for the ventilatory muscles. Except in very rare cases, this does not happen suddenly in CF. When respiratory failure does occur in someone with CF, it is in someone who has had severe lung disease for a long time.

Treatment of Respiratory Failure

Respiratory failure is another complication of CF in which the best treatment is simply a continuation and intensification of the usual treatments aimed at reducing bronchial obstruction, infection, and inflammation. In many cases, however, respiratory failure occurs only after the usual treatments have failed, and there is so little healthy lung tissue remaining that it cannot sustain the functions of bringing adequate amounts of oxygen into the body and eliminating enough carbon dioxide. If the oxygen level is low enough and/or the carbon dioxide level is high enough, this is clearly a life-threatening situation. (You may want to refer back to *Anatomy and Function of the Respiratory System*, at the beginning of this chapter, to review why this is so serious.)

In desperation, physicians and families may consider using a mechanical ventilator to do the extra breathing for the patient. In some special circumstances, this may be effective and may support the sick patient long enough for the lungs to improve, so that independent life is once again possible. These very unusual instances include respiratory failure that occurs suddenly ("acute" respiratory failure) and in a previously well patient, for example, as a result of an automobile accident or, rarely, as a result of a sudden serious viral infection like influenza. Respiratory failure in infants younger than 1 year is also a special circumstance in which temporary support with a mechanical ventilator may be helpful.

However, in most cases in which respiratory failure occurs, it is at the end of a long process, and the use of a mechanical ventilator does not reverse that process. The majority of patients with CF who are put on mechanical ventilators either die while still on the ventilator or are never able to come off it, despite weeks or even months of very intensive care. In order for a ventilator to work, a patient needs to have a tube in the trachea (either through the nose or the mouth, or as a tracheotomy tube, through an incision in the neck). These tubes are uncomfortable and make it impossible to talk. Ventilator support almost always means living in an intensive care unit, where there is usually little or no privacy, little differentiation between day and night, and constant monitoring by machines and people.

In some patients with CF, respiratory failure evolves more slowly and is called "chronic respiratory failure," or if less severe, "chronic respiratory insufficiency." Some of these patients may be treated with a ventilator machine that does not utilize a tube in the trachea but a nasal mask. This is sometimes called "noninvasive" ventilation, although patients that need this might not agree with that description! Nasal mask ventilation can decrease the work of breathing done by the fatigued respiratory muscles and in some cases may make those muscles function better even during times when the ventilator is not being used because they have been rested. Noninvasive ventilation has been utilized for patients in acute respiratory failure but is more frequently used for patients with chronic problems or who are awaiting lung transplantation.

Lung transplantation is a fairly new procedure in which a patient's lungs are removed from the chest and a new set of lungs and heart put in their place. With the first lung transplant being performed in the late 1980s, this procedure has now been performed in several thousand people with various kinds of lung problems, including almost 900 with CF (as of 2008). Some patients have done extremely well with this procedure and have been able to go back to work and resume a reasonably active life, whereas others have had many complications, and some have died. As with any new procedure, results are poor at first and improve as more experience is gained with them. This topic is discussed in Chapter 8.

Clearly, the best treatment for respiratory failure is prevention.

Cor Pulmonale and Heart Failure

Cor pulmonale literally means "heart disease caused by lung disease or breathing problems." Whenever the lungs are very severely affected (from almost any disease, including CF), or when the blood oxygen level is very low (from any cause), the blood vessels in the lung narrow, and it becomes difficult for the heart to pump blood through these blood vessels. Since it is the right side of the heart that pumps blood through the lungs, the right side of the heart gets a lot more exercise than usual. As with any other muscle, heart muscle will get bigger after it's had a lot of strenuous exercise. People who have had fairly severe lung disease for a period of time will commonly have a thick right-sided heart muscle, a condition called *right ventricular hypertrophy*. Not only will the muscle become thicker but the whole right side of the heart may also expand. This enlargement is the way the heart adapts to the excess work it's being asked to do. It is most often a *successful* adaptation. Since this is a successful adjustment by the heart to a difficult situation, it is not considered heart *disease*. Although there is an abnormal shape and size of the right ventricle of the heart, this is quite different from disease, which is, by definition, harmful. Right ventricular hypertrophy is the healthy adjustment to the abnormally great demands placed on the normal heart by the diseased lungs.

If the lung disease remains too severe for too long, the heart may no longer be able to meet all the demands placed on it. It may not be able to pump all the blood that's necessary, and some fluid may back up. This fluid can sometimes be noticed in the ankles and lower legs, and sometimes a feeling of fullness in the right side of the abdomen under the ribs signifies fluid buildup in the liver. When the heart muscle fails to pump its entire assigned load, we say that there is "heart failure," which is a frightening and misleading name for the condition, because it makes one think of heart *stoppage*, which it is not. Heart failure is the failure of the heart to do its full job. It is a serious problem but one that indicates a serious lung problem rather than a problem with the heart itself.

Treatment of Cor Pulmonale and Heart Failure

Once again, the most effective treatment for this complication of CF lung disease is the aggressive treatment of the lung disease itself. In some cases in which there is excess fluid, a diuretic medication may be helpful (see Appendix B).

Chest Pain

Chest pain is a fairly common complication of CF and has many different causes. The most serious cause is pneumothorax (see full discussion of pneumothorax, earlier in this chapter). The pain from pneumothorax is usually a sharp pain that occurs suddenly, is limited to one side, and is accompanied by shortness of breath. Other problems, while not as dangerous as pneumothorax, can be just as bothersome. The musculoskeletal system can be the source of chest pain in CF, especially when someone is coughing a lot: strained muscles, pulled tendons, and bruised or even broken ribs can occur. Infection involving the pleura (the membrane surrounding the lung) can be very uncomfortable, especially with deep breaths or coughs. This problem is called "pleuritis," or sometimes "pleurisy." Although anatomy books state that bronchi do not have pain-sensing nerves, some CF physicians think that pain may arise from large mucous plugs caught in small bronchi: clearly, some patients experience pain that disappears after they have coughed up a large plug of mucus. In younger people, the chest tightness that may accompany an asthma attack or a pulmonary exacerbation may seem like pain. Finally, there are nonpulmonary causes for chest pain in CF (heart attack is not among these): inflammation of the esophagus from acid reflux (see Chapter 4, *The Gastrointestinal Tract*) can cause "heartburn," which may be accompanied by difficulty in swallowing; and psychologic stress can certainly cause chest pain.

Clubbing

People with CF who have absolutely no lung problems will not have any skeletal problems that can be attributed to CF. However, almost everyone with CF who has even the slightest degree of lung involvement (and that means almost everyone with CF) will have a condition called "digital clubbing." This is an unfortunate name for this condition, since it sounds rather grotesque, and while in its most extreme form it can be very noticeable, in most cases it affects only slightly the shape of the fingers and toes. As shown in Figure 3.15, two features distinguish clubbed fingers from nonclubbed fingers: the first is the angle at which the base of the nail meets the finger. This angle becomes progressively flatter as clubbing increases. The second characteristic of a clubbed finger is that the thickness of the tip of the finger, the part beyond the last joint, when measured from the base of the nail to the bottom of the finger pad, becomes thicker than the finger at the joint itself.

The cause of digital clubbing is not known. In general, as lung disease worsens, so does clubbing. However, many people with fairly mild lung disease may also have pronounced clubbing, and some with advanced lung disease may have only minimal clubbing. Therefore, clubbing itself does not precisely reflect the degree of lung involvement.

There are other conditions aside from CF that are associated with clubbing, including some forms of liver disease, inflammatory bowel disease, and heart

FIGURE 3.15 Digital (finger) clubbing. The clubbed finger is flattened at the angle where the nail meets the skin, and the tip of the finger is thicker than usual.

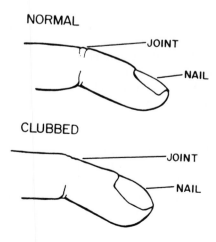

NORMAL

JOINT

NAIL

CLUBBED

JOINT

NAIL

diseases in which the blood oxygen level is too low. Clubbing is a very helpful diagnostic clue when a child with lung problems is being evaluated, since clubbing is found in most patients with CF older than 1 or 2 years, and is very rare in children who do not have CF. Any child with chronic or recurrent respiratory problems and digital clubbing should be tested for CF.

The degree of digital clubbing roughly corresponds with the degree of lung involvement, so treating the lungs may indirectly lessen the amount of clubbing. There is no treatment for clubbing aside from treatment of the lungs. Fortunately, a specific treatment is not required for clubbing, since it is not a painful condition. The only problem with clubbing is the embarrassment it can cause to some people in adjusting to having fingers that look different from normal.

TESTS

Several kinds of tests can give important objective information about the lungs in someone with CF. These tests may be useful to confirm the physician's or patient's assessment of the patient's condition, to guide treatment, to measure the response to treatment, or in some cases to identify a problem before it has become evident to family or physician. Since most problems can be treated best if they are discovered early, many CF centers employ these tests on a regular basis and not just when there is obvious trouble.

Pulmonary Function Tests (PFTs)

PFTs are tests that measure various aspects of lung function. They can determine lung size and presence and degree of bronchial obstruction. They can even give a good idea of which bronchi are blocked (the smallest bronchi or the larger central airways). They can identify asthma in children and adults, and they can measure the amount of oxygen circulating in the blood.

PFTs are a sensitive tool for following the condition of someone's lungs, showing subtle changes that might not have been detected otherwise. Most PFTs require the understanding and cooperation of the patient, and children older than 6 or 7 years are usually able to cooperate. Specialized testing is available for infants and toddlers who are not able to cooperate (see later).

Spirometry

Spirometry ("measuring breathing") is the simplest PFT and is available in most hospitals and clinics. In this test, the patient breathes in and out through a tube while a machine records the amount of air breathed and the speed at which it is blown out. This test is useful because how fast the air can flow is related to the size of the airways; small or obstructed airways result in reduced airflow rates. Many of the tests are very reproducible within subjects, making them useful for determining response to treatment or progression of lung disease over time.

The patient performing spirometry breathes through a mouthpiece connected to a flow-measuring device (pneumotachometer) while wearing noseclips. After taking a maximum inhalation, the patient is coached to blow out rapidly and forcefully for as long as possible. Patients older than 10 years are coached to exhale for a minimum of 6 seconds (which may feel like an eternity!), although younger children may not be able to blow out as long. This coaching is very important and requires a good bit of enthusiasm. A minimum of three efforts is required with two efforts being close to each other.

Several parameters can be calculated from these maneuvers. First, the total exhaled volume is termed the "forced vital capacity (FVC)." The volume exhaled in the first second is termed the FEV_1. Although the FEV_1 is far from a perfect measurement, it is very reproducible and is used as an "outcome measure" in almost all clinical research trials for CF. The airflow rate between 25% of the exhaled volume and 75% of the exhaled volume is termed the $FEF_{25\%-75\%}$ (or occasionally the maximal midexpiratory flow [MMEF]). This measurement is thought to reflect airflow in the smaller airways. The actual volume (or flow rate) of air that is measured is then compared with an expected amount (the predicted value), which is dependent on the patient's age, sex, ethnicity, and height. Using the measured value and the predicted value, we can calculate a percent of predicted value, which is like a test score. The lower the percentage predicted, the worse the patient's lung function is.

Figure 3.16 shows two kinds of graphs that the spirometer can produce. The first (Figure 3.16A) records the amount (volume) of air blown out after the largest possible inhalation, and the time it takes to exhale it forcefully. The solid line is from someone who has CF and normal lung function and the dotted line is from someone who has CF and a moderate amount of obstruction. You will note that for the patient with CF and obstruction, the vital capacity and FEV_1 are both smaller than in the patient with normal lung function.

These tests (FVC, FEV_1) are useful but they have one important drawback, namely, they are very "effort-dependent," meaning that a half-hearted breath will give worthless information. Experienced technicians can very often tell from the shape of the curve whether the patient has given as good an effort as possible.

Another way of looking at the information from spirometry is the flow-volume curve (Figure 3.16B), which shows how quickly air flows out of the lungs at different points during a maximum expiratory effort. This gives valuable information because air comes out much faster at the beginning of a breath, when the lungs are fully inflated, than it does later on in the breath, when the lungs are nearly empty. The flow-volume curve relates the flow rates to precise portions of the breath. The shape of the curve can identify the location of obstruction (for example, in the larger central airways or in the more peripheral airways) and also gives the technician feedback about the patient's effort during the test. Another reason this information is so useful is that the flow rates during the second half of a breath depend very little on

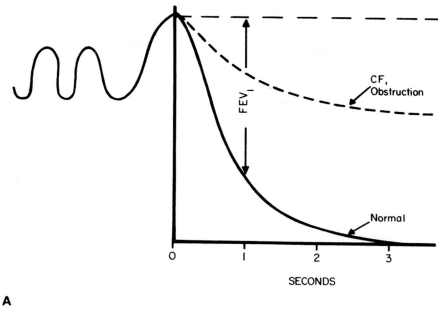

A

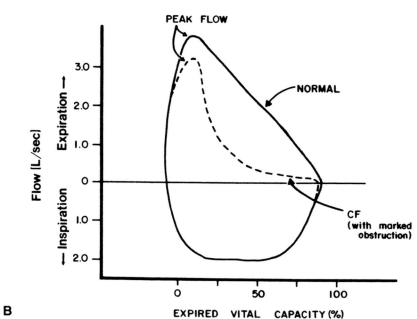

B

FIGURE 3.16 Pulmonary function tests. **A:** Volume-time curve. **B:** Flow-volume curve (see text for discussion).

how much force is used to exhale; that is, these flow rates are relatively effort-independent (compared to FVC and FEV_1) and are therefore valuable even in someone whose cooperation is less than perfect. Finally, the flow rates at the end of a breath seem to be a good reflection of the amount of obstruction in the smallest bronchi: during the first part of the exhalation, the air quickly empties out of the larger bronchi, and during the last half or quarter of the breath the air empties out of the smallest bronchi. Therefore, a slower than normal second half of a breath can indicate some blockage in the smallest airways, even when the larger bronchi are unobstructed and the first half of the breath is perfectly normal.

Lung Volumes

Lung volumes are measured by two different methods and require complex machinery, which may not be available in every hospital or physician's office. Yet they can give valuable information that cannot be obtained with spirometry. Spirometry measures the air that moves in and out of the lungs but indicates nothing about the actual size of the lungs or the amount of air left inside the lungs after a person has finished blowing out.

The helium dilution method for measuring lung volumes uses the "Iced Tea Principle." If you place a teaspoon of sugar into a full glass of iced tea and mix it thoroughly, the sweetness of the tea will depend on the size of the glass. Clearly, an 8-oz glass will be much sweeter with a teaspoon of sugar than a quart jar. Another way of saying this is—the smaller the glass, the greater the concentration of sugar. In fact, if you had tools precise enough to measure the exact sweetness or the exact concentration of sugar, and you knew the exact amount of sugar you put in (one teaspoon, in this case) you could calculate the size of the glass.

For measuring lung volumes, the sugar substitute is helium, a gas that is very safe to breathe in and which is not absorbed into the bloodstream. If you breathe in a known amount of helium for a few minutes, until it is thoroughly mixed with the air in your lungs, the concentration of helium in the air you breathe out can tell the size of your lungs. This method works fairly well for determining the size of your lungs at their largest (with the biggest breath in) and at their smallest (after you've breathed out all you can). These are the total lung capacity and residual volume, respectively. The method is not perfect because it requires that all of the bronchial tubes be open so that the helium can mix completely with all areas of the lung. If a portion of one lung is blocked off, the helium won't mix with the air in that part of the lung, and it will seem that the lungs are smaller than they actually are. What is measured by this method is the volume of lung which freely communicates with the mouth; that's the same as the total lung volume if the airways are healthy, but in obstructed lungs the volume will be underestimated.

The "body box" (total body plethysmograph) solves the problem of obstruction. It is an expensive piece of equipment that looks something like a space capsule or telephone booth (you may remember telephone booths, perhaps from Superman comic strips). Not many hospitals are equipped with body boxes suitable for testing children. The person being tested sits inside the box and breathes through a tube. When the box is shut, it is completely airtight, which allows changes in pressure within the box to be measured very precisely while the person breathes. The changes in pressure reflect the changes in chest size. A mathematical formula is then applied that translates the pressure changes into accurate lung volume calculations, which include all of the lung volume, whether the bronchi are blocked or open. If someone does have bronchial obstruction, the total lung capacity will not be affected very much, but since obstruction (especially of small airways) makes it difficult to empty the lungs, the residual volume (the amount of air left in the lungs after a maximum exhalation) will be larger than normal. Normally, the residual volume is less than 25% of the total lung capacity, but in someone with severely blocked small airways, it can be as much as 70% of total lung capacity.

Testing in Infants and Toddlers

Most of the tests described above have been adapted to infants and toddlers, with the obvious challenge being that we cannot ask the infant to "blow, blow, blow"! Infants are usually sedated using a medication called chloral hydrate, which is taken by mouth and works much more slowly than anesthesia medications used in the operating room. Once the child is asleep, he or she is placed on a special bed with a mask over the mouth and nose to measure airflow and pressure at the mouth.

In order to get the infant to exhale rapidly, we utilize a balloon inside a plastic jacket that encircles the chest and abdomen and which can be inflated rapidly from a pressure tank, gently but rapidly squeezing the chest, and forcing air out. Exhaled flow and volume are measured through the face mask. The infant's lung is first inflated to a predetermined pressure which results in a lung volume very close to total lung capacity. From this raised lung volume, the jacket encompassing the chest is rapidly inflated from the pressure tank, generating a full expiratory flow-volume curve which can look just like a curve obtained from a cooperative adult! As the lungs of small infants empty very quickly, we usually measure an $FEV_{0.5}$ (the volume exhaled in ½ second) rather than FEV_1, but most other measurements (FVC, FEF_{25-75}) are strictly comparable to those from older children. Lung volumes can also be measured with an infant body plethysmograph, using the same principles as apply to older children.

While these tests can be very informative, they are not available at all hospitals, and require specialized equipment and staff. The tests take much longer than in a cooperative child and do require sedation, so they are typically not performed as often as in older children.

Asthma Testing

Asthma is a condition in which bronchi are blocked because of inflammation within bronchi and contraction of the muscles in the bronchial wall (this contraction of bronchial wall muscles is sometimes called "bronchospasm").

While the flow rates and lung volumes from the tests just described can tell whether an obstruction is present, they can't tell what has caused it. However, if someone inhales a fast-acting bronchodilator, the bronchial muscle quickly relaxes and the obstruction decreases. If the PFTs are repeated, the flow rates will show dramatic improvement within a few minutes. Since it's important to know how much obstruction is reversible, many laboratories will automatically schedule a bronchodilator inhalation and repeat spirometry as part of routine PFTs.

Some laboratories may go one step further and try to identify people whose bronchi aren't yet blocked by bronchospasm but are susceptible to such blockage. These are people with reactive airways, which is another term for asthma. These people may have completely normal pulmonary function at a given time, but if they inhale certain chemicals, their bronchial muscles may contract much more readily than the bronchial muscles of someone with normal airways. To test for this, people may be asked to breathe in these chemicals (methacholine is the one most commonly used in this country; histamine is another), starting with a very dilute solution, and increasing step by step to a stronger solution, repeating the spirometry after each new challenge. The test is completed when the PFTs worsen. Someone has reactive airways disease if his or her PFTs get worse with a dilute (weak) solution of the chemical. These tests that measure airway reactivity are called "bronchial provocation" or "inhalation challenge tests." Other bronchial challenge tests involve PFTs before and after exercise or before and after inhaling cold dry air.

Blood Gases

Since the major job of the lungs is to bring oxygen into the bloodstream and to eliminate carbon dioxide, it may be important to know the blood oxygen and carbon dioxide levels. To find this out, a sample of blood from an artery (the most accurate) or capillary is obtained. An arterial sample is performed by inserting a needle into an artery and drawing out blood. Since a needle inserted into an artery can be much more painful than one inserted into a vein, a small amount of lidocaine (Xylocaine) may be injected into the skin first or the skin prepared with EMLA® cream, which numbs the skin and makes the test more tolerable.

Oximetry

Over the past years, painless, noninvasive monitors have been developed which decrease the need for arterial blood gases. These monitors are called "oximeters" (either ear oximeters or pulse oximeters), and they work through a computerized method: a light is shined through the fingertip or earlobe to a sensor on the other side of the finger or ear; the amount of light that can pass through the tissues is determined partly by the amount of oxygen that is bound to hemoglobin in the blood in those tissues. The oxygen saturation of the blood (the percentage of hemoglobin that is bound with oxygen) is calculated almost instantaneously by computer and is indicated on a digital display. A normal oxygen saturation is at least 95%.

Exercise Tests

Standard PFTs measure lung function while a person is resting. It may be useful in some situations to see how the lungs (and heart) function when they are put under stress, as with exercise. Exercise tests can range from very simple (listening to someone's lungs after he or she has been running in a hallway) to very complex (measuring the precise amounts of oxygen consumed, carbon dioxide produced, oxygen exhaled, time it takes to inhale and exhale, rate of breathing, heart rate, etc.). Many physicians feel that the exercise test is more successful than regular PFTs in detecting mild problems. This is because a mild problem will not present itself unless the system is stressed, as when people exert themselves to the limit. For most exercise tests, the person being tested pedals on a stationary exercise cycle or walks/runs on a treadmill. The test begins with an easy pace and gets increasingly difficult. While the test is going on, you may have to breathe through a mouthpiece like a scuba diver, so that the air you breathe in and out can be analyzed. In other tests, you may have electrocardiogram electrodes taped on your chest. In some tests, oximeters may be used, with a light taped to your finger or ear. In very special tests, there may even be a small plastic tube placed in the artery at your wrist. In other tests, none of those monitors may be used.

Exercise tests can show how physically fit a person is, and one study has shown that fitness level (as measured on an exercise test) was the test that correlated most closely with a CF patient's likelihood of surviving the next 8 years or more.

Chest X-rays

X-rays are generated by a machine that functions similarly to a camera. The x-ray machine is directed at the object to be studied and generates x-rays, which pass through that object, in varying amounts and intensity. The x-rays then strike and expose photographic paper which is situated behind the object. When there is no object in the way, and the x-rays hit the photographic paper directly, it becomes completely black. When an object such as lead is in the way, which totally blocks all the x-rays, the paper becomes completely white. The thicker or more dense a material, the more rays it absorbs and the whiter the image of that material on the resulting x-ray film. (These days, most radiology departments don't use photographic paper but rather use the same x-rays, with the images recorded digitally, by computers.) When the object in question is a person's chest, there will be recognizable white/black/gray patterns determined by the bones, lungs, heart, and so forth. The bones are quite dense and therefore will appear white on the final x-ray. The heart, because it consists of thick muscle and is filled with blood, also appears fairly white. The lungs are much less dense, since they are relatively delicate tissues largely filled with air, and therefore appear much blacker or at least a darker shade of gray. The lungs do contain some dense tissue, including blood vessels, so they are not totally black. The diaphragms mark the lower edges of the lungs and are white since they are fairly solid muscles.

Chest x-rays can give important information about the condition of the lungs. If, for example, a lobe of the lung is collapsed because it is filled with mucus, that lobe will appear much denser (whiter) than normal. If thick scar tissue has replaced healthy lung tissue, that too will be whiter than usual. Bronchial walls swollen by fluid or inflammation may have a similar appearance. In many cases it is possible to see "increased markings," meaning more white (dense) markings than normal, but it is not possible to tell whether the increased density is caused by inflammation or mucus (which can get better) or by scar tissue (which cannot get better).

A pneumothorax, in which air has escaped through a leak in the lung but is still within the chest, will show up on the x-ray as a totally black area outside the lung, while the lung itself will be whiter than normal (see Figure 3.12). The totally black area is air, and the lung will appear denser (whiter) than normal since it is partly collapsed, with the solid parts of the lung closer together than normal.

Lungs that are obstructed and difficult to empty will be larger than normal and will push the diaphragms downward (Figure 3.17). These overinflated (hyperinflated) lungs may not only push the diaphragms down into a flattened shape (compared with the normal dome shape) but also actually push the sternum (the front of the chest) forward. This is called "sternal bowing" (since the shape of the sternum comes to resemble an archery bow).

Computed Tomographic (CT) Scans

A CT scan is an x-ray technique in which many different x-ray images, of "slices" of parts of the body, are taken and organized by computer to give a more detailed view of the parts of the body in question. CT scans (also called "CAT" scans) of the chest show much greater detail than traditional x-rays. They also use considerably more radiation than standard chest x-rays and are more expensive. Chest CT scans have not yet replaced standard x-rays in the monitoring and care of patients with CF, but there are instances in which a chest CT scan can be useful.

Cultures and Sensitivities

It is important to know what bacteria are in the bronchi of someone with CF, in case antibiotic treatment becomes necessary. To identify bacteria, small samples of mucus are sent to a bacteriology laboratory where they are placed in different

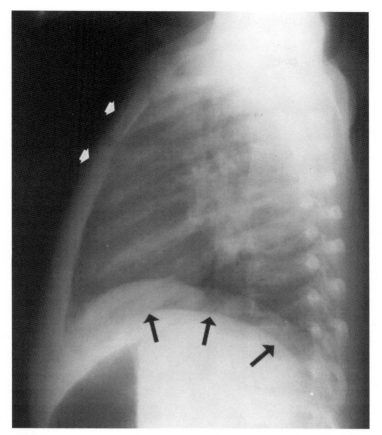

FIGURE 3.17 X-ray appearance of overinflation of lungs. These are lateral (side) views of the chest of two different children with CF. **A** shows normal lungs, with nicely domed diaphragms (*black arrows*), a normally straight breast bone (sternum—*white arrows*), and little air directly behind the sternum. (*continued*)

substances called "media." These samples of mucus can be obtained in several different ways: 1. Throat cultures: these can be done easily (for most people; some children really dislike them) in clinic: the child opens his or her mouth, and the nurse (isn't it always the nurse who does stuff like this?) will tickle the back of the throat with a long cotton swab. The results from a throat culture in patients with CF are pretty good in telling what bacteria are in the lungs (pretty good, in that bacteria on the culture were probably in the lungs, but not perfect in that some bacteria in the lungs might not show up on the throat culture.) 2. Sputum cultures. These are very easy for people who can spit out mucus that they've coughed up: no mean old throat swab, and the cultures from these specimens reflect lung

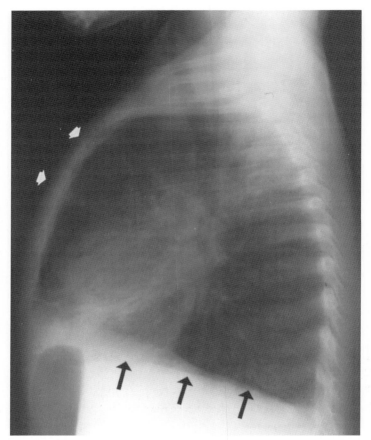

FIGURE 3.17 (*Continued*) In contrast, **B** shows severe overinflation of the lungs, with the diaphragms pushed downward and flattened (*black arrows*) and the sternum "bowed" outward (*white arrows*) and excessive air (*blacker*) behind the sternum. Note, too, that the overall depth of the chest from the sternum to the spine is much greater in the overinflated chest. This is referred to as an *increased AP* (anterior–posterior) *diameter*.

bacteria very well. 3. Bronchoscopy specimens. In some cases, physicians aren't satisfied that the throat or sputum cultures are telling the whole story, and they might want to perform a bronchoscopy, in which they pass a lighted tube down through the mouth into the trachea and large bronchi in order to suction a specimen directly from the lower airways. Most physicians do these procedures in the operating room or a special procedure room, with the patient under deep sedation or general anesthesia. However the specimen is obtained, it is then processed in the bacteriology lab: Some media are good environments for all types of bacteria to grow in, and others will allow only certain bacteria to grow. After the bacteria have grown they are analyzed and identified, with the entire process taking several days.

Once the bacteria are grown and identified, the task remains of determining which antibiotics are the most effective in killing those bacteria. To find this out, various antibiotics are added to the cultures and their effects are observed. One method of introducing antibiotics is through the use of paper discs that have been soaked with the antibiotic. These discs are placed at intervals around the plate where the bacteria are grown. If the antibiotic kills the bacteria, there will be a clear area around the disc, where the bacteria have not been able to grow (this clear area is called the "zone of inhibition"). If the bacteria are not killed by the antibiotic, they continue to grow right up to the disc, leaving no clear zone. Sometimes there will be a very small zone and sometimes a larger one. Most laboratories will define the response to the antibiotic based on the size of the clear zone. For example, when the antibiotic gentamicin is used in cultures of *Pseudomonas*, the bacteria are proclaimed *sensitive* to the antibiotic if the clear area is 15 mm or larger; if the clear area is 13 to 14 mm, it is considered *intermediate,* and if it is 12 mm or less, the bacteria are said to be *resistant* to the effects of the antibiotic. "Resistance" is thus a relative term, since the presence of even a very small clear space indicates that some bacteria have been killed. This also means that the laboratory might report a culture back as showing the bacteria to be "resistant" to a particular antibiotic, and your doctor might decide to use it anyway. Frequently in this kind of situation, the antibiotic has its desired effect despite the laboratory report.

SUMMARY

The respiratory system accounts for more than 95% of illness and deaths from CF, and therefore keeping it healthy is the most important thing that can be done for anyone with CF. Fortunately, there is much that can be done toward this end, and the tremendous improvement in life expectancy of patients with CF can be attributed largely to better prevention and treatment of lung problems. Most of the problems that develop in the lung are the result of bronchial blockage caused by thick mucus and of infection that follows the blockage. Physical means, such as PD and percussion treatments, and medications, including bronchodilators and mucus thinning drugs, help prevent and reverse bronchial obstruction. Antibiotics, given by mouth, aerosol, or injection, are very successful in treating bronchial infection.

The Gastrointestinal Tract

4

Douglas S. Lindblad, Daniel J. Weiner, and David M. Orenstein

THE BASICS

1. Cystic fibrosis (CF) affects several organs of the gastrointestinal (GI) tract, including the pancreas, the intestine, the gallbladder, the liver, and the esophagus.

2. Most people with CF need to take pancreatic enzymes with their meals and snacks to help digest their food.

3. People who skip their enzymes (or whose enzymes are not working right) have abdominal pain and frequent, large, smelly, loose bowel movements. They may also have trouble gaining weight and may sometimes develop serious deficiencies in certain nutrients.

4. With help from the CF center, anyone can learn how much enzymes to use.

5. Weight gain and nutrition are important to the health of the lungs in CF and to long-term survival.

6. Some patients with CF have episodes of intestinal blockage, which require prompt treatment. Signs of this problem include "stomach aches" and fewer bowel movements than normal. If your child has no bowel movement for 24 hours, call the CF center right away.

7. Some babies and children with CF have gastroesophageal reflux (acid moving backward from the stomach into the esophagus). Treatment with medications and changes in diet may be helpful.

8. Some CF experts recommend putting your baby to sleep on its stomach to minimize reflux.

9. A few patients with CF have serious liver problems.

THE NORMAL GI TRACT

The GI tract consists of a group of organs which function to digest and absorb foods and eliminate unwanted parts of the food as waste. Each organ of the digestive system, which includes the esophagus, stomach, small intestine, large intestine (colon), liver, gallbladder, and pancreas (Figure 4.1), has specific functions in this process.

In order for the body to use the food that we eat, the food must be broken down (digested) into basic elements that are small enough to cross through the wall of the intestine (absorption) into the bloodstream. It may be helpful to think about what happens to parts of a meal when they are eaten. For this purpose, we can use a (not completely well-rounded) meal consisting of meat, potato with butter, a glass of whole milk, and a dessert of hard candy. Each of these foods has a mix of nutrients: protein, fat, and carbohydrate. For this discussion, however, the meat will represent its main component, protein; the butter, fat; the potato, starch; and the candy, sucrose (a carbohydrate, or sugar, that is simpler than starch). The milk contains another simple carbohydrate, lactose, as well as fat and protein.

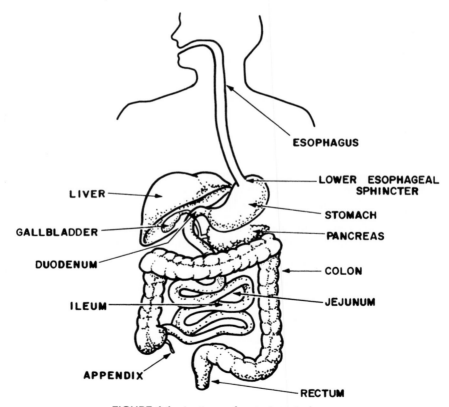

FIGURE 4.1. Anatomy of gastrointestinal tract.

The process begins with the sight or smell of food, which reflexively stimulates the GI system to be prepared for food intake. Digestion begins immediately when food is placed into the mouth. In the mouth, food is chewed and mixed with saliva, which contains digestive enzymes called amylase and lipase. The amylase begins to break down the starch of the potato. The lipase starts to break down the fat of the butter and milk. You will notice that most enzymes that break down food usually end in "-ase" or "-sin."

The chewed food is then swallowed, passing through the throat and entering the esophagus. In the throat, the food passes close to the opening of the airways; under normal circumstances, a reflex closes this opening to prevent food from traveling into the lungs (aspiration). This enables the esophagus to serve as a conduit, moving food safely from the mouth and into the stomach, without letting excessive air move down with the food. Yet, it also must let air or food come back up when the need arises to belch or vomit. A muscular region of the lower portion of the esophagus, known as the lower esophageal sphincter (LES), spends most of the time squeezed together in a closed position, which prevents stomach contents from coming back up, even if you're upside down. The LES relaxes only to let swallowing occur.

The chewed-up foods have now entered the stomach. Here, the protein in the meat and milk is acted upon by the enzyme pepsin, which is secreted by the stomach. The stomach also produces acid that helps in the process of protein digestion. The wall of the stomach contains muscle, which contracts, and makes for more mixing and helping to grind the food into smaller particles.

The food is slowly released from the stomach into the duodenum, the first part of the small intestine. Within the duodenum, one or two small openings bring digestive juices from the liver and pancreas into the intestine. This juice is carried from the liver and pancreas to the intestine by a system of very small tubes known as ducts. This juice, known as bile, contains large amounts of important digestive enzymes made by the pancreas. Bile also contains large amounts of bile salts (also called bile acids) made by the liver. Among the pancreatic enzymes are proteases such as trypsin, chymotrypsin, and elastase, which break down the protein in the meat and milk. Two other important pancreatic enzymes are amylase and lipase. Pancreatic amylase, like salivary amylase, continues to digest the starch in the potato. Enzymes located in the lining of the intestine also help to digest starch and sugars in the potato and the milk. Pancreatic lipase is a particularly important enzyme because it is the major fat-digesting enzyme in the GI tract. It is also very fragile and is destroyed in the presence of too much acid. The acid is normally neutralized by bicarbonate secreted by the intestine and also found in the bile. To function well, pancreatic lipase also requires the presence of bile salts from the liver and co-lipase produced by the pancreas.

Once the digestion of food is complete, the products can be absorbed through cells lining the small intestine. These ingredients can then pass into the bloodstream to be used where they are needed. While digestion is taking place, the muscles of the small intestine gradually churn and mix the contents and propel the contents forward toward the large intestine. In the large intestine, salts and water are gradually absorbed from this mixture. The leftover contents, which include non-digestible food products such as fiber and products from bacteria that normally live in the colon, are passed out of the body as a bowel movement.

In a person whose digestive tract is working properly, nearly all of the nutritious food that is eaten is digested by the pancreatic and other enzymes and absorbed by intestinal cells into the bloodstream. In particular, very little of the carbohydrate and protein and less than 7% of the fat is wasted. In conditions leading to malabsorption, such as CF, digestion and absorption are incomplete, and substantial amounts of fat and other nutrients can escape into the stools.

THE GI TRACT IN CYSTIC FIBROSIS

The remainder of this chapter is devoted to problems that may occur in the GI tract in patients with CF, with each problem being reviewed under the affected organ. Table 4.1 lists the problems and the frequency with which they occur. Nutritional issues in cystic fibrosis (CF) are covered separately in Chapter 6.

Pancreas

The pancreas has two distinct functions. The *endocrine* pancreas helps to regulate blood sugar (glucose) levels by producing hormones such as insulin. When this

TABLE 4.1

Incidence of Gastrointestinal Conditions in Cystic Fibrosis

Organ	Condition	Patients with cystic fibrosis with condition, %
Pancreas	Pancreatic insufficiency	85–90[a]
	Pancreatitis	1
Liver and Gallbladder	Cirrhosis	1–4
	Gallstones	10
Esophagus and Stomach	Gastroesophageal reflux	10–20
	Ulcers	1–10
Intestines	Meconium ileus	10
	Meconium peritonitis	1
	Distal intestinal obstruction syndrome	10–30
	Rectal prolapse	10–20
	Intussusception	1

[a]At birth, only about 50% are pancreatic insufficient.

function is lost, diabetes results; this topic is discussed further in Chapter 5. The *exocrine* pancreas supports digestion and absorption. Glands within the pancreas produce enzymes that digest fats (including lipase and co-lipase) and proteins (including trypsin, chymotrypsin, elastase, and carboxypeptidases). These enzymes travel through small tubes (ducts) to reach the intestine and support digestion. The normal pancreas also secretes fluid that is rich in bicarbonate, a substance that can neutralize acid coming from the stomach. The ability of the pancreas to secrete bicarbonate and transport digestive enzymes depends on the normal functioning of the **c**ystic **f**ibrosis **t**ransmembrane conductance **r**egulator (CFTR) gene and properly functioning CFTR protein in the cells lining the pancreatic ducts.

Pancreatic Insufficiency

In most patients with CF, abnormally thick and acidic pancreatic juice leads to blockage of the pancreatic ducts and damage to the glands that generate digestive enzymes. The damaged pancreatic tissue is gradually replaced by fat and scar tissue. As a result, the pancreas becomes progressively less able to support digestion within the intestine. This process begins prior to birth and continues after birth. When more than 90% of the enzymes are lost, digestion of fats and proteins is significantly compromised, a condition known as **p**ancreatic exocrine **i**nsufficiency (or PI for short). People with PI need to take pancreatic enzyme supplements in order to digest their food.

About 85% to 90% of patients with CF will eventually develop PI. The risk of this occurrence is closely related to the genetics of CF. Patients with most of the known CFTR mutations (including the most common, Δ*F508*) are very likely to develop PI. Those with "mild" mutations, with more intact CFTR protein, are more likely to remain pancreatic sufficient (PS). The prevalence of PI in CF increases in the first few months to years of life. About half of infants with CF will already have PI at birth and require pancreatic enzyme replacement. Most of the remaining children gradually lose pancreatic function with time. Up to 79% of 6-month-olds and 90% of 9-year-olds will have developed PI.

The intestine has some ability to digest carbohydrates (starch) and protein when the pancreas is not functioning properly. However, the digestion of starch is incomplete and may lead to symptoms of distention (bloating) and gas. The digestion of proteins is also incomplete and may lead to loss of proteins in the stool. When severe, this process may lead to low protein in the blood and puffy skin (edema).

The ability of the intestine to digest and absorb fats is highly dependent on a functioning pancreas. In patients with PI, fats are poorly digested and absorbed. As a result, they are passed through the intestine into the bowel movements, which are large, greasy, and more smelly than normal. The loss of fat through the stools represents a significant loss of calories to support the energy needs of the body. A given amount of fat has more calories (9 calories per gram) than any other kind of food (4 calories per gram of protein or sugar); so losing an ounce of fat means losing more than twice as many calories as would be lost in an ounce of carbohydrate or protein. The "textbook picture" of a youngster with undiagnosed CF is someone who is scrawny, has a huge appetite, and has frequent, large, smelly, greasy stools. This person is scrawny because much of the nutrients in the food go directly into the toilet. The apparently huge appetite is really a way of compensating for losing half of what is eaten in the bowel movements—it's as if you've been fed a half portion, so you eat another portion to make up for that. The poor fat absorption may also lead to a lack of certain nutrients, including essential fatty acids and fat-soluble vitamins (vitamins A, D, E, and K). This topic is discussed further in Chapter 6.

Before effective treatment was available, most children with CF die in infancy from problems that include malnutrition. In spite of an increased appetite, infants are not able to absorb sufficient calories and nutrients to meet their needs. With the availability of effective replacement pancreatic enzymes, most children with CF can achieve normal weight gain.

Diagnosis of Pancreatic Insufficiency

There are several ways in which a physician can determine if a patient with CF has pancreatic insufficiency. Knowing the CF genotype can be helpful, as most patients with all but a few "mild" mutations will eventually develop PI. Symptoms such as frequent greasy, smelly, large stools and difficulty gaining weight may suggest the possibility of fat malabsorption. When PI is suspected, a physician may select from several types of tests discussed below.

The most direct method, known as pancreatic function testing, is more invasive and only rarely used. This involves collecting a sample of fluid from the duodenum and measuring the content of pancreatic enzymes. This can be done either by passing a tube through the nose, esophagus, and stomach to the duodenum or during a procedure known as endoscopy, when a tube is passed through the mouth, esophagus, stomach, and duodenum while the patient is under anesthesia.

Several indirect tests for pancreatic function are available. A stool sample may be examined for the presence of fat droplets, which are not normally present in any significant quantity. A positive result suggests that some fat malabsorption has occurred, but this test is not very specific for pancreatic insufficiency. A more accurate test is the 72-hour fecal fat collection. This test involves collecting all of the bowel movements that are passed over a 3-day period into a container (the laboratory may supply a container such as a large paint can). The patient or his/her family also carefully records all of the food that is eaten beginning one day before the collection and extending until the end of the test. The patient should be consuming a high-fat diet and should avoid fat substitutes such as olestra. The dietician can then calculate the amount of fat consumed from the dietary log. The amount of fat collected in the stools is measured, and the fraction of stool that was absorbed can be determined. Absorbing less than 93% of the fat that was consumed implies fat malabsorption which may be due to pancreatic insufficiency. This test is also sometimes used to measure the effectiveness of pancreatic enzyme replacement therapy (PERT).

A newer, simpler, and much more convenient test involves measuring the amount of elastase-1, a pancreatic digestive enzyme, in a single stool sample. In patients with CF, there is a good correlation between a low elastase-1 measurement and pancreatic insufficiency. Other enzyme levels, such as trypsin and chymotrypsin, have also been used for this purpose.

Another test that is sometimes used is known as a "therapeutic trial." In this test, the patient is treated with PERT, and the patient is observed for a change in symptoms. A decrease in malabsorptive bowel movements or an improvement in growth suggests that the enzymes are helpful. Since the enzymes in small doses are not harmful and not very expensive, this can be a good, sensible test. It may not always give the most accurate information in the fastest time, however.

One further test that forms the basis for most newborn screening programs for CF also relates to pancreatic function. This blood test is performed on the first or second day of life. A dried spot of blood is analyzed for *immunoreactive trypsinogen* (IRT), a substance that is found in higher quantities in the blood of newborns with CF than in those without CF. It is not known why this is so, but it may be that the trypsinogen (which is a precursor for the enzyme trypsin) is partly blocked from getting out of the pancreas and into the duodenum "back up" into the bloodstream. One problem with this explanation is that even most CF babies with pancreatic sufficiency have an abnormal IRT. (Perhaps these pancreatic-sufficient babies have *some* pancreatic blockage—not total, and enough trypsin and other enzymes get into the duodenum to bring about normal digestion and absorption—but enough blockage that some trypsin backs up into the bloodstream and is detected by the IRT.) This test is discussed a bit more in Chapter 2, *Making the Diagnosis*.

Treatment of Pancreatic Insufficiency

Treatment of pancreatic insufficiency is simple, and the results are dramatic, now that PERT is available. Although it may seem complicated when families are first introduced to enzymes, virtually everyone who has CF or who has a child with CF soon becomes an expert in using enzymes. These enzymes are often enteric-coated, meaning that they are protected from stomach acid by a coating that only dissolves when it is in the nonacidic fluid usually found in the intestine. Since the raw enzymes (especially lipase) are easily inactivated by acid, the introduction of enteric-coated enzyme preparations in 1978 was revolutionary and made a huge difference in the effectiveness of this very important part of CF treatment. The quantity of enzymes to be taken is determined by evaluating such factors as bowel movements, appetite, and weight gain. In 2010, all companies producing enzymes were required by the Food and Drug Administration to perform clinical trials using their drugs and to re-label them with the exact amount of enzyme in each capsule. Many enzyme brand names changed to reflect this, some new brands emerged, and some brands were discontinued.

The amount of enzymes taken must be adjusted by your CF specialist. Too not enough enzymes may lead to malabsorption of nutrients and symptoms mentioned above. Usually, taking too much enzymes has no medical consequences, including no change in bowel habits, appetite, or growth. The only consequences are the financial ones associated with a paying for more enzymes. On occasion, too much of enzyme can cause a change in bowel habits, most commonly occurring as loose stools but occasionally as constipation. This problem usually resolves with decreasing the enzyme dose. Rarely, a more serious problem known as fibrosing colonopathy may occur. This problem was recognized in the 1990s when some patients taking very high doses of enzymes developed scarring of their large intestines. The scarring was associated with symptoms such as abdominal pain and bloody diarrhea. Many of these patients required surgery. This problem has never been seen except in those patients taking extremely high doses of enzymes and has become extremely rare since enzyme manufacturing changed in the late 1990s. Most patients with pancreatic insufficiency and CF do well with less than 2,500 units of lipase per kilogram of body weight per meal (or less than 10,000 units per kilogram per day). A 20 kg (44 lb) child may use 50,000 units of lipase per meal or less. Depending on the strength of the particular enzyme preparation, this means 5 to 10 enzyme capsules per meal or fewer. The risk of fibrosing colonopathy at this dose is extremely low.

Acute Pancreatitis

Pancreatitis is an inflammation of the pancreas that causes severe abdominal pain and, usually, vomiting. It occurs in people without CF, sometimes due to gallstones blocking secretion of the pancreas, due to drinking alcohol, as a side effect of medications, as a result of a viral infection, or due to other, less common, causes. Pancreatitis is uncommon among patients with CF, probably in part because most patients with CF do not have enough intact pancreatic tissue to become inflamed. In fact, patients with CF and pancreatic insufficiency virtually never develop pancreatitis. Among the few patients with CF and pancreatic sufficiency, a few (about 10%) will get pancreatitis. Blood tests and radiologic studies such as an abdominal ultrasound, computed tomography (CT) scan, or magnetic resonance imaging (MRI) may be helpful in the diagnosis. Most patients with acute pancreatitis are unable to eat or drink for a period of time, because doing so stimulates the pancreas and increases symptoms. Treatment usually involves a stay in the hospital during which intravenous fluids may be provided, and pain may be treated with medications. There is some evidence that giving pancreatic enzymes may help in this condition, but not all physicians are convinced by this. Nutrition during this time may be provided either via a tube that is passed through the nose, stomach, and duodenum into the distal intestine, or sometimes intravenous nutrition may be provided. Tube feeding into the distal intestine is much less likely to stimulate or irritate the pancreas than feeding by mouth. When feeding resumes, the physician may recommend a low-fat, low-protein diet for a certain period of time, since fat and protein in the diet are the main signals for the pancreas to secrete, and avoiding those elements may give the pancreatic inflammation more time to subside. Although the condition is rare, it often recurs in those unfortunate enough to have it.

Small and Large Intestine

Meconium Ileus

Meconium is a baby's first bowel movement, formed in the intestine while the infant is still in mother's womb. Since the baby has had nothing to eat, this bowel movement is formed from bile and bits of mucus and intestinal cells that have been shed into the stool. It is usually a dark colored and sticker stool than those passed subsequently as the infant begins feeding. A healthy infant will usually pass a meconium stool within 48 hours after birth.

In infants with CF, the meconium is much thicker and sticker than usual. This is thought to be related to the effect of the basic defect on the intestine, which produces thicker, more dehydrated intestinal secretions. In about 10% of infants, the meconium is so thick that it clogs the end of the small intestine, known as the terminal ileum. This condition, known as meconium ileus, prevents the baby from having a bowel movement. This may lead to a distended (swollen) belly, belly pain, and vomiting of bile, which may appear green or yellow. Sometimes the blockage leads to a tear in the lining of the ileum, and meconium escapes into the abdomen. This is called meconium peritonitis, and can make the baby quite sick. It occurs in about 10% of infants with meconium ileus, or in 1% of infants with CF.

Meconium ileus can sometimes be relieved with a special radiographic procedure called a Gastrografin® enema. This involves placement of a tube into the rectum and the instillation of Gastrografin® or a similar product into the rectum. Gastrografin® is a liquid with three characteristics that make it ideal to use in this situation: (a) it is very slippery and can get through just about any obstruction; (b) it is very concentrated and acts like a dry sponge, pulling fluid into the intestines and watering down the thick meconium; and (c) it appears on a radiograph (x-ray film) so the progress of the whole procedure can be followed. The Gastrografin® is carefully infused through the colon and into the terminal ileum in order to try to relieve the obstruction. When this procedure is carried out by radiologists experienced with its use in infants (ideally with the cooperation of surgeons and CF specialists), it is safe and very effective. However, in some infants, these enemas do not relieve the obstruction and surgery becomes necessary.

All infants with meconium peritonitis require surgery. When the surgery is performed by surgeons with experience in infants, it is usually successful. Babies who have surgery have a slightly higher likelihood of developing intestinal obstruction later in life because anyone who has abdominal surgery may develop scarring ("adhesions") which may narrow or block the intestines. Occasionally, babies with meconium ileus or peritonitis and a very sick intestine may need to have a portion of their intestine removed at the time of their operation.

Meconium ileus is a serious problem, but most infants who have it do well after treatment. If they make it through the first few weeks, their outlook is similar to that for other CF babies who have not had meconium ileus. Meconium ileus occurs almost exclusively in infants with CF; therefore, a baby with meconium ileus should be diagnosed immediately, and general CF care should begin right away. A sweat test should be performed. Despite a commonly held misconception that babies do not sweat enough for a valid test, most babies do give plenty of sweat for analysis and diagnosis. In those few infants who do not produce enough sweat, the baby should be treated as though he or she has CF until a definite diagnosis can be made, perhaps with genetic testing, or perhaps with a repeated sweat test (see the introduction and Chapter 2 for more discussion of the tests used to diagnose CF). There seems to be an increased risk of meconium ileus in patients carrying the 621+ G->T mutation and in children born to families with a history of meconium ileus.

Distal Intestinal Obstructive Syndrome (DIOS) and Constipation

Some patients with CF develop a syndrome of intestinal blockage similar to meconium ileus which occurs later in life. This problem usually occurs in patients with PI but occasionally happens in patients with PS. It is thought to result from thickened, dehydrated intestinal contents accumulating as a collection in the terminal ileum or sometimes the beginning of the colon (known as the cecum).

DIOS usually starts with as a brief period (a few days or less) of worsening crampy belly pain and bloating (abdominal distention) with decreased passage of stools. The blockage may lead to vomiting of bile which is green or yellow. Physicians may be able to appreciate a collection of stool in the right lower abdomen (by gently feeling the abdomen) or may see evidence of blockage on abdominal radiographs. DIOS has been classified as "complete" when a blockage is present and "incomplete" when the accumulated collection of stool and symptoms of distention or pain are present without the vomiting or obstruction.

If a person with CF has severe abdominal pain and no bowel movements, he or she should be evaluated for this problem. No bowel movements for 24 hours should prompt an urgent call to the CF center.

Milder cases of DIOS may be treated by oral lavage solutions such as polyethylene glycol 3350 (Miralax® or Golytely®). With complete obstruction, a Gastrografin® enema or surgery may be required.

The rate of occurrence of DIOS has decreased with the use of enteric-coated microsphere pancreatic enzymes. A recent study reported that DIOS occurs about six times per 1,000 patient-years. In other words, if you observed 1,000 people with CF over a year, there would be six episodes. Risk factors for DIOS include having a history of meconium ileus (especially with surgery), becoming dehydrated (for example by not drinking enough fluid and salt during exercise or hot weather), taking too few enzymes (which will make the stools large and bulky), dietary changes, some medications, and occasionally excessive enzyme use. In some patients DIOS can be a recurring problem.

Constipation is also a common symptom in patients with CF. General symptoms of constipation include an increase in the firmness of bowel movements, straining to pass bowel movements, and a decline in the frequency of bowel movements. These symptoms generally improve with the use of laxatives such as Miralax® (polyethylene glycol 3350). In children, constipation may be related to CF or may be due to other common causes such as stool holding.

Some CF patients with abdominal pain and a change in bowel movements suggesting constipation may notice lessening of their pain with treatment of constipation. If the abdominal pain does not improve with treatment, diagnoses other than simple constipation should be considered.

Intussusception, Volvulus, and Appendicitis

Intussusception is a rare problem that occurs when part of the intestine is pulled along inside another part of the intestine in much the same way that a telescope collapses on itself (Figure 4.2). It can be a complication of DIOS. The most common form involves the ileum being pulled into the colon. What probably causes this action is the sticky stool and mucus, which adhere to the insides of the intestine, are pulled along by the powerful waves that pull the food along, drawing the intestine with them. This "telescoping" may decrease the flow of blood to the intestine, which may damage or even kill a portion of the intestine, leading to bleeding or perforation (a hole in the intestine), which may make the patient very ill. Symptoms include intermittent or constant belly pain, vomiting, decreased

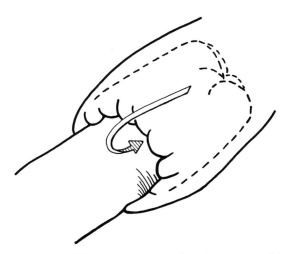

FIGURE 4.2. Intussusception. This condition occurs when the intestine slides within itself, like a telescope.

stools, belly tenderness, and blood in the stools. Radiographic studies may be helpful in the diagnosis. Treatment may include radiographic enema therapy in which the thick enema fluid can actually push the telescoped portion of the bowel and "untelescope" it, relieving the obstruction. Patients with this problem tend to do well if treated promptly. Other problems which may require surgery include appendicitis (inflammation of the appendix, a small tube attached to the beginning of the colon) and volvulus (a twist of a portion of the intestine which may damage the intestine).

Small Bowel Bacterial Overgrowth (SBBO)

In healthy individuals, the large intestine normally contains large numbers of bacteria, in the neighborhood of a billion bacteria per milliliter. A similar number may be found in the terminal ileum at the end of the small intestine. However, the duodenum, which is the first part of the small intestine or is usually a comparatively sterile environment, with generally fewer than a million organisms per milliliter. The types of bacteria found are also different, and are predominated by "oral flora" organisms normally found in the mouth with few or no "fecal" organisms normally found in the colon. A number of factors help to maintain this relative sterility, including the stomach acid, the intestinal mucus barrier, the immune function of the intestine, digestive enzymes, and the "motility" function (or movement function) of the intestine in propelling contents forward toward the colon.

When excessive numbers of bacteria inhabit the small intestine, this is known as SBBO. Signs and symptoms may include bloating, belly pain, diarrhea, fatty malodorous bowel movements, poor weight gain or weight loss, and nutritional problems including deficiency of vitamin B12.

In people with CF, the movement of contents through the small intestine is slowed by about 50% compared to people without CF. The reason for this slowing is not well understood. One factor may be the presence of undigested fat in the terminal ileum, which slows the small intestine by something called the "ileal brake." The mucus coating of the intestine is abnormally thick and dehydrated due to the basic defect. The interaction between intestinal bacteria, the mucus layer, and the CF intestine may also have effects on motility.

SBBO has been reported to occur in up to 30% to 50% of patients with CF. Several different types of tests may suggest the diagnosis. The most rigorous test is a quantitative culture of the duodenal fluid to determine numbers of anaerobic and aerobic organisms. Anaerobic cultures are difficult to perform and are not available at all centers. The method is also more invasive, with duodenal fluid being obtained through the placement of a tube or by endoscopy, as discussed regarding direct pancreatic function testing above. Noninvasive breath testing, in which the patient has breath samples collected before and several times after drinking a test solution is also available at some CF multispecialty centers. These tests do have some limitations, and are not 100% accurate. In some cases, blood tests or radiographic studies can also be helpful. Treatment generally involves intermittent treatment with antibiotics designed to decrease the bacterial load in the intestine.

Fibrosing Colonopathy

Fibrosing colonopathy is a very unusual problem that affected a few patients with CF, especially in the 1990s. It was seen only among patients taking very large doses of pancreatic enzymes with each meal. People who developed the problem had abdominal pain and some had bloody diarrhea. It is a serious problem that may require surgery. It has practically disappeared in the 2000s.

Persistent Abdominal Pain and Diarrhea in CF

Abdominal pain and diarrhea are relatively common symptoms in patients with CF (as well as in those without CF). In some cases, symptoms may be related to CF itself and may improve with simple measures such as adjustments in the pancreatic enzyme dose or the treatment of constipation. In other cases, symptoms may be due to a different intestinal condition not related to CF. Some of these non-CF conditions that might still affect patients with CF are discussed further below.

Celiac Disease

Celiac disease, also known as gluten-sensitive enteropathy, is an intestinal disorder associated with an intolerance to wheat, rye, and barley. In susceptible individuals, exposure to the gluten ingredient found in these products leads to damage to the lining of the small intestine. Some patients with untreated celiac disease may have abdominal pain, chronic diarrhea, difficulty gaining weight, vomiting, lack of progression through puberty, constipation, an itchy painful skin rash, or other symptoms. The presenting symptoms vary greatly, and some patients with the disease may have few or no apparent symptoms. A simple blood test can be used to screen for this problem. If the result is abnormal, an additional test known as upper endoscopy is generally recommended.

Celiac disease is a much more common problem than CF, affecting roughly one in 130 persons in the United States. Since celiac disease occurs relatively frequently, some patients with CF are also affected by this problem. Distinguishing the two on the basis of symptoms is challenging, since both can be associated with abdominal pain and malabsorptive symptoms. A 2009 Danish study of patients with CF found one in 83 patients also to have celiac disease, and an Italian study showed fewer patients affected. It is unclear whether the risk of celiac disease is increased in CF. However, it is prudent to consider this diagnosis in patients with persistent, unexplained GI symptoms.

Giardiasis

Giardia is a protozoan parasite capable of infecting the small intestine. It is frequently acquired by consuming water from a contaminated well or stream. It may also be acquired from contaminated food or an infected person. Symptoms of infection may include watery or smelly stools, bloating, crampy belly pain, difficulty eating, and difficulty gaining weight. Infection with Giardia occurs over four times more commonly among patients with CF than healthy persons. A simple stool test can identify the infection. In most patients, a course of an appropriate antibiotic is an effective treatment.

Clostridium difficile Infection

Clostridium difficile is a bacterial organism which can infect the large intestine, leading to inflammation known as pseudomembranous colitis (PMC). The symptoms of infection may include belly pain, diarrhea, and bloody stools. This infection almost always develops after exposure to various antibiotics, which leads to proliferation of this organism because the antibiotics have killed good bacteria in the intestines, as well as the bad bacteria they were intended to kill. It is also possible to be colonized with the organism, meaning that this bacterium is present in the colon but not in sufficient numbers to cause illness.

Patients with CF receive antibiotics on a frequent basis for lung infections. Colonization with *Clostridium difficile* is common in CF, occurring in 32% to 50% of patients, compared to 2% of healthy adults. Fortunately, most CF patients never develop symptomatic disease in spite of being colonized. It has been speculated that the environment of the CF intestine may tend to inhibit the growth of the organism. Rarely, CF patients may develop severe PMC. The treatment may involve hospitalization, antibiotics such as metronidazole or vancomycin directed against the organism, and sometimes surgery. Severe PMC in CF may be associated with the N1303 K mutation.

Rectal Prolapse

Rectal prolapse is a condition in which a small section of the intestine telescopes outward from the anus so that the inner lining of the rectum (end of the large intestine) becomes visible (Figure 4.3). This usually happens during a bowel movement. It is a common problem in young children with CF and occurs in up to 20% of patients. Although it is frightening for a parent to see, it is seldom dangerous or painful.

Rectal prolapse may be the first CF-related problem to appear before CF is diagnosed in a child. It may occur repeatedly. Several factors related to CF may contribute to rectal prolapse. Malnutrition may weaken the structures that usually support the rectum. Coughing and straining during sticky bowel movements may increase the pressure on the rectum, pushing it out.

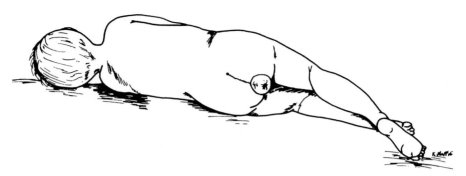

FIGURE 4.3. Rectal prolapse. This condition is similar to intussusception in that the bowel turns partly inside out. In rectal prolapse, the last part of the bowel (the rectum) turns inside out and protrudes from the anus.

Treatment usually consists of gently pushing the rectum back into place by hand. If this is difficult to perform or if the prolapsed rectum is darkly discolored, painful, or bleeding, immediate help should be obtained from a physician. The prolapse usually resolves with treatment of the CF and improvement in nutrition, bowel movements, and coughing. Rectal prolapse rarely may require surgery.

Rectal prolapse can sometimes happen in children with other conditions, such as severe constipation or diarrhea. Worldwide, rectal prolapse is common in malnourished children with intestinal parasites, fortunately rare in the developed world. Since rectal prolapse can be the initial symptom of CF, some experts recommend testing for CF in any child who develops rectal prolapse.

Esophagus and Gastroesophageal Reflux

Gastroesophageal reflux occurs when contents of the stomach (acid and partially digested food) come back up into the esophagus ("gastro" refers to the stomach, and "reflux" indicates a fluid going backward from the way it's supposed to go). This usually occurs during intermittent periods in which the LES, which would otherwise prevent reflux, temporarily relaxes. A certain amount of this is normal, and most episodes do not produce any symptoms. Reflux events are often quite frequent during infancy and tend to decrease in frequency after this. We may notice symptoms when contents come all the way up into the throat (or occasionally through the nose) or when the acid coming up leads to pain in the esophagus (that's what heartburn is). In most healthy people, the acid that comes up quickly travels back into the stomach without causing any problems. In some people the net exposure of the esophagus to acid is increased, leading to gastroesophageal reflux *disease* (GERD). This may be related to more frequent reflux episodes, prolonged episodes, delayed clearance, or some combination of these. In this circumstance, the lining of the esophagus may become inflamed (reflux esophagitis). Over time, this inflammation may lead to additional problems, such as bleeding, precancerous changes in the lining of the esophagus (Barrett's esophagus), or occasionally scarring and narrowing of the esophagus (stricture).

A separate problem is that gastroesophageal reflux can sometimes be associated with pulmonary (lung or breathing) problems. This may occur in two different ways: (a) refluxed material may reach the back of the throat and be aspirated into the lungs; or, more commonly, (b) nerves in the esophagus may become irritated by stomach acid, sending a signal down the bronchial tubes, which makes the bronchial muscles squeeze down and narrow the tube. In certain cases this is actually a protective mechanism. In other cases, the reaction of the bronchi may cause breathing difficulties similar to asthma and may make the breathing problems of CF worse.

Acid reflux is probably more common in people with CF, for several reasons. Some medications and treatments have the side effect of relaxing the LES, leading to more reflux. Patients with CF spend more time upside down or on their back (for treatments) than other people. Coughing increases the pressure within the belly, which may propel contents up into the esophagus. People with CF may also produce more stomach acid than usual, which may aggravate reflux disease.

Treatment for reflux is divided into three categories: simple measures, medications, and surgery. The simple measures include positioning and dietary modifications. Studies have shown clearly that babies have much less reflux when they sleep on their bellies than when they sleep on their backs. The prone (belly down) sleeping position has also been associated with an increased risk of sudden infant death syndrome (SIDS). Nevertheless, some CF experts do recommend that infants known to have reflux be placed to sleep on their bellies in order to limit gastroesophageal reflux, which itself has been associated with SIDS. Other options include elevating the baby's head with a wedge or a pillow under the mattress or blocks under the crib legs. The use of thickened infant feedings (generally with one tablespoon of dry rice cereal per ounce) is associated with a slight reduction in the number of daily visible episodes of reflux. Exposure to tobacco smoke should be avoided, as this may increase reflux, and is also directly harmful to the lungs. Reflux symptoms may increase with certain foods, including acidic foods (tomatoes, soft drinks, acidic fruit juices), spicy foods, chocolate, and caffeine (contained in tea, cola drinks, Mountain Dew, coffee, and other beverages). Older children with CF should eat meals at least 2 hours before bedtime, and they may wish to avoid the above foods if these cause symptoms. Tight fit jeans may increase pressure on the belly and push contents into the esophagus.

The main medications used to treat GERD are those that decrease acid production by the stomach. There are two main classes: "histamine 2 (H2) blockers" and "proton pump inhibitors." The most commonly used H2 blockers include ranitidine (Zantac®) and famotidine (Pepcid®). Frequently used proton pump inhibitors include lansoprazole (Prevacid®, which has the advantage of being available in a dissolving tablet which may be easier to take in by young children), omeprazole (Prilosec®), pantoprazole (Protonix®), and esomeprazole (Nexium®). Antacids such as Maalox®, Mylanta®, and TUMS® do not block acid production but may provide temporary symptom relief by neutralizing the acid already present within the stomach.

Occasionally, symptoms of GERD are not relieved or adequately controlled by these measures. In this case, a surgical procedure known as a Nissen fundoplication can be performed. This procedure involves wrapping the upper portion of the stomach around the lower portion of the esophagus to create a mechanical barrier to reflux. When performed by a surgeon experienced in children's problems, this procedure is frequently successful in treating reflux. The operation also changes the mechanics of the stomach in a way that can sometimes lead to additional symptoms or problems. As with any surgical procedure, careful consideration of the risks and benefits, sometimes in consultation with a gastroenterologist, may be helpful to decide when this procedure is an appropriate option.

Liver, Gallbladder, and Bile Ducts

The CF gene plays a role in the normal function of the liver, gallbladder, and bile ducts. The CFTR chloride channel is normally found in the cells lining the gallbladder and bile ducts. The channel helps to bring fluid into the bile ducts and also enriches this fluid in bicarbonate. The lining cells also secrete substances known as bile salts. This mixture known as bile travels through the tubes or bile ducts toward the duodenum. Some of the bile is stored temporarily within the gallbladder; when a meal is consumed, the gallbladder contracts and propels additional bile into the intestine. The bile salts have an important role in the normal digestion and absorption of fat.

When the CFTR channel is not functioning well in CF, abnormally thick and acidic fluid is found within the gallbladder and bile ducts. This fluid flows more slowly through the bile ducts, and the backup of bile can lead to inflammation (irritation) within the liver.

In about 1% to 2% of babies with CF, the decrease in bile flow leads to a problem known as neonatal cholestasis. The yellow bile cannot get out of the liver, and a substance known as direct bilirubin builds up in the bloodstream. This leads to a yellow discoloration of the skin called jaundice and yellow discoloration of the eyes called icterus. This problem occurs more commonly in infants with meconium ileus. It usually resolves on its own within a few weeks. Knowing that a baby in this situation has CF can be important to your doctor in understanding the reason for the cholestasis.

The abnormal bile in CF can lead to variable degrees of scarring resulting from irritation within the liver. About 10% of infants and up to 70% of adults will have small areas of scarring known as focal biliary cirrhosis. This is usually not associated with any symptoms or health problems. Occasionally, more extensive scarring occurs throughout the liver. Extensive scarring, termed multilobular cirrhosis, is usually accompanied by increase in pressure within the veins of the belly, known as portal hypertension. Fortunately, this is a relatively uncommon problem, occurring in fewer than 7% of patients with CF. It usually develops by around 15 years of age and is somewhat more common in boys than in girls. Some of these patients may be a carrier for a gene mutation known as alpha-1-antitrypsin Z, which may have contributed to the liver problem. In most patients, the reason for the development of a more significant liver problem is unknown.

CF-related multilobular cirrhosis and portal hypertension is a serious and complex form of liver disease which usually requires care by a liver specialist. Although rare, it has a significant impact as it accounts for over 2% of all deaths from CF. Patients with cirrhosis and portal hypertension typically have a small, firm liver (due to scarring) and an enlarged spleen. Under normal conditions, a significant portion of the blood from the intestine and spleen travels through a large vein to the liver (the portal vein) and then through the liver before returning to the heart. In a cirrhotic liver, the scarring causes resistance to the blood flow through the liver, which increases the pressure in the veins of the abdomen. This increase in pressure (portal hypertension) leads to enlargement of the spleen (splenomegaly), as blood cannot drain normally from the spleen through the liver and backs up into the spleen. The spleen is an organ found on the left side of the belly. One of the spleen's main functions is to filter old and damaged cells out of the circulation. As the spleen enlarges it filters more cells than usual, called hypersplenism, which may lead to low white blood cell counts and low platelet counts. An enlarged spleen is at increased risk of rupture, which can cause serious blood loss, so that patients with significant splenomegaly are generally advised not to participate in contact sports. Other abdominal veins may be enlarged, including those in the lower portion of the esophagus. Enlarged esophageal veins, known as varices, may sometimes rupture and bleed dangerously. The increased pressure in abdominal veins can also lead to leakage of fluid into the abdomen, known as ascites. A belly that is full with an enlarged spleen or significant ascites may lead to difficulties with breathing due to the inability to take a deep breath.

There is no direct treatment for CF-related liver disease yet. Treatment with ursodeoxycholic acid (UDCA) has been associated with improvement in certain blood tests related to liver and bile duct irritation. While these results are encouraging, the overall effectiveness and safety of this medication in CF are not known.

Portal hypertension and its complications can be managed with close follow-up with a GI or liver specialist. For example, ascites (the collection of fluid in the abdomen) can be treated by changing the amount of salt and water that a person consumes and by diuretics that increase urination. Bleeding due to portal hypertension can be treated by several procedures. Endoscopic variceal ligation, which involves the placement of a small rubber band around an abnormally large vein, can be used to eliminate sources of bleeding. This procedure is done by a physician, usually a gastroenterologist, who passes a flexible, lighted tube down the throat and into the esophagus.

Sometimes, varices and the other problems caused by elevated portal pressure may be treated by a surgical procedure, by the creation of a shunt, which directs blood flow away from the varices and liver into low-pressure veins. These are major abdominal surgeries and may make subsequent liver transplantation difficult or impossible. In a non-surgical approach, the transjugular intrahepatic portosystemic shunt (TIPS) procedure, a specialty radiologist places a tube into the jugular vein in the neck, and then down through the liver to create a similar diversion of blood flow. The TIPS procedure does not usually prevent a future liver transplantation. Splenectomy and partial splenectomy have also been performed in a few patients with significant symptoms related to their enlarged spleen. As with TIPS, liver transplantation can still be a future option for a person whose portal hypertension has been relieved by splenectomy or partial splenectomy.

With close follow-up of their condition, many patients with CF-related cirrhosis and portal hypertension may remain stable for many years. In most of these patients, the liver continues to perform its normal functions fairly well in spite of the presence of scarring. In a few (1% to 2%) of those patients, the function of the liver fails. Since the liver is an essential organ for life, liver failure may lead to death or the need for a liver transplant.

Liver transplantation can be performed for a person with CF-related liver disease whose liver has failed or for someone with difficulty in managing portal hypertension. As of 2010, more than 40 liver transplants have been performed in children with CF. Any transplantation procedure is an extremely serious undertaking, often with unpredictable consequences, and should not be done if the risks are not fully understood by the patient and family. Liver transplantation is discussed in greater detail in Chapter 8.

Many patients with CF have mild abnormalities on blood tests without any overt liver disease. When blood tests of the liver are obtained, it is quite common to see mild abnormalities related to liver irritation. These may be evident in 20% to 50% of individuals with CF at any one time. Over 90% of patients with CF will have had an abnormal test of this type by the age of 20. An increase in fat within the liver tissue (steatosis) is common in malnourished patients with CF but may also occur in apparently well-nourished children and adults. Variable degrees of scarring are present in the CF liver, as discussed above. A liver ultrasound may detect abnormalities such as liver enlargement, steatosis, or scarring in about 35% of patients with CF. Other radiology tests (such as CT and MRI scans) may also detect similar changes in the liver. A newer technique known as elastography, which offers the possibility of quantifying the degree of scarring within the liver, is under development. The search for markers which might be useful to detect and follow CF-related liver diseases is an active area of research.

The gallbladder is a pouch connected to the bile ducts, which accumulates and stores bile between meals. When a person eats, the gallbladder contracts and releases additional bile into the intestine to help digestion. Several abnormalities related to the gallbladder are associated with CF. In about 30% of patients the gallbladder is unusually small, but this does not generally lead to any problem. Prior to 1990, about 10% of patients with CF developed gallstones. The risk of gallstone development in CF is thought to be related to fat malabsorption, such that with the advent of modern PERT, the rate of gallstone disease has decreased to around 1%. Gallstones may sometimes move into and block the bile ducts, leading to abdominal pain, vomiting, jaundice, and other symptoms. When gallstones cause symptoms, surgical removal of the gallbladder is usually necessary.

Other Systems

Daniel J. Weiner and David M. Orenstein

5

THE BASICS

1. Diabetes is a problem that is recognized more as people with cystic fibrosis (CF) get older. Although it requires more care, treatment can improve your nutrition and pulmonary function.

2. Sweat glands make sweat that is very salty in people with CF, and occasionally babies with CF lose excess salt in hot weather. The salty sweat also gives us the sweat test.

3. Thick mucus in the reproductive system means that most men with CF are sterile (although their sex life is completely normal), and women have a harder time getting pregnant than other women.

4. Both boys and girls with CF may go through puberty later than their classmates, but most will develop normally, a year or two later.

DIABETES

In addition to producing digestive enzymes and acid-neutralizing juices, the pancreas produces hormones, especially insulin. Insulin *is an essential hormone that allows proper utilization and storage of energy.* It helps move glucose, the body's main simple carbohydrate used for energy, from the blood into the body's cells, and it also prevents the breakdown of glycogen (that's what we call glucose stored in the liver). In addition, insulin also prevents the breakdown of stored fats. Patients with cystic fibrosis (CF) may develop insulin deficiency, as discussed below. They may also have "insulin resistance." Insulin resistance means that the cells, especially muscle and liver cells, require more insulin than normal to transport glucose into them and perform other activities. Insulin resistance increases with inflammation, infection, and steroid use. Both insulin deficiency and insulin resistance interfere with the utilization of energy by cells, and contribute to nutritional and lung problems in individuals with CF.

When not enough insulin is produced, blood glucose (sugar) levels rise (we call this "hyperglycemia"), and less glucose (and energy) enters the cells. There are various degrees of insulin deficiency and hyperglycemia, but even mild forms tend to progress with time to diabetes. The diagnostic criteria for diabetes are blood glucose value greater than 200 mg/dL 2 hours after a standard oral glucose challenge, or a fasting blood glucose value greater than 126 mg/dL on two occasions. Some individuals who have abnormal glucose values, but do not meet the diagnostic criteria for diabetes, are classified as having "impaired glucose tolerance." Diabetes involves many complicated processes in the body. When the blood sugar level is above 200 mg/dL, sugar spills into the urine. Sugar in the urine pulls extra water with it, so people with diabetes lose water in addition to sugar and calories. They urinate a lot, drink a lot, may lose weight, and may feel "dragged out." The loss of glucose and water from the body produces other changes that can make people with diabetes malnourished, dehydrated, and quite ill.

Nearly one-half of all people with CF have some limitation in the ability of their pancreas to produce insulin, which is often detectable with oral glucose tolerance tests. Although cystic fibrosis related diabetes (CFRD) is relatively uncommon under the age of 10 years, recent information from the United States indicates that as many as 26% of individuals with CF between the ages of 10 and 20 years may have diabetes. From the ages of 20 to 30 years, another 10% to 20% develop it, and so forth, with an additional 10% to 20% developing diabetes with every additional decade. Stresses such as pregnancy, worsened lung infection, or some medications—most notably, steroids, which are sometimes used to control CF lung disease—can bring on CF diabetes. Diabetes that appears during these stresses often improves or goes away when the stress is removed. The diabetes in CF patients differs from type 1 insulin deficiency diabetes mellitus (T1DM). Rather than a complete insulin deficiency (as in T1DM), patients with CF have delayed as well as decreased insulin responses to a glucose challenge. Yet, they secrete enough insulin that the fasting blood glucose or the glucose before meals may be within the normal range in the early stages of CFRD.

Recent information obtained from the United States, Denmark, the United Kingdom, and France indicates that CFRD is associated with poorer health outcomes. These health problems can include poor weight gain, poor linear growth, and pulmonary deterioration. The onset of CFRD is often insidious (sneaks up on you), which is why your doctor recommends periodic screening tests. Oral glucose tolerance tests or continuous glucose monitoring provide the most valuable information regarding glucose control. Measurement of hemoglobin A_{1c} (HbA_{1c}) may be used to monitor blood glucose control, but it is not a reliable screening test for diagnosis. This test, which measures the amount of glucose in red blood cells, and is thought to be an indication of average blood sugar levels over a period of weeks or months, is often normal during the early stages of CFRD.

Treatment for diabetes involves several procedures. Regular monitoring of blood glucose is performed using a home glucose monitor. Complex carbohydrates (pasta, rice, potatoes, grains, etc.) are preferred over "simple sugars" (candy, soda pop, cake frosting, juices, etc.) because simple sugars are associated with high glucose values. The food choices for children with CFRD differ from those recommended for children with T1DM because of the increased caloric needs of children with CF. Insulin treatment is often beneficial. Insulin must be administered by injection, often several times a day. Some children with CFRD benefit from continuous sub-cutaneous insulin pumps. Oral medications to treat CFRD are not currently recommended. Interdisciplinary care with pulmonologists and endocrinologists can facilitate care for individuals with CFRD.

PUBERTY

Many children with CF have delayed onset of puberty. Typically, bone maturation as assessed by a bone age x-ray (x-ray of left hand) is also delayed. Potential reasons for delayed onset of puberty include inadequate caloric intake, increased metabolic needs, calorie loss through malabsorption, liver disease, and diabetes mellitus. Inadequate caloric intake can be due to picky eating habits, poor appetite because of being sick, poor appetite because of being undernourished (it seems strange, perhaps, but there is a condition known as "the anorexia of malnutrition," meaning that people who are badly undernourished often do not feel hungry—perhaps this is helpful to prevent suffering in starving people with no food available, but it's not helpful when there is food available!), or in some cases, inadequate food availability because of poverty. Malabsorption can occur because of inadequate enzyme intake or poor enzyme functioning (see Chapter 4). Active lung disease and inflammation increase metabolic needs and may require additional increases in caloric intake for adequate compensation. Coughing and hard breathing also burn up calories. Coughing or inflammation (or both) can decrease appetite. Delayed puberty can be emotionally difficult for young people, too, if all their friends are shooting up in height, and filling out, growing into physical adulthood, and they are left behind, with the body of a child. It may soften the blow somewhat if they know that the majority of young people with CF eventually go through puberty, although it may be a year or two behind their friends. For some children, treatment with low doses of an appropriate sex steroid can be helpful. Optimal caloric intake is the most effective treatment to promote linear growth and progression through puberty.

REPRODUCTIVE SYSTEM IN CF

Although the reproductive systems of people with CF are basically normal, the thick mucus found in so many other places in the body also affects this system. (The reproductive system is discussed at greater length in Chapter 14.)

The Male Reproductive System in CF

In boys and men with CF, the reproductive system is completely normal, with one exception. In 98% of boys and men with CF, the vas deferens is incompletely formed or totally blocked. The vas deferens is the tube that carries sperm from the testicles to the penis. This is the tube that is cut and tied when a man has a vasectomy. The sperm are formed normally in the testicles, but because of the blockage, they cannot get out. Men with CF have completely normal sex lives, but the 98% of men with CF who have this blockage are sterile. It is very much as though everything had been normal, and they had gotten a vasectomy. A small proportion of men with CF (about 2%) are not sterile, and some have fathered children.

It is possible to test whether a teenager or an adult with CF is one of the 98% who are sterile, or one of the 2% who are not. The patient simply gives a semen specimen to the laboratory, where it is analyzed for sperm. In addition, CF is one cause of infertility that is investigated in men who want to but haven't been able to father a child.

The Female Reproductive System in CF

In women with CF, the problems related to the reproductive system are more subtle than in men. The main problem is that the mucus lining the cervix (the opening to the uterus, or womb) is thick, just like mucus elsewhere. As a result it is harder for women with CF to get pregnant than for women without CF. It certainly is possible though, and several hundred women with CF have gotten pregnant, and many of these women have delivered babies.

Women whose lungs are in excellent shape when they get pregnant usually do well during the pregnancy. Women with CF lung disease may have a very hard time during the pregnancy. There are many women with CF who have been in fairly good health before they became pregnant, but whose health deteriorated during the pregnancy.

BONE HEALTH

Low bone mass (also referred to as low bone mineral density) is common in elderly people, especially women, but can also be seen in patients with CF. This condition is referred to as osteopenia, and if it's more severe it's called osteoporosis. Either condition can increase a person's risk for fractures, and both have been observed in individuals with CF. These problems are less apparent in young children, but develop during adolescence and adulthood. Malabsorption of vitamin D and other fat-soluble vitamins, poor nutritional status, severe disease, physical inactivity, chronic infection, and glucocorticoid (steroid) therapy can all impair bone mineralization. Delayed puberty, with lower sex steroid hormone levels, may also interfere with bone mineralization. **D**ual energy **x**-ray **a**bsorptiometry (DXA) is the gold standard method to measure bone mineral content. This is a special kind of x-ray with a very low amount of radiation which takes a picture of the bones. However, the interpretation of DXA in children and adolescents, particularly if they have below average height and weight, may be inaccurate, such that the bone mineral density appears to be lower than it actually is. Treatment of osteopenia and osteoporosis begins with prevention. Children with CF should be encouraged to participate in physical activity (particularly weight-bearing activities such as walking or jogging), eat a calcium-rich diet, and take adequate amounts of vitamin D. Serum vitamin D levels should be maintained in the normal range (between 30 and 60 ng/mL). Prompt treatment of inflammation and pulmonary exacerbations is also important. Some medications called "bisphosphonates" have been used to treat or prevent osteoporosis in adult women, but long-term information regarding the safety and efficacy of these medications in children is not available.

OTHER BONE AND JOINT PROBLEMS

Another complication of CF which may affect the skeletal system is one that causes bone or joint pain in the legs, particularly the knees. This problem is called **h**ypertrophic **p**ulmonary **o**steoarthropathy (HPOA). As the name indicates, it is seen in people with pulmonary problems, and refers to "something wrong with" (-opathy) the bones (osteo) and/or the joints (arthro). The term "hypertrophic" refers to x-ray findings in this condition, which include an elevation of the periosteum (the membrane covering the bone). This periosteal elevation makes it appear as though there is extra (hyper) growth (-trophy). The condition can be painful. It is not very common, and occurs mostly in people whose lung disease is severe. It usually improves as the lungs improve with treatment, but specific treatment for the bone/joint problem can also be helpful.

Finally, there is an uncommon and poorly understood arthritis—most often involving the ankle or knee, but sometimes affecting a few joints at the same time—that some people with CF get. The joint is tender, and may have a skin rash associated with it. It usually gets better with anti-inflammatory drugs, such as aspirin or ibuprofen. Episodes typically last 5 to 7 days.

CLUBBING

Clubbing of the fingers or toes is discussed more in Chapter 3 (Respiratory System). Clubbing is seen in almost all patients with CF and involves changes in the angle between the fingers and nails, as well as increased thickness of the finger tips. It is not painful and does not require specific treatment. The cause of clubbing is not known, but it is associated with CF lung disease.

Treating Bone and Joint Problems

Osteoarthropathy may cause some physical discomfort, and people often do not mention it to their CF physicians, being unaware that leg or knee pain could be related to CF. As with clubbing, osteoarthropathy improves when the lungs improve. Regardless of the condition of the lungs, osteoarthropathy responds very well to aspirin, ibuprofen, and other similar anti-inflammatory drugs (see Appendix B).

SKIN

Aquagenic Wrinkling of the Palms. Some patients with CF can develop increased wrinkling of their skin on their hands after soaking in water (during swimming, or a bath). This is called "Aquagenic Wrinkling" and is not a serious health problem (usually not requiring any treatment). The cause is not understood but may have something to do with the CF protein affecting movement of water in skin cells. Not all patients with APW have CF, but some patients have been diagnosed with CF only after noticing this problem (and then had a sweat test ordered by an astute dermatologist).

SWEAT GLANDS

Normal Sweat Glands

Sweat begins in the coil of the sweat gland, below the surface of the skin (Figure 5.1), as a fluid that is chemically very similar to blood. As it makes its way toward the skin, sodium—with its positive electrical charge—is pumped out of the duct, and eventually back to the bloodstream. Whenever a positive charge leaves any tube or duct in the body, a negative charge accompanies it in order to maintain the same total electrical charge. In the case of sweat, it is chloride and its negative charge that are carried out of the sweat fluid to follow the positive charge of sodium. By the time the fluid reaches the skin surface in the form of sweat, it still has some salt, but the sodium and chloride contents are very low compared with those in the blood. This helps the body conserve sodium and chloride, especially in hot weather or when someone is exercising heavily.

Sweat Glands in CF

It has been known for many years that people with CF have an extremely high salt content in their sweat. You've seen in Chapter 1 that CF cells set up a roadblock to chloride trying to pass through their membranes. This block in the cells of the sweat duct means that chloride is stranded within the duct fluid. Because the negatively charged chloride can't leave, it holds sodium and its positive charge back as well. This means the fluid that emerges from the skin surface as sweat has abnormally large concentrations of sodium and chloride (salt).

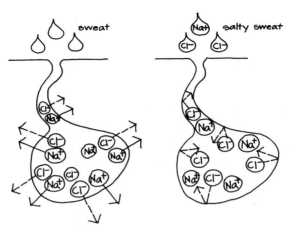

FIGURE 5.1 Sweat abnormality. In the normal (left) and CF (right) sweat glands, fluid begins in the base of the duct with salt (sodium chloride) content close to that of blood. Then, in the normal sweat gland, as the fluid moves up the gland toward the skin, sodium (Na^+)—with its positive charge—leaves the gland, and chloride (Cl^-)—with its negative charge—follows, in order to keep electrical neutrality (same number of positives and negatives in all body compartments). But, in the CF sweat gland, because of the missing or blocked CFTR (see Chapter 1), chloride cannot leave. Since chloride can't leave, it holds the sodium back too, and the fluid that emerges from the skin as sweat has a much higher concentration of sodium and chloride than normal.

This sweat abnormality is important for two reasons: (a) firstly, it allows the diagnosis of CF to be made through the sweat test, and (b) secondly, it means that some patients, especially babies, may become sick by losing more salt than they take in during the summer (see the section "Salt Loss" below).

Over 99% of people with CF have abnormal sweat. They produce a normal amount of sweat, but there is an excess of salt (sodium and chloride) in the sweat that they produce. People without CF have less than 40 milliequivalents per liter (mEq/L) of chloride in their sweat (and a similar concentration of sodium), whereas people with CF have more than 60 mEq/L (and usually more than 80 mEq/L). This means that an analysis of the sweat can tell physicians whether someone has CF or not. Once the result of a test is positive (abnormal), it will always be abnormal (meaning that if someone has CF, he or she will always have it). Also, a "positive test" is positive. Period. There are no differences between someone whose sweat chloride concentration is 83 mEq/L and someone whose is 115 mEq/L. Both have CF. The higher number does not mean a worse case of CF.

The Sweat Test

Much of the following information can also be found in Chapter 2.

Informal sweat testing has been done for centuries. There was a folk belief in Europe in the Middle Ages that "a child who tastes salty from a kiss on the brow…is hexed, and soon must die." Modern-day parents of children with CF frequently notice that their babies taste salty when they are kissed and that their older children have salt crystals on their faces and in their hair when they are active in the summertime. However, not everyone's taste buds are sensitive enough to distinguish between CF sweat and non-CF sweat. Fortunately, although a positive result of a sweat test means a child has CF, it is no longer true that he or she "soon must die." (Nor do we believe that he or she is "hexed"!)

Since the 1950s, a more accurate method of sweat testing has been available. The Gibson-Cooke method is a sweat test method that is highly accurate. When sweat testing is done by any other method, mistakes frequently arise, resulting in false positives (children who do not have CF but whose tests indicate that they do have it) and in false negatives (children who do have CF but whose tests indicate that they do not have it). The correct (Gibson-Cooke) method of sweat testing employs pilocarpine iontophoresis, and the quantitative analysis of sodium and/or chloride, as explained below:

The Gibson-Cooke method employs the chemical pilocarpine to stimulate the sweat glands to produce sweat. Pilocarpine reaches the working part of the sweat gland by first being placed on the skin, and then being driven into the sweat gland by a small electrical current; this process is called "iontophoresis." The sweat is then collected on a cloth or paper pad, or in a tiny coiled tube. It is then weighed carefully, and the sodium and/or chloride concentrations are measured very precisely (quantitatively).

To perform the test and collect the sweat takes 30 to 60 minutes. The laboratory analysis takes another 30 minutes or so. Therefore, it's usually several hours between the time someone comes into the laboratory and the time the results are ready.

The first step in the test is that the forearm (or occasionally, in a small baby, the lower leg, or even the back) is washed off to remove any salt that might be on the skin. Then some pilocarpine is placed on the skin. Pilocarpine is colorless and odorless, and looks and feels like water. Two flat metal electrodes are placed on the skin and are connected to a small box that sends a slight electrical current (approximately 5 mA) into the skin, driving the pilocarpine into the vicinity of the sweat gland, where it can "turn on" the sweat gland. The electrical current is usually not felt at all, but some people feel a mild tingling, and a few may even feel a harsher tingling or burning. It should not burn, and if it does, one should tell the technician, so that the current can be turned down.

After 5 minutes, the electrodes are removed, the arm (or leg or back) is again wiped off, and a piece of absorbent material (gauze or filter paper) or a tiny coiled tube is placed on the skin. The technician then wraps the arm, covering the gauze or filter paper with a dressing that is airtight and watertight, so that no sweat will evaporate or leak out. During the next 30 minutes, the dressing is left in place while the "revved up" sweat glands are making sweat. The technician then removes the dressing with tweezers or forceps, taking care not to touch the gauze or filter paper with his or her fingers, puts the gauze or paper (now soaked with sweat) into a bottle, and takes it to the laboratory. In the laboratory, the technician weighs the bottle to see how much sweat is there, rinses the sweat out of the gauze or paper or squirts it out of the coiled tube into a container, and then puts it through the chemical analyzers to find out precisely how much chloride is in the sweat.

When the test is performed by this method, by a laboratory experienced in performing this test, the result should enable the physician to make a definite and accurate diagnosis.

Positive tests from any other method should be confirmed with a test by the Gibson-Cooke method.

Problems with Sweat Testing

In an experienced laboratory, not getting enough sweat is the only major problem that can interfere with obtaining a reliable result. Most laboratory experts say that they must have 100 mg of sweat in order to be able to do an accurate analysis. Some people, especially some very young babies (under 1 month old), may not make enough sweat to analyze. There is a common (incorrect) belief that sweat testing cannot be done in very young babies. However, it can be done, and should be done in any baby for whom the possibility of CF has been raised. If enough sweat is collected—as it will be for the majority of babies—the results will be valid, even within the first weeks of life, and even in a premature infant.

Adults have higher sweat sodium and chloride levels than children, but even in adults, a sweat chloride concentration greater than 60 mEq/L is abnormal.

There are a very few conditions which give elevated sweat chloride or sodium levels, and these are usually readily distinguishable from CF. Similarly, there are very few people with CF whose sweat sodium and chloride concentrations are below 60 mEq/L. Finally, there are very few people whose sweat sodium and chloride concentrations are between 40 and 60 mEq/L. These few people are said to have test results in the "gray zone," or the "intermediate range," meaning neither definitely positive nor definitely negative. Tests in this range are discussed in the introduction to Chapter 2.

That a hospital or laboratory says they can perform a sweat test is not adequate assurance that they can do it correctly. Nearly one-half of all the patients who come to CF centers having had sweat tests done in outlying hospitals have received incorrect results from these tests.

Salt Loss

In addition to making the sweat test possible, the sweat abnormality can also affect the health of some people with CF. For each drop of sweat made, considerably more sodium and chloride are lost from the body than would be lost in someone without CF. In most children and adults with CF, the body is able to regulate the amount of salt in the bloodstream amazingly well. When more salt is lost, people want and take in more salt, and the kidneys reduce the amount of salt lost through the urine. Under most circumstances, even including active exercise in hot weather, if adequate salt is available, children and adults with CF should take in the proper amounts. Toddlers can have pretzel sticks and other salty snacks, whereas older children and adults can have access to the salt shaker, and no further supplements are needed. Salt tablets are not useful.

Infants with CF may lose too much salt in their sweat, and they are not able to tell their parents that they feel like having a pickle or pretzel or other salty food. Each year, especially during summer months, some infants with CF become ill because of having lost too much salt. They become lethargic, their appetite falls off, and they seem sickly. If this happens, they may require hospitalization and intravenous fluids containing replacement sodium and chloride. In order to prevent this problem, it's advisable to give infants a tiny bit of salt in their bottles during hot summer months. An amount as small as 1/8 teaspoon, once or twice a day, is probably adequate. This small amount is approximately the amount found in a salt packet in many fast food restaurants. Since too much salt can cause problems, it's best to provide moderate, regular supplements.

Some older children and adults who are very active during hot weather need to be careful about replacing lost fluids and salts. The only immediate danger for a teenager under extreme exertion, such as marathon running or a long, tough football practice in full uniform in hot weather, is fluid loss. Athletes should drink more water than they feel they need, since thirst is not as sensitive a guide as is the taste for salt. All children underestimate their need for fluid when they exercise in the heat, and young people with CF underestimate their fluid needs even more than other children. Salt replacement does not need to be immediate, and will be accurately guided by taste.

Nutrition

6

Judith A. Fulton, Iris Yann, Daniel J. Weiner, and
David M. Orenstein

THE BASICS

1. Nutrition is important for people with cystic fibrosis (CF) for growth and overall health, including the health of their lungs.

2. Good nutrition for patients with CF has three parts:
   a. High-calorie diet
   b. Pancreatic enzymes with every meal and snack containing fat and protein
   c. Vitamins

3. If someone can't gain weight on a regular diet, oral high-calorie supplements may help; if not, tube feedings may be helpful for weight gain.

THE IMPORTANCE OF NUTRITION IN CYSTIC FIBROSIS

Malnourished people do not grow well, and often they do not feel well. Malnutrition prevents the immune system, which is the body's defense against infection, from functioning properly. In someone with cystic fibrosis (CF), this may contribute to the pulmonary disease and hasten death. Patients with CF who are better nourished grow better, have better pulmonary function, and live longer than patients with poor nutrition.

MONITORING GROWTH AND NUTRITION

In an adult, generalized malnutrition shows up first as weight loss. In children, who should grow and gain weight steadily, a slowing down of weight gain may be the first sign of malnutrition. This is most easily detected by plotting a child's weight on a growth chart (Figure 6.1), which compares an individual's growth to

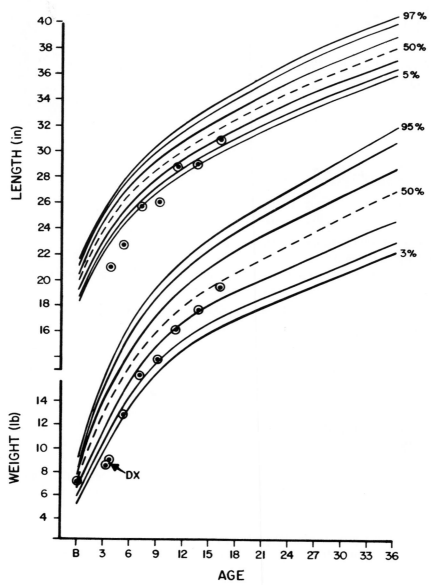

FIGURE 6.1 Growth chart. The solid lines represent the length and weight growth curves for healthy children at various ages (in months). The "3%" line refers to the length and weight of healthy children in the lowest 3% for their age, that is, 3% of healthy children will have a weight that falls on or below the 3% line, whereas 97% will be heavier. The "50%" dotted lines represent the 50th percentile or the average length and weight for healthy children. The circles represent the specific measurements for one youngster with cystic fibrosis. This child's weight was near average at birth and fell below the third percentile by the time of diagnosis (*Dx*). Treatment began after diagnosis, and the child's weight reached just below the average for age by 18 months.

that of other children of the same age and sex. If the child's growth does not keep up with the curves, malnutrition may be the cause. This growth curve should not be used as a "grade" where you strive to attain a high number, but as a form of tracking a child's growth over time. The growth curve shows the child's individual growth pattern over the years and is an indication of how the child is doing nutritionally. The growth charts include the standard measurements for height and weight, and in addition, a chart for body mass index (BMI), which looks at *weight in relation to height.* It can be calculated by dividing the weight (in kilograms) by the square of the height (in meters). The BMI (in kg/m^2) can be used to identify individuals who are under- or overweight better than just the weight alone.

When malnutrition affects growth, it usually affects the weight first. When weight has been severely affected, the poor nutrition can affect height in a similar fashion, and a child may begin to show signs of falling behind on the height curves (that is, he or she may not grow tall as fast as a healthy child of the same age). Finally, if severe malnutrition affects a very young child at a time when the brain is actively growing (up to about 36 months old), the head circumference may grow more slowly than normal. Weight, height, and head circumference should be plotted regularly for babies, and weight, height, and BMI for all children and adolescents.

Another method of assessing a person's nutritional state is called anthropometrics ("measuring people"). Measurements of skinfold thickness give an estimate as to how much fat is stored in the body, and midarm circumference gives an estimate of the amount of muscle protein. It is important to have both fat and muscle protein. When someone is not eating well, fat stores can be broken down to be used for energy, sparing the muscle protein so that the person does not become too weak. When the fat stores run out, the body is forced to use protein for energy, and muscle wasting takes place. Low muscle mass may also result from the lack of use (not enough exercising). Diet and exercise recommendations can be made when measurements of fat stores or muscle mass are low.

Many aspects of a person's nutritional state can also be measured by blood tests such as albumin, total protein, glucose, liver function tests, fat-soluble vitamins, and hemoglobin/hematocrit levels. These blood tests are typically obtained annually in people with CF.

CAUSES OF MALNUTRITION IN CF

At one time, it was assumed that the malnutrition that affects so many children and adults with CF was entirely due to the poor digestion of food, which, in turn, was due to the lack of pancreatic enzymes and bile salts, as was discussed in Chapter 4. Although enzyme deficiency is a major cause of malnutrition in CF, there are additional factors contributing to malnutrition: (a) malabsorption, as enzyme supplements do not work perfectly; (b) not ingesting enough calories; and (c) burning more calories because of inflammation in the lung. In addition, some patients with CF-related diabetes may also lose calories (sugar) in their urine.

Enzyme Deficiency

Although pancreatic enzyme supplements help a great deal, they do not work perfectly. The digestion of most patients with CF is not complete, even with enzymes, and some degree of malabsorption of foods still occurs. (Remember that digestion is the process of breaking down food into particles tiny enough for them to be absorbed into the bloodstream from the intestines, enzymes are needed for digestion, digestion is needed for absorption, and absorption of food is needed for growth and energy.) The imperfection of oral enzyme supplements is due to the difficulty of mimicking perfectly the body's finely tuned system for trickling the pancreatic enzymes into the duodenum just as the food arrives from the stomach. When pancreatic enzyme capsules are swallowed with meals, they may not arrive in the duodenum at the precise time to meet up with the food. The oral enzyme supplements can also be inactivated in the stomach by stomach acids. We do not usually supplement bile salts (similar to those naturally produced in the gallbladder), and the possible lack of bile salts may prevent the oral enzymes from acting optimally. Finally, with CF, the secretion of bicarbonate from the pancreas is also limited, causing incomplete neutralization of stomach acid, which may prevent the enteric coating on the oral enzymes from dissolving. All of these factors may contribute to malabsorption and poor nutrition, even in patients who take all of their enzymes as prescribed. Not taking the prescribed enzymes can also be a problem, and it is not unheard of for patients with CF to "forget" to take enzymes because of not wanting their classmates to see them.

In addition to interfering with good nutrition, malabsorption of food can also cause bothersome side effects. Some signs of malabsorption include the following:

- Gas and bloating
- Stomach cramps
- Frequent stools
- Greasy or floating stools
- Larger and looser, bulky stools
- Bad-smelling stools
- Light-brown or yellow stools

Often, malabsorption can cause the child's appetite to increase to make up for the food he or she is not absorbing. In fact, the "textbook picture" of a baby or a child with untreated CF is someone with a voracious (huge) appetite but poor weight gain. If you see a large increase in your child's appetite, you should watch for the other signs of malabsorption listed above. If you suspect malabsorption, discuss with the CF team how to adjust the oral enzyme supplements.

Intestinal infections can cause diarrhea with an increase in the number of stools that become watery instead of bulky and greasy. Diarrhea is different from malabsorption in that it is not treated by adjusting oral enzymes. To treat diarrhea that persists for more than 1 day, contact your doctor.

Inadequate Caloric Intake

It is commonly believed that people with CF have a large appetite, and some do. But, many children, teenagers, and adults with CF actually eat less food than their friends do. Malnutrition itself may decrease a person's appetite (this is called "the anorexia of malnutrition"). Feeling sick and coughing a lot can also decrease a person's appetite. This may be especially true for those who swallow lots of mucus. Many years ago, patients with CF were prescribed a low-fat diet, because it resulted in less fat in the stools. Having less fat in the diet meant less fat in the stools; unfortunately, it also meant fewer calories for the body to use for growth. The low-fat diet attempted to make up for the lost fat calories by increasing calories from carbohydrates. However, a gram of fat has more than twice as many calories as a gram of carbohydrate; so, if you are on a low-fat diet, you have to eat a lot more to get the same number of calories for growth. On low-fat diets, many people with CF were unable to eat enough calories and became malnourished. With the right amount of oral enzymes, even a high-fat diet can be digested and absorbed, giving more calories with less food. A low-fat diet is no longer recommended except under very special circumstances. Instead, a high-fat, high-protein diet is recommended for almost all patients with CF. Even so, it simply may be impossible for some patients with CF—try though they will—to eat enough to supply their needs. In this case, it is still possible to reestablish good growth, with one or more of the available additions to a well-rounded diet (see later in the chapter).

Increased Caloric Demands

The third main reason for malnutrition in CF is an increased use of calories. Coughing, breathing hard, and fighting an infection all require additional calories. If you are using more calories in these ways all day, the need for extra calories accumulates. It may be difficult for the person with CF to keep up with this high calorie demand. The caloric intake required to maintain good growth in someone with CF may be 30% to 50% *more* than that required for a person of the same age and sex without CF.

SPECIAL DEFICIENCIES IN CYSTIC FIBROSIS

Hypoalbuminemia (Low Blood Albumin Levels)

Albumin is the main protein in blood. One of its primary roles in the blood is to keep water in the arteries and the veins. If there is not enough albumin in the blood (hypoalbuminemia), water leaks out into the skin and other organs and produces skin puffiness called "edema." Hypoalbuminemia and edema may occur in infants with CF before they are diagnosed and may be the clue that leads to the diagnosis of CF. Hypoalbuminemia is treated by giving pancreatic enzymes and plenty of protein in the diet.

Essential Fatty Acid Deficiency

Essential fatty acids are fatty acids the body needs that it cannot make from other nutrients; therefore, they have to come from the diet. Two essential fatty acids, linoleic acid and α-linolenic acid, are found in breast milk, fresh-water fish, and vegetable oils such as canola and safflower. Linoleic acid is further metabolized (processed) in the body to arachidonic acid; α-linolenic acid is metabolized to docosahexaenoic acid (DHA). DHA has gotten a lot of publicity recently, with speculation that abnormal fatty acid metabolism is a primary problem in CF and that DHA supplements may be helpful. More research needs to be done in this area before we can recommend jumping on the DHA bandwagon. All of the essential fatty acids are used for a number of complex and necessary functions, including the manufacture of cell membranes. They also appear to be needed for optimal lung function. The difficulties in fat digestion and absorption in untreated patients with CF can show up early in life as deficiencies of these essential fatty acids, since the body's need for them cannot be met by making them out of other nutrients. In addition, the essential fatty acids that do get absorbed may get used for other caloric needs: For example, they may get "burned up" to supply energy for breathing. With newborn screening and infants being diagnosed and getting started on enzymes at a younger age, fewer infants may have this problem.

Iron Deficiency

Iron is concentrated in the blood, but some is present in every living cell of the body. Iron's main function is to carry oxygen from one body tissue to another via the blood. Most iron is present in the hemoglobin molecule of the red blood cell. Iron deficiency will lead to low hemoglobin levels and anemia (low red blood cell concentration). Symptoms of iron deficiency include weakness, fatigue, decreased resistance to infection, and irritability. To screen for iron deficiency, blood levels of hemoglobin are measured.

Good dietary sources of iron are fortified cereals, meats, dried fruits, and deep-green vegetables. Iron in meat, poultry, and fish is absorbed better than the iron from vegetables. Iron-deficiency anemia is the most common nutritional deficiency in children in North America, affecting almost 40% of young children. It is most common after 1 year of age (between 12 and 36 months) when children stop taking breast milk or iron-fortified formulas and begin taking whole milk, which is low in iron. It also occurs in adolescent males and females from adolescence through adulthood. Iron deficiency may occur from inadequate iron intake, impaired absorption, or blood loss. It is important during times of higher iron needs to encourage the intake of iron-rich food sources or to supplement the diet with a multivitamin with iron. These times of high iron needs include times of blood loss through healthy causes (especially menstruation), bleeding from injury or disease, or times of multiple blood tests.

If anemia is detected, an oral iron supplement will be prescribed and to improve iron absorption, take the supplement with a beverage that contains vitamin C (orange or grapefruit juice).

Fat-Soluble Vitamins (Vitamins A, D, E, and K)

Vitamins A, D, E, and K require fat to be absorbed and, since patients with CF have trouble digesting and absorbing fat, the bloodstream levels of these vitamins are often low in patients with CF. As part of their daily medical therapy, patients with CF are put on a "standard CF dose" of fat-soluble vitamins, on the basis of age. This dose is higher than that recommended for people without CF. It is important that the vitamins prescribed are taken daily to prevent deficiency of those vitamins. To make vitamins easier to absorb, they should be taken with meals when oral enzymes and food are supplied. Blood tests can then tell whether more vitamins are required. If a vitamin level is low, this could be from not taking the prescribed dose daily or not taking the dose with enzymes. Whatever the reason for the low vitamin level, extra vitamins may be prescribed to help improve the blood levels.

There are vitamin supplements especially made to meet the fat-soluble vitamin needs of patients with CF, and for most patients these are more convenient. Some of the CF vitamin preparations include AquADEKs™ (Axcan Pharma US, Inc., Birmingham, AL) and SourceCF® multivitamin (Eurand Pharmaceuticals, Huntsville, AL).

Some people may want to take more vitamins and minerals than have been prescribed, thinking that more may be better. Actually, the body uses only a certain amount of each vitamin and mineral, and a large excess cannot be used. For some vitamins (water-soluble vitamins), the extra amount just ends up in the urine. (Some public health experts who laugh at Americans' overzealous use of vitamins say that "Americans have the most nutritious urine in the world!") The fat-soluble vitamins are not excreted in the urine, and taking an excessive amount can be dangerous.

Vitamin A

Vitamin A is needed for fighting infections, preventing night blindness, and general growth and maintenance of the body. Retinol and carotene are two types of vitamin A. Vitamin A is found in animal products, particularly liver, egg yolks, and fortified milk. Carotene is found in dark-green, deep-yellow, and orange vegetables and fruits and is converted to active vitamin A in the body. Vitamin A is normally absorbed from the intestine and then stored in the liver to be used when it is needed. Two proteins made by the liver—prealbumin and retinol-binding protein—are needed to extract vitamin A from the liver. Blood levels of vitamin A have been found to be below normal in some people with CF, even when supplemental enzymes and vitamins are given. The abnormal fat digestion is part of the problem with vitamin A in CF, but even when vitamin A is absorbed and stored in the liver, it will not be available to the body if there are low levels of prealbumin and retinol-binding protein (two forms of albumin). Zinc is a mineral that helps retinol-binding protein extract vitamin A from the liver, so it is important that patients receive zinc in their diet and multivitamins. Vitamin A levels can be decreased with acute illness, so levels measured during an illness may yield misleading low results.

A CF multivitamin should be given daily to help prevent deficiency. Vitamin A is better absorbed when it is taken with a meal and enzymes. β-carotene is a precursor to vitamin A and functions as an antioxidant in fighting inflammation. It is uncertain whether a β-carotene deficiency exists in patients with CF, but this question (and others about β-carotene in CF) is being studied.

Vitamin D

Vitamin D is needed for growth of strong bones and teeth and for normal functioning of many other organs. It may be important in regulating inflammation, including in CF airways. It is important for the absorption of calcium and phosphorus from the diet into the bloodstream. Vitamin D has taken on added importance over recent years with our increasing awareness of problems with bone health in older patients with CF. Severe vitamin D deficiency causes a bone disease called "rickets," in which the bones are abnormally soft. This problem is unusual in CF. More subtle vitamin D deficiency can contribute to problems that are much more common, especially in older patients and those who have received many steroid medications. These more common bone problems are *osteopenia* and *osteoporosis*. *Osteopenia* means a decreased bone mass or density; *osteoporosis* is osteopenia that is bad enough to reduce the bone strength so much that fractures are more likely. Vitamin D is found in fortified milk and dairy products. It is also made in the skin by the action of sunlight, but in areas of limited sunlight, in people who stay indoors, or who use sunscreen with sun-protection factors of greater than 8, the exposure to the sunlight might not be enough to meet the vitamin D needs. Vitamin D from the diet or the skin must be activated by the liver and the kidneys, which means that people with liver or kidney disease are more susceptible to vitamin D deficiency. The Cystic Fibrosis Foundation recommends checking vitamin D levels annually to screen for deficiency. If deficiency does occur, the diet should be reviewed for adequate calcium and vitamin D intake and additional vitamin D will be needed to correct the low blood levels. Plenty of sunshine is also helpful to keep an adequate amount of vitamin D in the body, and weight-bearing exercise (like walking or jogging) is also important to maintain bone strength.

Vitamin E

Vitamin E is important for the functioning of a number of important body parts, especially nerves. Good sources of vitamin E are vegetable oil, wheat germ, dried beans, and peas. Symptoms of vitamin E deficiency may include unsteadiness while walking. Vitamin E deficiency also causes an abnormal knee-jerk reflex, which the doctor checks by hitting the knee with the rubber reflex hammer.

Vitamin E deficiency can be detected by blood tests. Low vitamin E levels are common even with patients taking supplements and pancreatic enzymes. Standard multivitamin supplements do not contain the amount of vitamin E needed to maintain adequate levels. If you take a standard multivitamin, a separate vitamin E supplement is recommended. Vitamin E in the CF multivitamins is in a formulation that may make it easier to absorb and contains more vitamin E than in the standard multivitamin. If blood tests indicate a deficiency, a higher dose of vitamin E can be prescribed. Water-soluble forms of vitamin E are more easily absorbed than the more expensive health food store preparations of vitamin E.

Vitamin K

Vitamin K is needed by the liver for making some of the clotting factors that stop bleeding. When the vitamin K level is low, the clotting times are prolonged. Vitamin K is also important for bone formation. Green leafy vegetables and cauliflower are good food sources of vitamin K, and it is also found in dairy products. In addition, bacteria that normally live in the intestines make vitamin K. People with CF may need extra vitamin K, because both dietary and intestinal sources of vitamin K may be less than normal, for two reasons: First, vitamin K may not be well absorbed by the patient with CF; A second problem that someone with CF might have is that antibiotics given to treat infection in the lungs may kill the bacteria in the intestines, cutting down on the number of intestinal bacteria available to make vitamin K. This means that some people with CF who take a lot of antibiotics may need additional vitamin K.

Low blood levels of vitamin K can lead to serious bleeding. There are two blood tests for clotting factors to estimate vitamin K levels. These are the "PT" test (prothrombin time) and the "PTT" test (partial thromboplastin time). The PT becomes abnormal if levels of vitamin K are too low, and in more severe deficiencies, the PTT may also become abnormal. A newer test measures a protein that is increased when vitamin K levels are low (PIVKA, or protein induced by vitamin K absence) and may be more sensitive than the prothrombin time. Vitamin K deficiency can be corrected by adding oral or injected vitamin K supplements. Since the liver is needed to make clotting factors, even vitamin K given by injection may not be enough if the liver is failing to work (as in severe cirrhosis, discussed in Chapter 4). In this case, the already-made clotting factors may be administered by giving a transfusion of "fresh-frozen plasma." The CF multivitamins contain some vitamin K but more research needs to be done to determine whether they contain enough vitamin K. If you take an over-the-counter multivitamin, look for one containing vitamin K. Further studies need to be done to determine the optimal dose of vitamin K for patients with CF.

Hypomagnesemia (Low Blood Magnesium)

Magnesium, like calcium, phosphorus, sodium, and chloride, is one of the minerals the body needs. Good food sources of magnesium include whole grains, dark-green leafy vegetables, milk, soybeans, and molasses. Normally, magnesium is absorbed from the diet, and the kidneys get rid of any extra magnesium through the urine. When there is too little magnesium in the blood (hypomagnesemia), the signs include weakness, shakiness, and muscle cramps. In CF, there are a number of causes for hypomagnesemia. Maldigestion and malabsorption may prevent the magnesium from being absorbed from the intestine. Some antibiotics given for lung infections [especially the "aminoglycosides" (see Appendix B)—most of these end in "-micin" or "-mycin"] and diuretics given for heart or liver problems may cause too much magnesium to be lost in the urine. During a physical examination, hypomagnesemia can be checked for by assessing the knee-jerk reflex. If the knee-jerk reflexes are too brisk (the opposite of what happens with vitamin E deficiency), this could indicate low magnesium levels. The hands and face muscles can be examined for muscle spasms. Blood measurements of magnesium can confirm the diagnosis of hypomagnesemia. The treatment is by oral or intravenous (IV) magnesium supplements. Sometimes a large amount is needed to correct a deficiency.

Hypoelectrolytemia

The main chemicals in the bloodstream that carry an electrical charge, such as sodium, chloride, and potassium, are called *electrolytes*. People with CF lose a lot of salt in their sweat, and since salt consists of sodium and chloride, they may lose enough sodium and chloride to lower the blood levels of these electrolytes. This is especially likely to happen during exertion (exercise) in hot weather or in infants whose diet is low in salt, and who can't tell us they feel like having something salty to eat.

Once CF is diagnosed, the problem can usually be prevented, and most CF experts advise adding extra salt to the diet. Infants receiving formula and plain baby foods that are low in salt should have a small amount of salt added to the formula: about ⅛ tsp per day should be about right for an infant younger than 6 months and ¼ tsp for an infant older than 6 months. The small salt packets at many fast-food restaurants contain about ⅛ tsp of salt. This small amount of salt should prevent any problems from developing and will avoid the serious problems that could be caused by giving too much salt at one time. During hot weather or times of increased sweating, this amount of salt may need to be increased. Older children need no special treatment other than free access to salty foods or the saltshaker. Their taste will tell them how much salt they need. This is discussed more in Chapter 5 (*Other Systems*).

"Complementary" and "Alternative Medicine" Products

There are several "complementary" and "alternative medicine" or health food products available that make claims to cure or help CF. These products can be problematic for two reasons. First, these products are classified as nutritional supplements, and are not regulated by the Food and Drug Administration (FDA) nearly as carefully as medicines or drugs. No proof of safety or effectiveness is required. Furthermore, there is no assurance of purity or potency in most of these products. If you want to try one of these products, first discuss it with your CF team. Some products could interfere with the CF medicines that you take daily, others might not help, and some might actually be dangerous.

NUTRITIONAL TREATMENT

Basic dietary treatment of CF consists of a well-rounded diet with plenty of fat, protein, and carbohydrates, taken with enough pancreatic enzymes to provide maximum absorption. Tables 6.1 and 6.2 contain guidelines and suggestions for maintaining good nutritional intake. There is a whole section later in this chapter on how to use pancreatic enzymes.

NUTRITION THROUGH THE YEARS

For infants, either formula or breast milk is recommended. If formula is used, a milk-based formula fortified with iron is advised until 1 year of age. Since pancreatic enzymes are often given in baby food at a young age, it is fine for babies to start baby foods as early as 3 to 4 months of age. Remember, though, before going overboard with solids, ounce-for-ounce, formula usually has more calories than solid baby foods, so you want to avoid filling up with foods that are lower in calories than regular infant formula. If the infant needs to "catch up" on the weight

TABLE 6.1

Suggestions for Improving Your Child's Nutrition

1. Plan a definite eating schedule with three well-balanced meals and at least two snacks daily. Try to have the meals around the same time each day.
2. Meals should last 20–30 min. Young children have short attention spans and usually lose interest in eating after spending this amount of time at the table.
3. If the child refuses to eat for more than 10 min, remove him or her from the table and offer nothing to eat until the next scheduled meal or snack.
4. Scheduled snacks are important, but all-day snacking or "grazing" should be avoided. Grazing keeps the child full and he or she never really feels hungry.
5. Give a large, high-calorie snack at bedtime, unless the child has reflux (see Chapter 4).
6. Keep food offered simple. Children can be overwhelmed by too many foods at one meal.
7. Try to make foods attractive and appealing. Offer foods that the child can easily manage (cut-up meats, etc.).
8. Make the child's eating environment comfortable. Children should sit in sturdy chairs with their feet supported. The table and the food should be easily reached.
9. Avoid distractions at mealtime, such as television. Television provides too much stimulus and the child does not focus on eating.
10. Be sure that the child is not filling up on fluids. Do not give any beverage 30–60 min before a meal.
11. Reward positive behavior with verbal praise. Sticker charts may work well with younger children.
12. Parents should set good examples by eating nutritious meals with their children. If you don't eat well, you can't expect your child to eat well.

curve, the dietitian can give you special recipes to concentrate formulas or breast milk for higher calories. Babies who are tiny and cannot put gain before they are diagnosed often catch up on their growth curve and begin to look much healthier very soon after starting their oral enzymes and general CF care (see Figure 6.1).

Toddlers and preschool-aged children with CF should use whole milk (3% fat). Continual snacking or "grazing" is discouraged because it makes it harder to time the oral enzymes accurately and hard to make the diet nutritious. Three meals and two to three snacks a day work well for most children with CF.

Feeding problems are common in all children, with meals often becoming battlegrounds, and the problem can be worse in someone with CF—the parents know the importance of nutrition, and the child senses how important this is to the parent. Furthermore, it is one area of a child's life where he or she can exert a lot of control—you cannot force a child to eat if he or she truly does not want to.

TABLE 6.2

Ways to Increase Calories

1. Add margarine to the bread of sandwiches; grill sandwiches. Melt margarine on vegetables, waffles, and potatoes.
2. Add grated Parmesan cheese to spaghetti, casseroles, popcorn, and salads.
3. Melt cheese with scrambled eggs and casseroles and add to sandwiches. Order extra cheese on pizza.
4. Chopped nuts add lots of calories; add to cookie dough, breads, and pancakes. Buy breakfast cereals with nuts and dried fruit for higher calories per serving.
5. Drink whole milk instead of 2% or skim milk. Use whole milk cheeses instead of skim milk cheeses.
6. Add powdered nonfat dry milk to whole milk to increase the calories (¼ cup powder milk to 8 oz whole milk). Use the high-protein milk in cooking.
7. Use cheese sauce on vegetables, potatoes, pretzels, nachos, and french fries.
8. Use gravy on meats, potatoes, rice, noodles, and french fries.
9. Use top hot chocolate, pudding, gelatin, and milkshakes with whipped topping.
10. Use extra eggs in pancake, waffle, or french toast batter.
11. Add a package of vanilla instant breakfast to instant pudding mix.
12. Choose glazed doughnuts instead of cake doughnuts (275 cal vs. 105 cal) or chocolate-covered sandwich cookies instead of vanilla wafers (90 cal vs. 10 cal).

The parents' responsibility is to offer their children nutritious foods at mealtimes and snacks and encourage them to eat, but in the end, it is up to the child how much he or she will eat. Avoid force-feeding your child. By making the mealtime enjoyable, you can keep eating a pleasant part of CF care. A child may enjoy a picnic lunch outside, eating with a friend, or in another room of the house for a change. If you have a picky eater who is eating just a small amount of food, the goal is to make that small amount as high in calories as possible. Children at this age will start learning the importance of taking oral enzymes, and some will start swallowing the capsules.

School-aged children with CF will be learning to take more responsibility for their care as they start spending more time away from home. They will be responsible for deciding what foods to eat and when to take their enzymes. The frequent smelly stools caused by malabsorption can be embarrassing for school-aged children. They may find it hard to discuss their stools and symptoms, but it is important that they overcome this embarrassment so that they can learn to take care of themselves. The wish that most children have to be the same as all their friends is difficult to fulfill with the CF diet and enzyme capsules required for each meal. The routine of taking enzymes needs to be continued no matter where they eat, at home or away. With sports and other physical activities, children with CF will need to use extra salt and drink more fluids than their friends do.

Teenagers are in a category of their own (some people think that they are actually from another planet, but we'd like to deny those rumors here and now). Teens are often on the run, and don't seem to have time to sit still for their regular meals; they often like fast food. They need to remember (and sometimes need reminding) that food is important, and taking enzymes with their meals is crucial. Well-balanced meals are important. However, heavy reliance on fast food is not necessarily all bad. The same thing that makes much fast food bad for most people—big portions, lots of calories, lots of fat—can actually be helpful for the busy teenager with CF *if* he or she remembers to take enough enzymes.

HISTORY OF PANCREATIC ENZYMES

Pancreatic enzymes have been used for decades, and there are several brands of them on the market that vary in their strength. This determines how many pills need to be taken. The US FDA launched a rigorous review of pancreatic enzymes to help ensure that they were the most effective products. In April 2004, a new rule was issued requiring makers of pancreatic enzymes to get their drugs approved by the FDA by April 28, 2010. For the enzymes to receive FDA approval, companies needed to test them in clinical trials in people with pancreatic disease, including CF, to confirm their safety and effectiveness. Currently approved pancreatic enzymes are listed in Table 6.3.

TABLE 6.3

FDA Approved Pancreatic Enzymes Comparison Guide as of Spring 2011

Product	Lipase[a]	Protease[b]	Amylase[c]
Creon 6,000	6,000	19,000	30,000
Creon 12,000	12,000	38,000	60,000
Creon 24,000	24,000	76,000	120,000
Pancreaze 4,200	4,200	10,000	17,500
Pancreaze 10,500	10,500	25,000	43,750
Pancreaze 16,800	16,800	40,000	70,000
Pancreaze 21,000	21,000	37,000	61,000
Zenpep 5	5,000	17,000	27,000
Zenpep 10	10,000	34,000	55,000
Zenpep 15	15,000	51,000	82,000
Zenpep 20	20,000	68,000	109,000

Numbers refer to content in USP units.
[a]Lipase, fat-digesting enzyme; most important for patients with cystic fibrosis; one capsule with 8,000 units of lipase is roughly equivalent to two 4,000-unit capsules of lipase (if all are enteric-coated or all non–enteric-coated).
[b]Protease, protein-digesting enzyme.
[c]Amylase, starch-digesting enzyme.

The goal of this requirement was to make sure that the enzymes have the right amount of active ingredients to digest and absorb foods and prevent inconsistency in products that can lead to problems in digestion. The CF Foundation has supported getting the FDA approval for pancreatic enzymes as it is seen as a step forward in improving the quality of care for people with CF.

How to Use Pancreatic Enzymes

See Also Appendix B

Remember from the previous discussion of how pancreatic enzymes work that, normally, these digestive chemicals are released from the pancreas into the duodenum (the part of the intestine right after the stomach) just as the food passes into the duodenum from the stomach. We try to duplicate this process by using oral pancreatic enzyme supplements. These enzymes should ideally mix with the food in the duodenum, just as happens in people without CF. This means several things. First, enzymes need to be taken with meals (and with *each* meal): These are not a once-a-day or a three-times-a-day medication. If someone has two meals, the enzymes should be taken twice; if someone has three meals and two snacks, the enzymes need to be taken five times, directly with the food. Some physicians recommend taking the whole enzyme dose at the beginning of each meal, whereas others think that it's better to take one-half the enzymes at the beginning and the rest halfway through the meal. Once you take the oral enzymes, they are effective for about 45 minutes to 1 hour. This means that if you are a slow eater, or are eating over a long period, then the dose should be split and some enzyme given later in the meal. If you finish eating and have a snack 5 minutes later, no more enzymes are needed, but if you have a snack 1½ hours after your last enzyme capsule, you need to take more enzymes.

Most enzymes are enteric-coated and come in capsules with small beads inside. These beads are a bit like an M&M: There's a thin coating, and the good stuff (in this case, the enzyme itself) is inside the coating. The coating protects the enzymes from stomach acid, since acid destroys the enzymes. The coating is designed to dissolve when it's in a nonacid environment, which is usually the case in the duodenum. So, it "melts in your duodenum, not in your stomach," like the M&M melts in your mouth and not in your hand. This works beautifully, because it means that when the system works as designed (most of the time), the coating dissolves and the enzymes are released in the duodenum exactly where the body's own pancreatic enzymes are designed to enter the intestine and mix with the food to begin digesting fat and protein. When enteric-coated enzymes were introduced in the 1970s, they provided a revolutionary change in the ability of patients with CF to digest and absorb food.

The enzyme capsules can be swallowed whole (that's the most convenient way, once a child is old enough to swallow capsules) or opened up and the beads taken separately. The beads can be mixed with some soft food, such as applesauce. This is the most common way for babies to take the enzymes. Applesauce is a good food to mix the beads in, because applesauce is acid, and therefore the enzyme's coating will not dissolve while it's sitting in the food waiting to be eaten. The applesauce or other food should not be heated, because the heat will dissolve the coating. Even with cool applesauce, the beads should not be allowed to sit in the applesauce (or other food) for long: They should be mixed in just before the meal. If they sit too long and the coating does dissolve, the enzyme will start to digest the food and may make it less tasty. It won't be dangerous, but it just won't be quite as attractive or effective. The beads can also be just placed on a baby's tongue and rinsed right down with a bottle or breast-feeding. For older children and adults, beads can be taken alone, in their capsules, or mixed mostly with any foods, but it's important that they not be chewed, because that will break the protective coating, with two bad results: The patient will get a bitter taste (and possibly some lip or mouth irritation), and the enzymes will likely be destroyed by acid once they get to the stomach.

It's a good idea for anyone using enzymes to practice good mouth care and be sure that all the beads are out of the mouth at least by the end of the meal. Breast-feeding mothers will need to clean their breasts carefully to avoid nipple irritation. In some babies, enzymes passing out with the stools can cause a burn to the buttocks if the diapers are not changed frequently or the bottom not cleaned thoroughly.

Who Needs Enzymes?

Most people with CF (85% to 90% of all patients with CF) need to take enzymes with their food in order to digest that food. As many as one-half of all newborn babies with CF do *not* need to take enzymes, but most of these babies will gradually develop a need for enzymes over the first months or years.

How Much Enzyme Is Needed?

There is no rule for how much enzyme a patient will need, and the amount varies tremendously among patients and even changes a bit for each patient depending on what is in the particular meal or snack. The amount of enzyme needed for a particular meal depends on several things including:

1. The person's age and size
2. Amount of pancreatic blockage
3. Amount of fat in the meal or snack

A tiny snack, or one with no fat, will require no enzymes, whereas enzymes will be needed for a meal or snack with fat in it, and more enzymes will be needed for an extra large meal or for one with a lot of fat. A plain potato is virtually all carbohydrate, and therefore doesn't require enzymes for digestion. However, if you eat your baked potato loaded with butter and sour cream, then you would need to take enzymes with it. Many patients know that they will need more enzymes for pizza or their dad's chili than for most meals.

How Do You Know How Much Enzyme to Take?

At first, it seems that it will be very difficult to learn how to adjust the enzyme dosages, but most families become experts very quickly. Here's how: Some people say that the digestive system is a long tube that leads from the kitchen to the bathroom (food in the top, bowel movements out the bottom). There is a certain truth here, and it's the key to knowing how much enzyme you need. Undigested fat ends up in the stool, making for frequent, bulky, smelly bowel movements that will sometimes have oil or grease droplets visible in them or leave an oily film on the toilet water. If you see bowel movements like that, you know that more enzymes are needed. Be careful not to make changes in the usual enzyme dosage on the basis of one messy stool; instead, make sure that there is a pattern. Everyone—with or without CF—has a sloppy stool on occasion, whether it's because of a little virus, some bad food, a medication, or other cause. These common sloppy stools are nothing to worry about and will get better on their own. Frequently, patients with CF get so used to increasing their enzymes for "sloppy" stools that they see a messy bowel movement, increase the enzymes, and find that the stools become normal quickly (which they might have anyway if it wasn't an enzyme problem that caused the one abnormal bowel movement in the first place). Then, since the stools have become normal, they keep the enzymes at the new higher dose. The next time there's another single abnormal stool, they increase the dosage again, and so on. In this way, many patients with CF end up taking much larger dosages of enzymes than they really need. So what? In most cases, the only problem with taking too much enzyme is the minor bother of swallowing extra pills, and cost: You're paying for more medicines than you need. For some people taking very high enzyme dosages, however, there is a small chance of a dangerous complication, with scarring of the colon (the large intestine), with the scary name *fibrosing colonopathy*. This condition almost always requires surgery (and is discussed in Chapter 4). Fibrosing colonopathy almost never occurs in anyone taking less than 2,500 units of lipase each meal for each kilogram they weigh (and, in fact, the condition has been seen only rarely since the mid 1990s).

Poor Response to Enzymes

There are several reasons that someone may not get the appropriate benefit from a usual dosage of enzymes. If stools continue to be loose, you should contact the CF center staff. Some causes of loose stools have to do with enzymes not working well, whereas others don't have anything to do with the enzymes. Some causes of loose stools are as follows:

- Excessive juice intake (very common with toddlers, no relation to enzymes)
- Introduction of solid foods to an infant (may need more enzymes)
- "Grazing"—eating makes enzyme dosing difficult

- Not taking extra enzymes with "fast foods" or other high-fat meals
- Not taking extra enzymes with milk or other beverages with fat
- Not taking enzymes with snacks that contain fat (e.g., candy bars and peanuts are high in fat)
- Lactose intolerance (inability to digest the sugar in milk) can cause malabsorption
- Chewing enzymes
- Excessive stomach acid
- Not taking enzymes
- Not taking enzymes in the beginning of the meal

HIGH-CALORIE NUTRITIONAL SUPPLEMENTS

Milkshakes and commercial high-calorie nutritional supplements can be prescribed if routine nutritional measures are not sufficient. Sometimes people who cannot eat enough calories in their regular diet can drink the supplements for enough extra calories to start gaining weight. Busy teenagers and active adults find the ready-to-drink nutritional supplements very convenient when they are away from home or in place of a meal. Examples of high-calorie supplements are presented in Table 6.4. Special high-calorie recipes are presented in Appendix D.

HORMONES AND APPETITE STIMULANTS

If patients do not eat enough regular food and high-calorie supplements, they are sometimes given medications to increase their appetite. Some examples of these are *dronabinol* (*Marinol®*), *megestrol* (*Megace®*), and *cyproheptadine hydrochloride* (*Periactin®*). None of these have been studied in large groups of patients with CF, so their overall safety and effectiveness are still unknown. Megestrol is a female hormone, and it has been used successfully in recent years in a very few patients with CF as an appetite and growth stimulant. It may cause or worsen diabetes and may suppress the normal activity of the adrenal gland, upsetting the body's own hormone regulation. Cyproheptadine hydrochloride (Periactin®) is an antihistamine that can be useful in combatting allergic reactions and has the *side effect* of increased appetite. Some physicians have prescribed it for patients with CF to take advantage of that side effect. It can also make you sleepy and cause a dry mouth. There is a concern that it might dry lung secretions excessively as well, so it should be used cautiously, if at all. Dronabinol (Marinol®) is in a class of medications called "cannabinoids" and is used to treat loss of appetite and weight loss. Side effects include fatigue, confusion/decreased mental alertness, anxiety, and euphoria.

Growth hormone (somatropin) occurs naturally in the body and is responsible for normal growth. Growth hormone injections have become popular as a way to cheat among strength and bodybuilding athletes. Patients with CF may

TABLE 6.4

High-Calorie Supplements

Product name	Serving size	Calories per serving
Boost®	8 oz	240
Resource® Breeze (juice)	8 oz	250
Boost® Kid Essentials	8 oz	240
Boost® Kid Essentials 1.5	8 oz	355
Boost® Plus	8 oz	360
Boost® Pudding	5-oz can	240
Carnation® Breakfast	1 package and 8-oz milk	300
Enlive® (juice)	8.1 oz	250
Ensure®	8 oz	250
Ensure® Plus	8 oz	350
Ensure® Pudding	4 oz	170
Jevity®	8 oz	250
Jevity 1.5®	8 oz	355
Nutren Jr®	8.3 oz	250
Nutren 2.0®	8.3 oz	500
Pediasure®	8 oz	240
Peptamen Junior®	8.3 oz	250
Peptamen 1.5®	8.3 oz	375
Polycose Powder®	As desired[a]	23 per tbsp
Pulmocare®	8-oz can	355
Scandical®	As desired[a]	35 per tbsp
Scandishake®	1 package and 8 oz milk	600
Two-Cal HN®	8 oz	470
VHC 2.25®	8.3-oz can	560

[a]The products whose serving size is listed as "as desired" are added to as much liquid (e.g., milk) as you like.

have low levels of this hormone, and supplements with manufactured growth hormone have been shown in a couple of studies with a very few patients to be safe and effective in increasing body size. The drug is very expensive and needs to be given by injection, usually once a day. Testosterone is the most important male sex hormone in the body, and it too has been found to be low in some patients with CF. If testosterone levels are low, supplemental testosterone may be able to help restore normal growth. Like growth hormone, it is given by injection and is very expensive. Some physicians worry that testosterone can hasten the aging of bones, which increases (height) growth initially but prematurely closes the *growth plates* of the bones, shutting off the possibility of further growth.

TUBE FEEDINGS

Some patients cannot take in enough calories by mouth to gain weight or to maintain weight. For these patients, calories (in the form of liquid formulas) can be given by tube feeding while they sleep. The tube used reaches directly into the stomach or the intestine. This has been done for patients with CF in a number of different ways. Some patients have used a **n**asogastric **t**ube (or NG tube) that passes in through the nose, down the throat, and into the stomach. Some young children who found this idea repellent at first have quickly become used to the tube, and older children have learned to insert the tube themselves each night before bed. The improvement in growth and appearance and feeling of well-being have made this extra effort worth to them.

A second—and much more common—method of tube feeding is through a gastrostomy (or G-tube). In this method, a tube is placed through the skin of the upper abdomen and into the stomach during a minor operation. In some centers, it can even be done in the radiology department with the patient sedated but not under general anesthesia. After the tube is placed, the patient is usually not allowed to eat large amounts for the first few weeks, while the small surgical wound heals. Once it has healed, the patient can eat as much regular food as he or she wants, and additional calories are fed through the tube while the patients sleeps. As with the NG tube, results from this type of feeding have been dramatic. See Figure 6.2 for an example of the kind of growth that can result from a G-tube. This tube has the advantage of not having to be replaced each night, and it does not involve the discomfort of a tube that goes through the nose. It also does not interfere with breathing or coughing. The G-tube is invisible under the clothes when it is not being used and can be hooked up to the supplemental feeding at night. When it is no longer needed it can simply be removed without an operation. Jejunostomy (or J-tube) feeding is similar to gastrostomy feeding, except that the tube goes into the second part of the intestine instead of the stomach. It is less commonly used but has the advantage of protecting against gastroesophageal reflux of the tube feeding (see Chapter 4). Predigested formulas are often used for the gastrostomy and jejunostomy feedings. These formulas may not need enzymes for digestion or absorption (depending on exactly what makes up the fat source in the formula—if the fat is fully predigested, no enzymes are needed, but if the fats are *long-chain* or even *medium-chain*, enzymes will still be needed).

No one likes the idea of tube feeding when he or she first hears about it. However, many people with CF have been converted when they see the dramatic growth that is often achieved with these tube feeds. Many patients have also felt that a big burden has been taken off them: They have usually been trying to eat enough to gain weight, and their parents have certainly been "on their case" continuously to eat more; now with the food coming in by tube feeds, they don't have to force themselves to eat. It is important not to wait too long if tube feeds are to be tried: Someone whose nutrition and overall health are too bad may not benefit.

2 to 20 years: Girls
Stature-for-age and weight-for-age percentiles

NAME _____

RECORD # _____

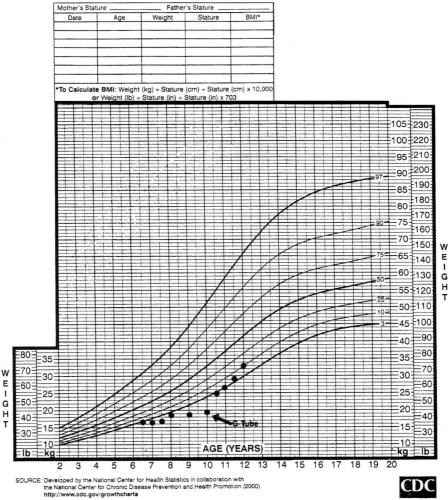

FIGURE 6.2 Growth chart showing weight of child before and after placement of gastrostomy tube ("G-tube") for nighttime supplemental feedings. Note the large weight gain after tube feedings were instituted.

Problems with Tube Feeds

Tube feeds require either the discomfort of placing the tube each night and removing it each morning or the discomfort and risks of a minor surgical procedure. Many people feel "full"—uncomfortably so for a few—in the morning after a night of tube feeds, and they may not want to eat breakfast. Some may even vomit from being overfull. These problems can usually be taken care of by slowing down the feedings toward morning or by medications that help the stomach empty faster. Some may also experience increased heartburn and reflux (see Chapter 4). In these cases, a G-tube can be converted to a "G-J" tube by threading a smaller tube through the G-tube into the stomach and then into the duodenum and finally leaving its tip in the jejunum (Figure 4.1). Occasionally the tubes will leak, causing some wetness and mess. This leaking can usually be taken care of by changing the tube. Finally, for many people, the weight gain is very good only while they get the tube feeding, and the benefits are lost if the feeds are stopped.

INTRAVENOUS NUTRITION

IV nutrition is rarely required, because nutritional supplements or tube feeding is usually sufficient to improve nutrition. IV nutrition (also called "parenteral nutrition") can be given through a long-term IV into a large vein, usually in the upper chest. As with the supplemental nutrition by mouth and by tube, IV nutrition can be given at home so that a person's life can be continued normally. This is a very expensive form of nutrition and should be used only if the patient is unable to tolerate tube feedings into the stomach or the intestine. There is a slight risk of serious infection of the IV line. If the line does become infected, it needs to be removed and another placed. Use of IV nutrition for a long time can also be harmful to the liver.

SUMMARY

In summary, there are three components of CF nutrition (high-calorie diet, oral pancreatic enzymes, and vitamin supplements). With aggressive application of all three components, most patients with CF should be able to grow well and maintain nutrition that is adequate to support their overall health.

Hospitalization and Other Special Treatments

7

Jonathan E. Spahr, David M. Orenstein,
Daniel J. Weiner, and Louise T. Bauer

THE BASICS

1. Some patients with cystic fibrosis (CF) need to be hospitalized, especially to treat worsened lung infection.

2. These hospitalizations often last 2 weeks, but can be shorter or longer.

3. During the hospitalization, patients get antibiotics through an intravenous (IV) line and have some blood tests.

4. There are ways to make the hospitalization less frightening than it might otherwise be.

5. Your CF center staff can help.

6. Some patients get IVs at home, usually after the IVs have been started in the hospital.

HOSPITALIZATION

In a given year, about 30% of patients with cystic fibrosis (CF) will have to be hospitalized. The most common reason for a hospital admission for someone with CF is the treatment of worsened lung infection, commonly referred to as *pulmonary exacerbation* (see Chapter 3, *The Respiratory System*), especially with intravenous (IV) antibiotics and increased airway clearance. The time needed for IV antibiotics is the time it takes to get back to the usual state of health, most commonly about 2 weeks. This chapter reviews what happens during such a hospitalization and includes general information about hospital routines and procedures, an explanation of the various treatments and tests, and an introduction to the different health professionals you'll see in the hospital.

Preparing for Hospitalization

Admission to the hospital upsets the daily routine of a family, and can be confusing and frightening. With the help of staff from the CF center (especially CF nurses and social workers), children and families can cope with the stress, straighten out the confusion, and be much less frightened. In fact, both child and family can learn from the experience and come away from it as stronger, more mature individuals. In order to accomplish this, the family must be well informed about what to expect.

Parents should ask questions they may wonder about in order to know what to expect in the hospital. Here are some examples:

- What are the visiting hours?
- May I stay overnight with my child?
- May brothers and sisters visit?
- Is a "pass" allowed, so I can take my child out of the hospital for a break?
- Can I assist with my child's care (baths, feeding, treatments) if I would like to do so?
- Are there any therapies or medicines that I need to bring to the hospital?
- Which doctor is in charge of my child's care? What other doctors will be working with him or her?
- Who are the other members of the health care team?

The best way to prepare your child for a hospitalization is to talk to him or her in simple, honest words about what will happen when he or she is in the hospital. What you say and *how you say it* are very important and will affect your child's understanding and comfort during his or her stay in the hospital. When possible, this should be done before admission. Some of the most common questions children may ask are:

- How long will I be in the hospital?
- When will I go into the hospital?
- When will I come home?
- Will I get any needle "sticks"?
- What will the other kids be like?
- Can mom and dad stay with me?

As you answer these questions, you will acknowledge that there will be some painful procedures (IVs, blood tests). These things need to be mentioned, but do not need to be dwelt on. Similarly, you can and should point out the "neat" things about the hospital (playrooms, etc.), without implying that all will be wonderful fun. Some children might not ask their parents questions about the hospital. They might choose to discuss their worries with another trusted adult in an effort to spare their parents additional concern. Developing relationships outside the family circle is a normal part of growing up, and this should be fostered as it occurs.

It is helpful for children to have descriptions of what the hospital rooms look like, and how daily life will differ from what they are used to. A prehospitalization tour is especially helpful so that the children can see for themselves, and see that things may not be quite as scary as they feared and that some things can even be fun. These tours can usually be arranged through the CF staff (especially nurses and social workers).

Encourage your child to pack personal items from home (toys, blanket, clothes, pajamas, school books, laptops, music) and perhaps pictures of family members. Parents should also plan to bring few things, including insurance information, a list of current medications, a list of allergies, important telephone numbers, money for parking and food (for parents), identification, legal papers (especially for adult guardians who are not the child's biologic parents).

Admission: Checking In

The following events occur just preceding most admissions to the hospital: The hospital admissions office will be notified by your physician of the date and reason for your hospitalization. The people in the admissions office will need to ask some general questions and get your insurance information. Your pediatrician or family doctor (or insurance company) will have to provide insurance authorization for the admission. This is done over the telephone before you come in or in the admissions office on the day of your arrival. After you "check in," in the admissions office, you will be sent to one of the inpatient floors. A member of the staff will orient you to the floor (show you how to call for a nurse; how the bed, phone, and television work; and inform you of the usual floor rules and schedules, etc.).

Soon after you arrive on the floor, a nurse or patient care assistant will check your "vital signs" (pulse—how fast your heart is beating, respiratory rate—how fast you're breathing, blood pressure, and temperature), and will weigh and measure you. This person will usually ask you about what medicines you take at home, and whether you are allergic to any medications or foods. He or she will ask things like nicknames, food preferences, and where parents can be reached. These things will enable him or her to help plan for your care during your hospital stay.

The next step is usually to meet a doctor who will ask more extensive questions about your medical history and then perform a physical examination. In a small community hospital, the doctor may be your own physician; in a large university hospital, the doctor is likely to be an intern or resident (see below for an explanation of the "cast of characters"). After the questions and examination, the physician will write orders for treatment and the necessary treatment will begin. Whoever the doctor is who does your admission paperwork, examination, and orders, remember that you should always have the right to talk to your CF physician anytime during your stay in the hospital. Remember, you are in the hospital to get better. Make sure that whoever comes into your room washes their hands. If they forget, they will appreciate the reminder.

Daily Life in the Hospital

Most often when patients with CF are admitted to the hospital for treatment of a pulmonary exacerbation, they are not terribly sick or disabled. The reason for these hospitalizations is to *keep someone relatively well*, not to cure someone who is dreadfully ill. Some people, including young doctors or nurses, may not understand that and may even say, "You don't look sick enough to be in the hospital." They miss the point that your health is suffering and that the reason for the hospitalization is to get you back to your normal state of good health. While you probably won't be so sick that you need to be in bed all day, it is important to remember that you are in hospital to improve your present and future health.

Most children's hospitals, and many general hospitals, encourage parents to participate in their child's care but to take care to remain *parents*, not *nurses* or *doctors* in the eyes of their child. Bathing, feeding, play, bedtime stories, and maintaining normal discipline standards are activities that promote normalcy in the hospital. While parents may want to be present as a source of support and consultation during painful or frightening procedures, some experts believe that they should avoid being enlisted to assist directly with such procedures (such as stabilizing an arm for blood test or injection). When this does happen, it may seem that the parent has given up his or her job as a *protector*.

Different Ages, Different Needs

Hospitalized children need different things from their parents at different ages.

The infant and toddler are too young to understand what is happening and cannot fully comprehend the parents' explanation. For an infant, the parents' trusted, nurturing presence can be comforting. Cuddling, rocking and singing, and playing are all familiar activities that bring security to a new, frightening environment.

As children advance to *the preschool years*, they begin to understand more of what is happening. Their primary fears in the hospital are abandonment and lack of mobility. They benefit from regular contact with parents and the presence of a stable group of caretakers when their parents cannot be there. They also enjoy active play, despite their IV lines!

Children in this age group may have many fantasies and develop their own reasons for why things happen. They may misinterpret hospitalization as a punishment. New sights, smells, and sounds may be particularly frightening. They benefit from simple, concrete explanations immediately before procedures about what they will sense (see, hear, feel, smell) during a new experience. They may also attempt to stall a nurse or doctor who is about to perform a painful procedure. As a rule, it is best to provide a simple explanation and then allow the staff member to proceed quickly and with confidence.

Older preschool and school-aged children have a greater understanding of events and benefit from explanations. They also benefit from participating in planning their daily care and being provided with choices about their schedules, meals, and therapy where applicable. They should be encouraged to maintain contacts with friends while in the hospital and to develop new friendships with other patients.

Teenagers with CF are faced with the complications of a chronic illness at a time when they are most concerned with a changing body, achieving independence from their family, and establishing relationships with the opposite sex. CF may thwart many of these goals by slowing growth and delaying puberty and by imposing a home-care regimen that perpetuates dependence on the parents. In addition, no teenager wants to be different from others, and the young man or woman with CF may appear different or have different needs, making it more difficult to establish new relationships. In the hospital, teenagers benefit from many of the same practices as their younger counterparts: explanations of what to expect, opportunity to participate in planning their care, making choices about some flexible areas of care, and contact with school friends. This assistance should be provided in the context of the special needs of the changing, developing adolescent who is seeking to establish some measure of independence.

Hospitalization can be upsetting. Sometimes it can be very upsetting if the child or teen will be missing something important while in the hospital. First day of school, prom, homecoming, birthday parties are all very important things for children and teenagers. Finding out that someone is upset about missing an important activity and figuring out whether it is possible for them to attend that activity can make a big difference. You may need to pry a little to get this information from children and teenagers.

What to Wear

Children will probably be up and around most of the day, so they should wear regular clothes. You might want to be sure they have roomy, loose sleeves to fit over IVs.

Activity

You should try not to let being in the hospital decrease your activity. Most hospitals, especially children's hospitals, will have playrooms and teen lounges, and you should take advantage of these facilities, while being careful about infection control at the same time (see section after next). You may be able to use a physical therapy gym or even to leave the hospital (on a pass) to get even more activity. This may be a chance to visit museums or other favorite places. You may be a bit tired, particularly at first, and you shouldn't push yourself too much, but you should try to be up and around most of the day. If you lie in bed all day, you will definitely get out of shape, and that will make it even harder to do stuff.

Schoolwork

Two or three weeks is a lot of time to miss from the school year, so it is very important to try to keep up with your schoolwork. Your doctor can help you arrange for work to be sent or brought to you in the hospital. Some hospitals have a schoolteacher on their staff to help students keep up with work. Some school systems have arrangements for home (or hospital) tutors for anyone who will be out of school a certain amount of time. It is very important that you do whatever is necessary to keep up with schoolwork while you're in the hospital.

Infection Control

Lung infection is of course one of the main things that cause deterioration of the health of people with CF. Worsened infection—particularly with bacteria such as *Pseudomonas aeruginosa*, *Burkholderia cepacia*, and *Staphylococcus aureus*—is the main reason for hospital admission. We are not sure yet how people with CF become infected with these different bacteria (this topic is discussed at greater length in Chapter 3), but increasing evidence shows that *one* way is "person-to-person" transmission, meaning you can get some bacteria from other people. These other people include patients with CF who might already have a particular kind of bacteria, and could include health care workers. Because of the possible risks of getting new—and perhaps more dangerous and difficult-to-treat—bacteria from other patients, many hospitals and clinics now have rules that separate patients with CF from each other. These rules may include the following:

- No rooming together
- No visiting in one another's rooms
- The necessity to cover mouth and nose during coughing spells
- Careful disposal of tissues that have mucus in them
- Not touching other patients with CF
- Wearing masks when moving through the hospital (this is to protect you)
- Health care providers will wear gowns and gloves (this is also to protect you)
- And so forth

Some hospitals have set aside separate floors of the hospital for patients with and without certain specific bacteria (especially *B. cepacia*). These restrictions can be annoying, and perhaps even frightening, but they seem to keep to a minimum the number of cases in which patients come down with new bacteria, and therefore should be followed. In fact, you can help, by suggesting good hygiene to other people coming into your room: Ask other patients to cover their mouths when they are coughing and to wash their hands after coughing spells. Demonstrate that you're not "picking on" anyone else by doing the same things yourself. And, don't be shy about suggesting to your nurses, respiratory therapists, or doctors to wash their hands before they touch you.

The Hospital Cast of Characters

You will meet many different people in the hospital in addition to other patients, and it can be confusing as you try to figure out who everybody is. Remember, with any problems or major questions, your doctor is in charge.

Nurses and Patient Care Assistants/Partners

Hospitals could not run without *nurses* and *patient care assistants* or *patient care partners*. Nurses are licensed professionals who collaborate with the patient's attending physician and other health care team members to evaluate, plan, implement, and coordinate the patient's care.

A patient care assistant (in some hospitals called "patient care partner") is a trained caregiver who provides basic, direct patient care and will be "partnered" with your nurse. They are often assigned by the nurse to administer appropriate aspects of your care, such as taking vital signs, assisting with feeding and bathing, and other supportive tasks. The nurses and partners will help you to communicate your needs and concerns to the appropriate staff, and in general help to make your stay successful and pleasant. They may be able to answer many of the questions that arise regarding treatments, schedules, and so forth.

Physicians

You are likely to see a number of different physicians in addition to your own doctor. Especially if you are in a children's hospital and/or a teaching hospital (one that has students, interns, and residents), you will also be meeting a number of people at the various levels of medical training. It is helpful to know the different stages of medical training.

Medical students have gone to college for 4 years and are now enrolled in a 4-year medical school. The first 2 years consist of classroom and laboratory learning. In the third and fourth years, students spend time in the hospital, learning various specialties such as pediatrics, general internal medicine, and surgery. After completing 4 years of medical school, students graduate and get their doctoral degree (M.D. or D.O.). They are now doctors.

The first step after becoming a doctor is internship. An *intern* is a doctor who is beginning to train in one specialty—pediatrics, internal medicine, family medicine, surgery, psychiatry, or obstetrics/gynecology. After the internship year, the specialty training continues with 2 to 4 years of "residency." (Most programs no longer call first-year trainees "interns," but rather "first-year *residents*.") After a resident has finished the 3-year residency, he or she is qualified to set up practice as a specialist (family doctor, pediatrician, etc.).

Some physicians choose to get even more specialized training and take 2- or 3-year subspecialty *fellowships*. Subspecialties include pulmonology (respiratory problems, including CF), cardiology (heart), and neurosurgery (brain and nervous system surgery). Some of the "trainees" you meet might be young students, whereas others may have had 4 years of college, 4 years of medical school, 3 years of pediatric or medicine residencies, and several years of fellowship.

As we've already mentioned, interacting with many different people at various levels of training and understanding can be difficult for patients and families, especially when several people ask you the same questions. It may also be frustrating to realize that you know more about CF than some of the nurses and physicians who will be taking care of you or your child. Remember, though, that your own physician is knowledgeable about CF and is in charge of your (or your child's) treatment.

In addition, you can view this as an opportunity to help in the education of the people who will be the nurses and physicians in the community. Many families with a child with CF have had very frustrating experiences of going from doctor to doctor trying to find out what was wrong until they found one who knew about CF. One of the best things that anyone can do to help future children with CF is to make a contribution to the education of physicians who will be seeing those children, so that eventually all family doctors, pediatricians, and even adult medical specialists will be knowledgeable about CF, will be able to recognize it, and will have an idea of how to begin treatment.

Consultants

Occasionally, your physician may ask a colleague to give an opinion about a problem or a possible treatment. The other physician will probably look through your (or your child's) chart, ask some questions, and do a physical examination. This colleague is likely to be a specialist or a subspecialist, possibly a *gastroenterologist* (stomach, liver, and digestive system specialist), *surgeon*, or *cardiologist*. These colleagues who are called in to give their opinion about one part of the treatment plan are called consultants. It is the job of the consultant to give an opinion and perhaps make suggestions. It is not the consultant's job to carry out treatments or order tests without your physician's approval.

Other Health Professionals

In addition to nurses and physicians, you are likely to have contact with other professionals, including *respiratory therapists* and *physical therapists*, who may be involved with aerosols and airway clearance treatments (ACT). Some hospitals will have *child-life workers* to help make the hospitalization a more positive experience. These people are trained in child development principles, and are frequently clever at finding just the right kind of entertainment for a child in the strange environment of the hospital. More importantly, they are sensitive to the signals children give through their play and talk, about things that are upsetting or threatening to them. Child-life workers and *child development specialists* often can give parents, nurses, and physicians important insights into what is going on in the minds of hospitalized children.

Nutritionists or *dietitians* may help with menu selection, recommendations about high-calorie supplements, special diets that might be needed (e.g., for someone with diabetes), adjustments to enzymes. *Social workers* will be available to help with a variety of problems, from very tough family adjustment problems (these are discussed in Chapter 12, *The Family*) to the day-to-day worries of insurance and transportation expenses. Other people you may come in contact with include people from a television service, hospital maintenance people, and janitors.

Parents play an important part in their child's health care and contribute their intimate knowledge of their child. Health care providers have experience with many different children over a span of years. Together, with a cooperative, positive attitude, parents and health care providers can educate one another about the needs of the child and effectively plan and carry out hospital care.

TREATMENTS AND TESTS

Intravenous Antibiotics

One of the main reasons for being admitted to the hospital is to get powerful antibiotics (especially those that kill *Pseudomonas* organisms) that are effective only when given directly into the bloodstream. A short, soft, plastic tube or catheter is inserted in the vein with a needle; the needle is then removed, leaving the soft catheter in place. (Some children seem to like to know that the dreaded "N-word"—needle—will be thrown away, leaving just a tiny straw-like tube in.) The end of the catheter is taped to the skin, and its end is closed off with a rubber cap or attached to more tubing through which fluid can be administered. When the needle is first inserted, it will hurt a little as it pierces the skin, but once it is removed, leaving the plastic catheter in place, it is rarely painful. Babies, children, and older patients alike can usually carry on with their daily activities with an IV in place. There is a medicated cream (EMLA or LET cream) that can be used to numb the skin where the IV will go. The only problem with this cream is that it needs to be in place for 45 minutes for it to work, so putting it on will delay things a bit while you wait for it to take effect.

The veins that are most often used are those on the back of the hands and on the forearms, but if these veins are difficult to find in an infant (as is often the case with a chubby baby), foot veins or veins in the scalp may be used. Foot veins should not be used in anyone who can walk, unless there is no other choice. Scalp vein IVs look as though they'd be very uncomfortable, and most parents are bothered by the idea of them at first, but they are no more painful than an arm vein IV and have the advantage of not requiring the immobilization of an arm. If a hand or arm vein is used, an arm board (which looks like a splint) helps to keep the hand or forearm stable, which in turn helps keep the IV within the vein. A plastic or cardboard cup may be taped over the needle to protect it and prevent it from being bumped.

When the IV is about to be started, it's a good idea to tell the person starting it if you have preferences about which hand or arm to use: If someone is right-handed, it's better to leave the right hand alone, so that it can be used for writing, playing video games, and so forth. Similarly, it's better to pick a spot that will leave the elbow free to bend. If a baby has favorite fingers or thumb to suck, he or she will be much happier if those fingers or that thumb are not taped out of mouth's reach.

IVs last only for a limited period, for they eventually go bad ("infiltrate") and need to be replaced: Antibiotics are powerful chemicals, and may irritate the vein, eventually weakening its wall so that it starts to leak, making the arm swell and become tender. When this happens, it is time for a new IV. Although IVs may occasionally last a couple of weeks, a few days is closer to the average. Fortunately, there is another kind of IV that can last safely and comfortably for a long time.

Intravenous Lines for Prolonged Use: The Central Line

In patients who require very long courses of IV treatment and, in fact, in patients who are getting the standard 2 or 3 weeks of IVs, it is not convenient or comfortable to keep using regular hand or arm vein IVs, which last only a few days before they have to be changed. In these cases, a "long line," or a "central line," can be lifesaving, or at least much more convenient. These lines are a special kind of IV that has its end in a very large vein or in the heart (the "central" in "central line" refers to the fact that the end of the tube, and therefore where the medicines go, is in the central part of the body—near or in the heart—compared to the regular old IVs—also called "peripheral" IVs because they are in the *periphery*, or on outside of the body, or on the surface, of the body). When this IV is used, the medication runs into an area of a very large blood flow, so that even powerful chemicals will be diluted quickly and will not irritate the veins the way they do with a hand vein. Long lines are either tunneled under the skin (and in some cases, placed entirely under the skin) or held in place with a stitch or two so that they will not be dislodged by accident.

The main types of central lines are: (a) "PICC" lines (percutaneously inserted central catheters, which are designed for temporary use for up to several weeks— "percutaneously inserted" means they're put in by sticking a needle through the skin; this is to distinguish them from the other lines, which usually require a bigger operation, with an incision (cut) made in the skin); (b) Broviac and Hickman catheters (permanent—or very long-lasting—central lines, with exit tubing tunneled under the skin, exiting through the skin on the chest); (c) Mediports, Infusaports, and Portacaths (also permanent—or very long-lasting—central lines that are *totally* under the skin); and (d) Hohn catheters (placed in the same way as a Broviac or Hickman, but much easier to remove).

PICC lines are very similar to regular IVs except that the tubing is much longer, and can be pushed into the vein far enough so that it follows the vein back to the large veins in the chest (such as the *superior vena cava,* the largest vein bringing blood back to the heart from the upper part of the body) or even back to the heart. These lines can stay in for weeks at a time.

The Hickman and Broviac catheters are similar to each other and are lines that are inserted through a small incision, usually in the skin of the neck or by the collarbone, with one end being placed in one of the large veins in the neck, and threaded down into the *superior vena cava* or into the heart itself, while the other end may be tunneled under the skin of the chest. In this way, the only part of the catheter that is in contact with the external environment (air, clothes, bath water, etc.) is the tip, which comes out from under the skin on the front or side of the chest. Once the original incisions have healed completely, it's safe to bathe, play sports, and pursue normal activities with the line in place. You should avoid getting hit directly in the chest, and some surgeons prefer that you do not swim with one of those long lines in place, but everyone agrees that most normal activities are perfectly safe.

Mediports, Portacaths, and Infusaports are used much more commonly nowadays and have virtually replaced Hickmans and Broviacs, mostly because of their greater safety and convenience. They are inserted similarly to the Hickmans and Broviacs, with the tip ending in the *superior vena cava* or the heart, but the end through which medicines are infused is *under the skin,* with no tubing sticking out. This means any activity (other than those in which the area would be hit hard) is safe with these devices, and the risks of infection are much less, since the end is not exposed. These totally implanted devices have a small reservoir just under the skin. It's the rubber top of this reservoir which is punctured with the needle for hooking up to antibiotic infusions. For most of the time, these devices—which can be placed under the skin of the chest, upper leg/groin, or arm—are just left in place and are out of the way. When antibiotics are needed, a small needle can be put into the rubber cap at the beginning of the 2- or 3-week antibiotic course, and the infusion tubing hooked to it. The skin does not need to be punctured for each dose of antibiotics. The skin will need to be punctured about once a month for flushing the tubing with saline and heparin, to make sure the line does not become blocked with blood clots.

Placement of Long IV Lines

Most of the long lines are placed by surgeons or radiologists with special skills in using x-ray or ultrasound to do procedures (interventional radiologists), but some particularly skillful pediatricians or internists might also do the line placement. Broviacs, Hickmans, Mediports, Portacaths, and Infusaports are intended for very prolonged usage—months or even years—and are usually placed in the operating room or the radiology suite, with the patient deeply sedated under general anesthesia. Recovery from the procedure is very rapid.

For PICC lines, general anesthesia is virtually never needed since their placement is not very much different from a regular IV; they are just longer, get gently pushed farther into the vein, and last much longer than a regular IV. Many times, if you can tolerate getting a regular IV placed, the PICC line can be placed by a skilled nurse or doctor at the bedside. That is, it can be done relatively quickly and easily without sedation, anesthesia, or special monitoring.

Removing Long Lines

Central catheters may be removed when they are no longer needed; they may *need to be* removed if they become infected or damaged. Mediports, Portacaths, Infusaports, Hickmans, and Broviacs require a formal operative procedure for removal.

The Hohn catheters and PICC lines do not stick as tightly to the tissue under the skin, so they can be removed easily, just by pulling (after removing any stitch that might have been used!). For this reason, they can be used in situations where they will be needed for just a couple of weeks.

Equipment

Some special equipment is needed for the proper care and use of the central lines, especially when patients are using them out of the hospital. Equipment for keeping them sterile is essential. Special pumps are helpful to push medications in at the proper rate because problems could develop with medications running in too fast or too slowly. Special needles and tubing are needed to attach the central lines to the bottle or plastic bag holding the medication. For Hickman, Broviac, and Hohn catheters, the needles pierce the rubber cap at the end of the line, but for the Infusaports, Portacaths, and Mediports, special needles are required to pierce the skin and stay firmly in the reservoir under the skin for the days or weeks of the course of antibiotics. Solutions must be on hand to flush the lines after use (these typically contain saline and heparin to keep blood clots from forming in the line while it's not being used).

Care of Central Lines

Exquisite care must be taken so that these lines do not become infected. Infection in these lines nearly always means that they must be removed. If they need to be replaced, another procedure is required and perhaps another session under general anesthesia, entailing additional risks. More importantly, these lines are in the heart or close to it, and infection in the lines means serious bloodstream infection in the patient. People can get extremely ill from bloodstream infection. With proper care, these lines seldom become infected, even out of the hospital, perhaps because the people who take care of the lines at home are usually the patients themselves or a close family member. Whenever the small dressing (often little more than a band-aid) is changed, and medications begun, the procedure used must be sterile (allowing no germs to enter). Sterile gloves are worn, the area is cleaned according to strict guidelines, using strong antiseptic solutions, and all tubing ends that would touch the end of the central line are kept scrupulously clean.

Care must also be taken to see that the lines are not pulled out or bumped hard. This protection is easy to provide: The tubes are quite thin and only a small portion sticks out of the skin, so the tubing can be coiled and covered with a small amount of gauze and taped in place. Care of the central lines that are totally under the skin (Mediports, Infusaports, Portacaths) is much easier between courses of medication than care of the lines with ends sticking out from under the skin. In fact, other than avoiding direct hits to the site of the implanted device, very few precautions need be taken; it's fine to swim, surf, and so forth. Unfortunately, every course of antibiotics requires that a needle pierce the skin to enter the central line whose reservoir lies just beneath the skin, and such a needle stick is also needed about once a month *between* courses of antibiotics, to keep the tubing open. Usually, people with these central lines do not mind the inconvenience of these few needle sticks, particularly compared to the many sticks they would have had with traditional IVs.

In deciding whether to have one of these lines, you have to decide where you'd like to have it. As with so many things, each location has advantages as well as disadvantages: On the chest, the reservoir is probably the most stable, and easiest to enter with the needle, but may interfere with chest physical therapy (CPT), or vest therapy for airway clearance treatments. In young women, the surgeon or interventional radiologist must take care to avoid breast tissue, or an area that would be rubbed by a bra strap when he or she places a reservoir under the skin on the chest. Newer Mediports have evolved to be small enough to fit on the underside of the upper arm. The advantage of this site is that it is protected and hidden from view. This site is possible only with the newer, smaller Mediports, as the older Mediports were just too large to fit comfortably under the upper arm. The upper leg has been a convenient place for many patients, and a few young women have given strict instructions that it be hidden by a bikini-bottom for their time on the beach. Some patients are a little shy with the placement meaning that any manipulations of the reservoir (like the every-month "flushing" of the line), done by a stranger, are in what is usually a private part of their body. Many others have liked the fact that lines placed in the upper leg are hidden from public view virtually all the time. One patient couldn't have this kind of line because it would have hit on the lower "uneven bar" when she did her vigorous gymnastics practice and competitions.

Complications

Infection is the most common serious complication that can occur with a central line. A central line infection can be a medical emergency, and at best usually means removing the infected line and replacing it with another one. There is a limit to the number of times this can be done because once a long line has been in a particular vein, it may be difficult to put another line back through the same vein.

A very rare complication—air embolism—can be fatal. This happens when the central line has been opened to the air (rather than clamping it before connecting it to the medication tubing) and the patient takes a big breath, allowing air to rush into the line, and then into the heart. A small amount of air in the line will do no harm, but a large amount can be extremely dangerous. This can be guarded against by not leaving the line open to air; older children and adults should be careful to hold their breath for the short period of time that the line might be open. The danger of air accidentally entering a central line does not exist with the

Mediport, Portacath, or Infusaport systems since they are not uncapped when hooked to the bottle or bag of medication.

In rare cases, a piece of the catheter has been known to break off and travel through the veins and lodge in a dangerous position, where it can block blood flow to an important part of the body.

Bleeding from accidentally uncapping the central line can be serious, since the tip of the line is in an area of very high blood flow.

Fortunately, most of these complications are quite uncommon when central lines are taken good care of.

Using Central Lines

Once the IV is in place, medicines can be given through it. The medications are mixed with saline (salt water) or dextrose (sugar) water and then either allowed to drip through tubing into the IV under the force of gravity or are pushed through the tubing by electric pumps that regulate precisely how much goes in and how fast. It usually takes 30 to 60 minutes for antibiotics to run into the vein. When the medications have finished going into the vein, the IV may then be connected to tubing through which simple saline or dextrose mixtures are passed until it is time for the next antibiotic. A much more convenient procedure is to flush the IV with a small amount of saline and heparin (a drug that prevents blood clots from blocking the needle) and then to leave a cap on the end of the IV. Once the IV line is flushed with heparin and capped, it can safely be left alone for many hours and will be ready for use when it's time to give the next dose of antibiotics. This means that the person does not have to be tied continually to the IV pumps, tubing, and bottles, and will be free to move about.

Two different antibiotics are commonly used. Each of the antibiotics must be given on its own schedule. Schedules range from a continuous infusion (meaning that the antibiotic is being infused 24 hours a day, 7 days a week) to one infusion every 24 hours, with the most common intervals being every 6 or 8 hours. If blood levels are checked, they may indicate that the dosage or schedule needs to be changed, for example, from every 8 hours to every 6 hours.

OTHER TREATMENTS

Other aspects of the treatment will vary at different CF centers, but will often include *ACT* (airway clearance; see Chapter 3), two to four times a day (or even more), and *aerosol treatments* (with bronchodilators, antibiotics, or both—also discussed in Chapter 3). It is not unusual for a patient (especially a teenaged patient) to get a bit cranky when he or she is awakened in the morning for an aerosol or ACT. It's important to remember that these treatments are a big part of the reason for the hospitalization, and the people who are giving you the treatments are trying to help you get better. *Anti-inflammatory medications* (e.g., prednisone) may be included in the treatment. *Exercise* may or may not be prescribed, and on admission, patients may be feeling a bit "under the weather" and need more rest than usual. In most cases, people come into the hospital having been very active. It is important to continue that level of activity to avoid deconditioning. In almost all cases, after the first few days, patients should be up and out of bed most of the day. In some hospitals, you may be able to attend school (your own school or an in-hospital school room) or work, on an altered schedule built around the medication schedules.

Nutrition is also an important part of in-hospital treatment, including *vitamins*, *pancreatic enzymes*, and plenty of *calories*. Food can sometimes be an issue because the hospital food is seldom as good as home cooking. Most hospitals give a choice of foods, and many even allow inpatients to order from a hospital cafeteria menu if they don't see something they want on the regular patient menu.

TESTS

The effectiveness of the antibiotics probably relates to the peak level of the drug (the highest level that is reached), and their toxicity (harmful effects) most likely relates to the "trough" (lowest level). Since the peak usually occurs within 30 to 60 minutes after the medication enters the vein, and the trough is hours later (just before the next dose), careful monitoring of drug levels will necessitate a double test, one just after the drug has gone in, and one just before the next dose. If the levels are too low or too high, the physicians will know that they must adjust the dosage. In this way, it is possible to get the maximum benefit from the medications and the minimum toxicity. This is good, but at the same time, it's a bother since blood levels may need to be checked again with the new dosage. An idea that occurs to many patients is, "Why not draw my blood from my IV, so you don't have to stick me?" This can be done for some tests, but not for antibiotic levels. The reason it can't be done for the antibiotic levels is that since the antibiotics were given through the tubing, there is often some extra left within the IV tubing itself, so the level within the tiny length of tubing will be higher than the real level in the bloodstream. Once the right dosage is found, it is not necessary to recheck the levels frequently.

Other Blood Tests

When someone is admitted to the hospital, several kinds of blood tests are usually done. Almost always, these admission tests can be done with one needle stick, even if several tubes of blood are needed (the total amount of blood needed will seldom be more than 1 tbsp). Different tests may be done, including blood counts and measurement of blood electrolytes (chemicals such as sodium, chloride, and potassium). It is also common to check the blood levels of chemicals that reflect kidney function because many antibiotics can affect kidney function.

Some of the tests are done only at admission, but others are repeated periodically through the hospitalization. For example, kidney function tests might be repeated once or twice a week to make sure that the drugs have not caused a problem. As we've already discussed, blood may be taken several times to measure antibiotic levels.

Other Tests

Chest radiographs ("chest x-ray") and *pulmonary function tests* (PFTs) may also be done shortly after admission and at intervals during the hospitalization to monitor the progress you are making (see Chapter 3 for a discussion of these tests). *Electrocardiograms* (ECGs) and *echocardiograms* are often performed to determine the heart's condition and see if it's showing evidence of having to do extra work. Other tests might also be done, depending on the circumstances. A *hearing test* might be performed if drugs that are being used might affect hearing. As always, if you do not understand what a test is, or why it's being done, ask.

LENGTH OF IV ANTIBIOTIC TREATMENT

The ideal length of time to get IV antibiotics to fight bronchial infection is the time it takes to get you back to your baseline pulmonary function, that is, the amount of time needed to get you back to your usual state of health. Most often, this is about 2 weeks, but it can easily take 3 or more weeks. It is rarely more than 3 weeks or less than 2. Most CF experts feel that it is a mistake to let the calendar determine the length of treatment without regard to the patient's progress; rather, it is the patient's response to treatment that should dictate the length of hospitalization. PFTs and a physical examination can often help in determining the length of stay, but often it is the patients themselves and their families who contribute most to this decision. They are the people who know best, for example, just how much the patient is coughing. The observations of the patient and family are very important in this regard. While several weeks on IVs can seem like a very long time, and it may be tempting to try to arrange stopping as early as possible, it is wise to remember that the time invested in achieving good health is time well spent. It is quite possible that a few extra days at the end of a hospitalization or course of IV antibiotics may mean several more weeks or months of good health.

BRINGING THE CARE HOME

There are many ways that complex kinds of treatment can be carried out at home, thus avoiding prolonged hospitalization. These include home IVs, various kinds of tube feedings, and different ways of giving oxygen.

Home IV Lines

In years gone by, IV treatments were usually done in the hospital. In recent years, partly because of pressure from insurance companies, IV antibiotics are frequently used at home, either after progress has begun in the hospital, or in some cases even starting at home. Whether you can do these treatments at home will be determined by your physician, in consultation with you. Insurance companies and HMOs (health maintenance organizations) are putting increasing pressure on families and physicians to use IVs at home instead of the hospital since it may be cheaper for these companies, whether or not it is as effective as the hospital. Families may push for home treatment as well, for obvious reasons: Travel back and forth between home and hospital to visit a hospitalized child is difficult and time-consuming. If there are other children at home, it's that much more difficult. Patients like the idea of being at home with family, friends, and pets, too. Families need to be absolutely clear about the disadvantages as well as the obvious advantages of home treatment. Several things must be taken care of before someone can be sent home with an IV: There must be someone at home to take care of the IV—to connect the tubing to the needle for infusing the antibiotics, to flush the tubing after the antibiotics have run in, and to keep the IV from clogging. The medications must be mixed and stored properly, and they must be run in at the right speed. Someone must be available who knows what to do if the IV comes out or goes bad. Arrangements also have to be made for regular checkups, including blood tests (antibiotic levels, etc., as would be necessary in the hospital) and physician examinations. This can be extremely tiring and—depending on how well the IV is working, and what schedule is needed for the particular antibiotics—time-consuming. For example, a common combination of two antibiotics includes one that needs to be given every 6 hours and another that is given every 8 to 24 hours. This is a schedule that leaves little time or energy for the parent (or adult patient) to do anything else, including good airway clearance.

Who Takes Care of the IV Line?

In many areas, home medical care companies or IV infusion companies have taken on many of the tasks of visiting homes, helping to restart IVs when necessary, working with families to run the IV medications, supplying electric pumps to regulate the speed at which the medication is run in, drawing blood for tests, working with pharmacies to supply the medications, and so on. If such a service is not available, public health personnel, such as visiting nurses, may help with these tasks. In other cases, families and physicians have been able to piece together a team of people to do the various things. Some emergency department nurses have volunteered to restart IVs when necessary, and helpful pharmacists may take care of preparing the antibiotics. Your CF center staff can help you make these arrangements. It is very important to check whether home IVs will be covered by your insurance.

Checking Up

Once someone is freed from the constraints of the hospital, by being sent home on IVs, it is easy to forget that if he or she were in the hospital, there would be physicians to monitor the progress of the treatment and to check for evidence of drug toxicity at least once a day. It is important to maintain close contact with your physician after hospitalization, particularly if you're still taking the powerful drugs that are traditionally given only under supervision in a hospital. Checkups once a week, or more or less frequently, may be necessary.

ENDING HOSPITALIZATION OR HOME IV TREATMENT

When leaving the hospital or finishing a course of home IVs, it is important to get written instructions about home care and whom to call with questions and when to return for a checkup.

Parents may notice some temporary changes in their child's behavior after hospitalization. Children may have nightmares, fear of strangers, fear of the parent's absence, may throw tantrums or may become aggressive or rebellious, or may try to avoid returning to school. Some children have "regressive behavior"—that is, they act babyish even though they had been quite "grown up" for their age before the hospitalization. These reactions are not unexpected, but should be brought to the attention of the pediatrician or CF center team for recommendations.

SUMMARY

A several-week course of IV antibiotics, whether in the hospital or at home, can cause anxiety and disrupt a patient's and family's life. Yet, with cooperation among patient, family, and health professionals, these treatments can be carried out with minimum discomfort and can help improve and sustain health for a long time.

Transplantation

8

Geoffrey Kurland, Jonathan E. Spahr,
Daniel J. Weiner, and David M. Orenstein

THE BASICS

1. Transplantation is taking a healthy organ from one person and putting it in another person, usually to replace a damaged organ. This has been done with the lungs for hundreds of people with cystic fibrosis (CF). It has also been done rarely with the liver in people with CF and severe liver disease.

2. Transplantation is very difficult and expensive, and requires as much or more care afterward than CF itself. Getting a transplant is much like trading one disease for another.

3. One major hurdle with lung transplantation is that there are more people needing lung transplantation than there are lungs to transplant. Recent changes in lung allocation procedures mean that patients with sicker lungs are placed at the top of the list and receive lung transplantations sooner than those whose lungs are not as sick.

4. Some patients with CF have done very well after lung transplantation, some have had months or years of problems, and some have died.

5. Medicines to prevent the body from attacking the transplanted organ are important after transplantation; getting too little of this type of medicine can cause rejection, while too much can allow infection to set in.

6. Approximately 75% of patients with CF who get a lung transplant will be alive 1 year later, approximately 50% to 60% after 2 to 3 years. Longer survival is certainly possible. More than 80% of children with CF who receive liver transplants will be alive 3 to 5 years later.

The term "transplantation" is commonly used in the daily newspapers as well as in the medical literature. Transplantation is surgically removing an organ from one person and placing it in another person. The person receiving the transplanted organ is known as the *recipient*. The person from whom the organ is obtained is known as the *donor*. In virtually all cases, transplantation is designed to replace severely damaged organs with organs that are healthier. In almost every case, the damaged organs are removed from the recipient at the time the new organs are put in.

The donor organ is removed from someone who doesn't need it. In the case of a kidney or a bone marrow transplant, this is often a living relative of the recipient. We have two kidneys, but can live healthy lives with only one kidney. Part of the bone marrow can be removed and the remaining marrow will grow back with no harm to the donor. In each case, the living donor can spare the transplanted organ for a sick relative. In many cases, though, the organ needed for transplantation is the one we can't live without—such as the heart, lung, or liver. In this case, the person from whom the donor organ comes is most often someone who is dead, particularly someone who has had severe brain damage from trauma (car crash, etc.), but whose lung (or liver or heart) has not been damaged. Later on, we'll discuss this further.

Several different types of organ transplants have been performed, dating back as far as 1906 when the first attempt was made to transplant a pig's kidney into a person. The first human-to-human kidney transplant was done in 1936, and the first successful kidney transplant was done in France in the early 1950s. (Some of the organs for these early transplants in France came from prisoners right after they had been executed by guillotine.) Since then, attempts have been made—with varying degrees of success—to transplant the liver, heart, pancreas, intestines, bone marrow, and lung.

The first human liver transplantation was performed by a team directed by Dr. Thomas Starzl on March 1, 1963. At that time, there were only a few drugs available to prevent rejection of a transplanted organ. Dr. Starzl persisted in his pursuit of liver transplantation, despite the fact that it was not until 1969, some 6 years after the first attempt (!), that a patient lived for more than 1 year after a liver transplantation. In June 1963, only 3 months after the first liver transplantation, the first human lung transplantation was carried out. That first patient survived less than 1 month after the transplant. Both rejection of the transplanted organ and infection were major problems in the early days of transplantation. They still are formidable challenges to successful transplantation and will be discussed later in this chapter.

A major advance in transplantation was the discovery of the powerful antirejection drug cyclosporine in 1978, which improved the ability of physicians to prevent rejection of transplanted organs. Recognizing this new drug as one that would be useful for organ transplants, Dr. Bruce Reitz of Stanford University successfully carried out the first combined heart–lung transplantation in 1981. Only a couple of years later, in 1983, the first heart–lung transplantation in a patient with CF was performed at the University of Pittsburgh by a team headed by Dr. Bartley Griffith.

The number of successful liver, lung, and heart–lung transplantations increases every year, but there are many more people awaiting transplants than there are available organs.

Some patients with CF may be faced with the possibility of a transplant because of their disease. In most of these cases, it will be a lung transplant; in a very few cases, it will be a liver transplant. The total number of patients with CF (adults and children) who received lung transplants in 2009 in the United States was 212. The total number of patients with CF (adults and children) who received liver transplants in 2009 was 15. This is out of more than 25,000 patients, meaning that fewer than 1% of CF patients got a lung or liver transplantation in 2009.

In this chapter, we'll describe transplantation, explain the reasons some people with CF might benefit from a transplant, and identify some of the more important problems with transplantation. In addition, we'll try to explain why transplants may sometimes have to be considered even if the patients don't feel sick enough to think they need a transplant. First, we'll discuss transplants in general, then, matters that are specific to lung transplants, and, finally, matters that pertain especially to liver transplants.

WHO NEEDS A TRANSPLANT?

With a treatment that is relatively new and as hazardous as transplanting an organ, it is difficult to say that anybody *needs* it. With a broken arm, it's easy to say, "you need to have that bone set, and the arm put in a cast," because we know that you will have much less pain, suffering, and long-term disability if the break is treated that way. With organ transplantation, particularly lung (or liver) transplantation for someone with CF, it's much harder to be certain of the outcome with or without the treatment. This uncertainty is related to the difficulty in predicting what will happen to patients with CF who do and don't get transplants. We will discuss this later in this chapter. Despite the uncertainties, most CF doctors agree on some broad guidelines for which patients should be considered for transplantation. These guidelines assume that to be a "good candidate" for a transplant, you need to be sick enough, but not too sick. If you're not very sick, it doesn't make sense to get a transplant because your chances of doing well for a long time are better without a transplant, and you would be using organs that could otherwise be used for someone who might die without them. However, if you are too sick, or have certain medical conditions that we'll discuss later, the chances of success with the transplant are small, and you and your family will have been put through a very hard (and expensive) ordeal, again using organs that would have had a better chance of helping someone else.

LUNG TRANSPLANTATION

Who Should Be Considered for Lung Transplantation?

For lung transplantation to be worth the risks, most experts believe that the patient's quality of life must be intolerable, with difficulty breathing and an inability to carry out the daily tasks of living (school, work, recreation activities). The experts also believe that lung transplantation should not be done if the person is likely to survive for more than 2 years without a transplant. One difficulty here is that there are no good tests to tell us when someone's life is intolerable or when someone with CF will die. People are amazingly different from each other in their ability to function under what seem to be the same circumstances. This is certainly true for people with CF and their lung function. Two patients with CF with equally good (or bad) lungs, as measured by their pulmonary function tests (PFTs) (see Chapter 3, *The Respiratory System*) may have very different lifestyles: one may be nearly bedridden, while the other carries a full load of college courses and works part time in a pizza shop. So, the PFTs cannot tell us if someone's quality of life is good or bad. One yardstick that is sometimes used is that if someone needs to use oxygen all the time in order not to feel short of breath, he or she should consider lung transplantation.

What about knowing when someone with CF will die from his or her lung disease? Just as the PFTs don't tell us exactly how well someone feels or what he or she can do, they also can't tell us how long he or she will live. As we discuss in Chapter 15, *Death and Cystic Fibrosis*, there are some rough statistics that say someone with CF with a PFT [specifically, the forced expiratory volume at 1 second (FEV_1)] below 30% of what it should be has a 50:50 chance of being alive in 2 years. Many physicians have taken this information to mean that if someone has PFTs that low, he or she should consider lung transplantation. Recent studies have suggested that using other factors such as weight, the presence or absence of diabetes, and the type of bacteria in sputum may all be useful at predicting survival. However, a lot of work must still be done before physicians can use this information to decide who should receive a transplant. Later in this chapter, we'll talk about how to make the final decision about whether or not to go for lung transplantation.

Who Should Not Be Considered for Lung Transplantation?

Just because certain organs, such as the liver or the lungs, can be transplanted, it does not mean that every patient will benefit from a transplant. For some people, the modern medical approach of "if it's possible, we should do it!" does not fit with their view of the world. For these people, the very high-tech (and high-cost) modern medical procedures are not appealing, especially if it means that they might lose control of their own destinies. Some patients have felt that, although a transplant might be the only way to prevent dying within the next few years, dying may not be the worst thing possible. There is no question that the possibility of transplants has changed the way people with CF die. In the past (or now, if someone is not considering transplantation) when patients' lungs had reached a certain point, and it was likely that a patient would die in the near future, the physicians', patient's, and family's efforts generally were directed at trying to keep the patient comfortable while providing care that might help make the patient better if that were possible. If there were ever a conflict between patient comfort and a treatment, the treatment would be skipped and patient comfort would be emphasized. Now, if someone is waiting for an organ to become available, there is often a level of desperation: we need to wait for the organ, so stay alive at all costs! Thus, a patient and family may not be able to deal with their own thoughts of losing each other and may not be able to say or do things that need to be said or done. Instead, all efforts are put into survival at all cost until the call comes saying that lungs are available. Losing the little peace and calm that previously was possible in contemplating death seems too high a price for some patients, and they choose not to consider transplantation. Patients, families, and physicians also now realize that getting new lungs does not guarantee that everything will be perfect afterward. Instead, many patients have as much trouble, and spend as much time in the hospital after transplantation as they did before the transplantation. So, some patients and families choose not to be considered for new lungs.

In some other situations, the likelihood of success of transplantation is very small and the known risk of the procedure is quite large. Such situations are known as *contraindications* to (reasons not to do) transplantation. Physicians must take into account all such factors before deciding whether a transplant procedure is indicated. Certain factors are associated with such a poor outcome that they are considered *absolute* contraindications to transplantation. Other factors may be associated with an increased risk, but this risk still may be acceptable in a sick patient; these factors are considered *relative* contraindications to transplantation. A single relative contraindication usually does not prohibit transplantation, but the presence of several relative contraindications may be adequate to disqualify a patient from receiving a transplant. Not all transplant centers agree on relative or absolute contraindications, although all transplant physicians must confront such issues in each patient they see. The decision to "list" someone for transplantation (see below for more on the transplant list) is often made by a team of physicians, nurse specialists, psychologists, and social workers, and their view of the relative or absolute contraindications in each patient becomes the basis for their final decision to proceed or not proceed with transplantation.

There are several absolute contraindications to lung transplantation. A severe infection that has spread into the bloodstream and caused alterations in the function of other organs, such as the kidney, heart, and brain, is one of the most important contraindications to transplant. Infections from HIV (human immunodeficiency virus) or other chronic infections such as tuberculosis are considered absolute contraindications to lung transplantation. A cancer that is not confined to the organ for transplantation is also an absolute contraindication. In many centers, severe kidney or liver disease is a contraindication to lung transplantation.

Because patients with CF commonly have bacteria such as *Pseudomonas* or *Staphylococcus* organisms in their airways, the mere presence of these bacteria is not a contraindication to transplantation. However, as is discussed in the next section, bacterial infection of the transplanted lung is a common complication in patients with CF. Over the years, several transplant centers have reported that CF patients who had airway bacteria already resistant to most antibiotics had more problems with serious infections following lung transplantation. In several of these reports, a specific type of bacteria known as *Burkholderia cepacia*, particularly if it was resistant to all antibiotics ("panresistant") was associated with a very high risk of death following lung transplantation. More recent studies have shown that the bacteria present in CF sputum before lung transplantation are the same organisms that cause lung infections following transplantation. This means that if a patient with CF has panresistant organisms (*B. cepacia* or others) before transplantation, then the infections after transplantation will be very difficult to treat. Because of the risk of severe and untreatable infections following transplantation, many centers now consider the presence of bacteria resistant to all available antibiotics an absolute contraindication to lung transplantation.

There are numerous relative contraindications to lung transplantation. These include previous chest surgery or pleurodesis (discussed in Chapter 3, *The Respiratory System*), poorly controlled diabetes, or a history of a psychiatric disorder. Malnutrition is a relative contraindication to transplantation, and many transplant centers are unwilling to consider performing transplantation in a patient who is too thin. As you will see, the surgery involved in transplantation is very extensive and there is a long recovery period. Patients who are weak because of malnutrition may not have the physical strength to recover from the operation. Most transplant centers suggest feeding tubes such as nasogastric, gastrostomy, or jejunostomy tubes to provide enough nutrition to allow the patient to be strong enough to survive the surgery.

Another relative contraindication is a history of what is referred to as "noncompliance." This means not taking prescribed therapy such as antibiotics or pancreatic enzymes, not doing regular airway clearance, or failing to be seen regularly by a CF physician. The importance of a patient and family being able to take medications, do treatments, and show up regularly for their appointments cannot be overstated. Transplantation is a complex process, and the treatments and medications following transplantation must be done exactly as prescribed. Because there are many more people who need new lungs than there are lungs available, it is important that the organs be transplanted into patients who will take care of them. Patients and families must be able to cooperate with the transplant team to maintain good function of the transplanted lungs; transplant physicians are less likely to believe that a patient will do what he or she is told after transplantation if the patient is unable (or unwilling) to follow instructions before the transplantation.

Transplant List

There is no shortage of people whose doctors believe they need a transplant. There is, however, a big shortage of donor organs for these patients. There are several reasons for the shortage, beginning with the fact that most donor organs have to come from people who have died—and died in a way that has not damaged the organ in question (for patients with CF, this means lungs or liver). In some circumstances, the donors have decided while they were alive that in the event of their death they wished to be organ donors. They may have signed a "donor card" and informed their families and clergy. Unfortunately, relatively few people have expressed such a desire. More often, the families of potential donors must be approached at the tragic and upsetting time when their loved one is dying. It is difficult for many families to agree to organ donation at such a time; therefore, many organs that would have been suitable for transplant are not made available.

Organs must be taken for transplantation before they are too damaged to help the transplant recipient. Once the heart stops beating and blood is no longer flowing into organs such as the lungs or liver, those organs rapidly become damaged. For this reason, organs are removed from the donor before the donor's heart has stopped beating. Many of us were taught from childhood that the heartbeat is the true sign of life, and life continues until the heart actually stops beating. Medicine, however, has advanced to the point of having ventilators that breathe for us and medications that stimulate the heart to beat strongly. The availability of transplantation as a science has raised the question of what constitutes life and what constitutes death. Most physicians, scientists, and clergy now believe that the true measure of life lies not in the heart beating or in breathing, as these can be artificially stimulated, but in the presence of brain function. Now, people with severe brain injuries, who are being kept alive with machines such as ventilators, can be tested to see if they have any brain function. If they don't have brain function and are not receiving medications that affect brain function, they are considered "brain dead." This term means that their brain will not recover any function and, although the machines may keep them "alive," they are not experiencing life, are not thinking, and have no brain function. (It may be more appropriate to think of the machines that keep air moving in and out of their lungs, and blood circulating, etc. to be "organ support," and not what they're usually called, "life support.") Such patients could serve as donors of organs for transplantation if those organs (heart, lung, liver, etc.) still function normally. This is the reason for the timing of when organs are taken from donors. It also helps to explain why many families find it difficult to agree to organ donation: their loved one appears asleep, rather than dead.

Once the organs are removed from the body of a donor, they are cleared of all blood by washing in a salt solution through the blood vessels that go to the organ. This preparatory phase before transplantation is known as preservation, and allows the organs to be transported to the recipient's hospital. A liver can be preserved for up to 24 hours after it is removed from the body, while lungs become hopelessly damaged within 4 to 8 hours. So, even if there is no difficulty with a family's agreeing to donate the organs from their family member, the organs do not survive very long at all. If they are to be transplanted, it needs to be within a matter of hours. You can't call the central supply department in the hospital to order up a lung or liver.

Soon after transplantation became a widespread medical technique, it was apparent that there were many more people who were waiting for transplants than there were organs available. Because physicians and politicians were worried that organs might actually be sold or not given to the most needy recipient, The Transplant Act of 1984 was passed by Congress to make sure that organ donation is fair and equitable. A private, nonprofit national organization known as the United Network for Organ Sharing (UNOS) was set up to keep track of transplant recipients and donors. As a part of their job, UNOS maintains a computerized list of patients awaiting transplantation and matches donor organs with appropriate recipients. In the UNOS system, the country is divided into regions served by local organ procurement organizations, which in turn are responsible for helping local physicians identify potential organ donors and helping transplant centers obtain the organs for transplantation.

Getting on the Transplant List

The first step in being considered for transplantation and getting on the transplant list is being referred to a transplant center by your regular physician. In the case of patients with CF, this physician would most likely be your CF physician. The referring physician sends information about you to the transplant center, and the transplant physicians then decide whether you should be seen and evaluated. The information your physician will send to the center will include your recent PFTs, chest radiographs (x-ray films), results of your sputum cultures, and laboratory reports about your kidney and liver function. In addition, your physician will usually speak with one of the transplant physicians about your illness, how many hospitalizations you've had, and how well you follow the physician's advice. The transplant physicians will look at the information and decide whether you should be evaluated more fully to see if you should be listed for transplantation. If the decision is made to evaluate you, then you travel to the transplant center and undergo more tests (radiologic tests, blood tests, exercise tests, etc.). You are seen by a number of physicians, usually including a transplant surgeon, a pulmonary specialist, an infectious disease specialist, and (in the case of liver transplantation) a gastroenterologist. You and your family are interviewed by social workers and, in many centers, a psychiatrist. This latter point is important and emphasizes the fact that transplantation is not only a difficult surgical and medical procedure, but is also a highly stressful circumstance for patient and family. If all the members of the transplant team agree that you are sick enough to require a transplant and that you do not have one of the absolute contraindications to the procedure (such as the presence of panresistant *B. cepacia* in your sputum), then you are "listed" on UNOS's computer as an "active" candidate for transplantation.

Your Spot on the List

The main reasons for UNOS to keep a transplant list are that there are more people waiting for transplants than there are organs to go around, and it is necessary to decide as fairly as possible who should get an organ when it becomes available. There are separate lists for different organs, and, although it may seem a bit odd, the "rules" governing the different lists are different.

The List for Lung Transplants

How long you will wait for lungs depends on very few things: your size (since lungs that are either too big or too little are more difficult to transplant successfully), your blood type, your disease (there are other diseases for which a person would need a lung transplantation) and, most importantly, how bad your lung disease is. Prior to 2005, people on the waiting list climbed to the top based on how long they had been on the list (first come, first served). In 2005, the rules changed to make lung allocation more similar to other organ transplantation. That is, those with sicker lungs get lung transplants sooner than those with healthier lungs. In the unusual circumstance when everything is equal between two people waiting for a lung transplantation (a tie), time on the waiting list will break the tie and the person on the waiting list longer will be offered lung transplantation first. This new rule for ranking people on the list by severity of disease, known as the Lung Allocation Score (LAS) went into effect for patients 12 years of age and older in 2005. The old system, in which length of time waiting for a transplant is the main determining factor, is still in effect for children younger than 12 years.

Prior to 2005, if two people on the list were the same size and blood type, and one had been on the list for 2 years and the other had been on for 1 and 1/2 years, the one with the 2-year wait would be offered the next set of lungs, even if she were not as sick as the other one. Obviously, that system seemed unfair. The other problem with the old system was that it made it very difficult for the lung transplant team and your CF doctor to decide when was the right time to list you for transplantation. The average waiting time for a lung transplantation was about 2 years. Therefore, doctors needed to make their best guess as to how bad someone's lungs would be in 2 years (but as we all know, most doctors are not good at predicting the future).

Many factors go into deciding the "LAS" that attempts to assign lungs to those people who need them most urgently; at the same time, some of the guesswork is taken out of the decision of when to list for lung transplantation. Preliminary data suggest that the system is working: people who are really in need of lung transplantation are getting it while those who are not as sick are not getting transplantation too soon.

Remember, this LAS rule is only in effect for people older than 12 years (although this may change very soon as there is discussion about making a scoring system for children younger than 12 years). Fortunately, it is rare for children with CF younger than 12 years to need lung transplantation. Of all lung transplants done for CF since 1995, only 3% have been in children younger than 12.

What makes up the LAS? Several factors combine to make a score that determines how sick (or healthy) someone is when contemplating lung transplantation. Those factors include PFT results, use of oxygen or other respiratory support, exercise capacity, and secondary complications such as diabetes, kidney disease, and pulmonary hypertension.

Waiting on the List

Once the patient is "listed" for transplantation, and he or she moves up the list (by time if younger than 12 years and by severity of disease if older than 12 years) he or she must wait until an organ becomes available. As we've just discussed, this can be as long as 2 years or more for patients waiting for lung transplants. In most cases, routine follow-up care is done by the referring physician (your usual CF physician and family physician), but the transplant physicians will often want to see you at their center at regular intervals (usually every 6 to 12 months). The visits to the transplant center will allow the transplant physicians to examine you, to look at your sputum cultures, PFTs, and radiographs, and to get an idea of how sick you are. In the case of the LAS, it also gives a chance to update your "score."

Some transplant centers require candidates for transplantation to become involved in specific exercise and nutrition programs, which are designed to strengthen the patient and improve his or her ability to withstand the stresses of surgery and recovery during the postoperative period. Several centers even require that patients and their families move to the city where the transplant will take place. Some of these demands on patients may improve their chances of surviving until the transplant can be done, and some of the demands placed on both patients and their families will show the transplant team that these prospective recipients are able to follow directions, take medications, and comply with all therapeutic measures. While this may seem unfair, we should remember that organs for transplantation are rare and valuable commodities. As we keep pointing out, there are many more patients seeking transplantation than there are available organs. A patient who does not take care of himself or herself after transplantation not only hurts himself or herself, but has also "taken" a donated organ away from someone else—someone who might take better care of themselves (and the new organ). Many centers doing transplantation are less willing to transplant organs into patients who have shown that they are not able to take care of themselves properly before transplantation.

"Active" and "Inactive" Patients on the List

The list of candidates awaiting transplantation is divided into *active* and *inactive* status. The status of any candidate can be changed from active to inactive (or vice versa) depending on a variety of factors that we'll discuss. People who are "active" move up toward the top of the list based on score and/or as people ahead of them go off the list (because of getting a transplant, dying, deciding against transplantation, or becoming inactive). Once the patient reaches the top of the list, the active candidate will be offered the next organ that becomes available. People who are inactive will not be offered an organ even if they have the highest score and/or are at the top of the list.

There are several reasons that a patient might change from active to inactive on the list. First, a candidate may be at the top of the list and receive a call to be transplanted at a time that he or she doesn't feel sick enough to have the transplant, or the candidate might be too frightened. The candidate may then turn down the offered organ. The lung will then be offered to the next person on the list, and the first candidate will not be penalized. If this happens several times, however, the transplant team can suggest that the candidate be changed to inactive for a while. If some time later the patient is ready to be considered for a transplant, he or she will become "active" again and the place on the list will be determined by the amount of time he or she had accumulated waiting while on the active list.

A second major reason for changing a candidate from active to inactive may be a change in the candidate that is an absolute contraindication to transplantation. An example of this might be the finding of a major new infection outside the lungs, such as an infection in a Mediport central line (see Chapter 7, *Hospitalization and Other Special Treatments*). This would have to be treated before the patient could get a transplant. Most of the time, the patient is not put on the inactive list while such an infection is being treated, but if organs became available during the treatment of the infection, those organs would have to go to the next person on the list. If the infection proved difficult to treat, the candidate might have to change his or her status to inactive at that time.

Sometimes the problem may not be in the patient's overall health, but in his sputum cultures. As we've already discussed, some centers will not allow transplantation in patients who have panresistant bacteria in their sputum. An example of this would be a patient who starts to grow *B. cepacia* in his or her sputum after being listed as active. If someone's culture begins to show those bacteria, the patient may be inactivated until the culture clears up. In many centers, such patients are not inactivated, but they will not undergo transplantation. This allows them to continue to maintain a spot on the list while efforts are made to get rid of the resistant bacteria in their sputum.

In some instances, candidates have been made inactive when they have not been able to follow through with their medical therapy. For example, patients who refuse to do prescribed chest physiotherapy treatments or who fail to be seen regularly by their CF physician are more likely to be inactivated by a transplant center.

Technique of Lung Transplantation

General Considerations

Transplantation surgery is complicated and difficult. It is done in specialized medical centers by highly skilled surgeons and anesthesiologists. The surgery involved in lung transplantation requires large incisions (cuts) through the skin and other tissues that make up the wall of the chest, which permit the surgeons to inspect, remove, and replace the damaged organs. The removal of the organ from the recipient must be done carefully, leaving the arteries, veins, and (in the case of the lung) airways (trachea and main bronchi; see Chapter 3, *The Respiratory System*) in place, for these must be attached to the donor organs in such a way as will allow the new organ to function normally. Each of these new attachments, in which a donor artery, vein, or airway is joined to the native (recipient's) artery, vein, or airway, is known as an *anastomosis* (pronounced a-nass-to-mo-sis) and is a crucial part of the surgery. The site of the anastomosis may be weaker than the rest of the donated organ and can come apart more easily. This breakdown of an anastomosis, known as *dehiscence* (pronounced *de-hiss-sense*), can result in severe bleeding or (in the case of the airway) sudden respiratory difficulty. Anastomoses are also subject to narrowing, known as stricture or stenosis. In blood vessels, this can lead to blood clots at the site of stricture. Stenosis of the anastomosis in an airway can result in difficulty breathing.

Although the transplant surgery is done while the patient is deeply anesthetized, there is a lot of pain and discomfort during recovery from these operations. While many patients do very well right after lung transplantation, full recovery from these procedures may take weeks or even months.

Specifics of Lung Transplantation Procedures

Until the late 1980s, most lung or heart–lung transplantations were done through what is called a median sternotomy, in which the breast bone is cut from top to bottom and the chest is opened by pulling the cut sides apart. Now, most lung transplant operations are done using what is known as an *anteroinferior transthoracic incision*, also known as the "clamshell" approach. This means the surgeon cuts across the lower part of the chest wall from one side to the other, allowing the entire upper part of the chest wall to be lifted up, much as you would raise the hood of a car (or open a clamshell). This gives the surgeon a better look at both lungs and makes the surgery somewhat easier. A good view inside the chest is especially important if the recipient has CF, because patients with CF often have scarring of the thin membrane (the *pleura*) that covers the surface of the lung. This scarring may also involve the lining of the chest wall, which is also a thin membrane and is also called the pleura. Normally, the space between these two membranes (called the *pleural space*) is lined only with a tiny amount of fluid, and the lungs can be pulled out of the chest cavity relatively easily, but in CF, there can be a lot of scar tissue between the pleural surfaces, making it difficult to remove the lungs. Furthermore, scar tissue bleeds easily when it's pulled apart.

The earliest operations for lung (and heart–lung) transplantation involved removing the donor lungs together, still attached to the lower part of the donor trachea. (In the case of heart–lung transplantation, the lungs still had their attachments to the heart, and the heart and lungs together, known as the "heart–lung block," were removed from the donor.) For those early lung transplants, the recipient lungs were also removed together, leaving behind most of the recipient's trachea, along with the pulmonary arteries coming from the right side of the heart and the pulmonary veins leading back to the left side of the heart. The top of the donor trachea was attached to the lower part of the recipient trachea and the donor and recipient arteries and veins were joined. This is known as double-lung transplantation, because the two lungs are placed into the donor as a single unit.

As you can imagine, this is very exacting, tedious, time-consuming work. The surgeons must use many tiny stitches in these delicate tissues, making sure there is not even a small hole left behind that would allow blood to leak out of the veins or arteries being sewn together or air to leak out of the ends of the trachea that were sewn together. The surgery takes hours, during which time the patient has no functioning lungs (and in the case of heart–lung transplantation, no beating heart). In order for this surgery to be possible, the patient's blood must be rerouted outside the body through plastic tubing to a "heart–lung machine," also called "cardiopulmonary bypass." This machine takes blood and oxygenates it, then pumps it back into the body. Blood going through cardiopulmonary bypass machines has the danger of clotting within the plastic tubing, or in the patient when it returns, so it needs to be treated with "anticoagulants," drugs that interfere with clotting. Like so many other things done in medicine, this can be a double-edged sword: along with preventing the bad clotting that might take place within the bypass machine or the patient's blood vessels, these medicines can also prevent good clotting that is needed to stop the bleeding of surgical wounds. Some of the early patients with CF who had this kind of surgery for lung transplantation had a lot of bleeding into the pleural space around their new lungs and many of them died because the bleeding would not stop. This is one of the reasons that previous *pleurodesis* (see Chapter 3, *The Respiratory System*) is considered a relative contraindication to lung transplantation at many centers. Pleurodesis is a procedure that purposely irritates the lining of the lung so that it scars to the chest wall and prevents problems like pneumothorax (air that escapes from the lung and causes a lung collapse). This scar tissue can bleed profusely. Another problem with this form of double-lung transplantation is that the anastomosis of the trachea may not receive good blood supply and the tissue may die, leading to dehiscence of the anastomosis, which can lead to sudden respiratory difficulty and death. In addition, the tracheal anastomosis is more likely to become narrowed (stenosed) if the tissue is damaged at the junction.

There is a newer technique for lung transplantation that has become more widely used. It is called "sequential single-lung transplantation." In this technique, each donor lung is removed as a separate entity, with its attached artery, vein, and airway. Each recipient lung is also removed one at a time, leaving behind small lengths of the artery, vein, and airway that can be joined to the corresponding donor artery, vein, and airway. One donor lung is transplanted into the recipient while the patient is breathing with the remaining lung. Once the first lung is transplanted, the recipient breathes with that new lung while the second lung is removed and the second donor lung is transplanted into position. The technique of sequential single-lung transplantation is considered safer and has a better survival record than double-lung transplantation. In many cases, cardiopulmonary bypass is not needed during sequential single-lung transplantation, so the risk of bleeding during and after the transplant surgery is much less. Patients with especially poor lung function may still have to go on bypass during the surgery because they don't have enough functioning lung tissue left in one lung to support them with that lung alone while the other lung is being removed and replaced. By reattaching each airway near the lung instead of reattaching both lungs as a unit to the trachea, this technique leads to a lowered risk of dehiscence of the airway anastomosis. However, the risk of stenosis of the airway with sequential single-lung transplantation is increased, because the airway near the lung is smaller than the trachea.

At the time of surgery, several plastic drainage tubes are placed through the skin into each side of the chest. These tubes will drain any air or fluid around the transplanted lungs and will help keep them inflated. They are usually removed within the first 2 weeks after the surgery.

"Living Donor Lobar" Transplantation

A relatively new and exciting development is the technique of "living donor lobar" transplantation for lung recipients. This procedure uses two live donors, each of whom donates a part of one lung. The donors are usually (but not always) related to the recipient. The part donated is one of the sections of the lung known as a "lobe" and serves as an entire lung for the recipient. Living lobar transplantation offers several potential advantages over transplantation using organs from people who are unrelated or who have died. First, since the donor organs are being given specifically to the recipient, there is no competition for those particular organs, and therefore no need to be on a waiting list. This means that someone who is too sick to survive the long waiting list time might be able to get a transplant anyway. Second, the operation can be scheduled, and can be done during the day with everything relatively calm and prepared. All too often, organs for the usual lung transplant recipient arrive on very short notice, in the middle of the night, perhaps when the chief surgeon is out of town or when the patient and family are not fully prepared to take the huge leap necessary for transplantation. Yet decisions must be made within minutes or hours to "go" or not. Finally, if the donors are closely related to the recipient, there may be a lowered risk for severe rejection. While the risk for rejection is always present (unless an organ is transplanted from an identical twin), transplantation under this circumstance may mean that the recipient will require lower doses of immunosuppressive medications.

There are, however, several potential disadvantages to living related donation. First, it involves three people who have major chest surgery: the recipient and two donors. All surgical procedures have some risk involved, and although the risk is greatest for the recipient, there is some risk to the donors. Second, there is the possibility that a donor might feel undue pressure to donate part of his or her lung even though he or she is not sure about doing it. In families with more than one patient with CF, the decision to consider living lobar transplantation can be agonizing: if you donate a lobe to one patient, you will not be able to do so for anyone else. Finally, this type of lung transplantation is not very common and so many lung transplantation centers do not have much experience performing this type of procedure. With the relatively recent use of the LAS, it is suggested that the need for living donor lobar lung transplantation may be reduced, because sicker patients will have a better chance to receive the few available donor lungs.

PROBLEMS (COMPLICATIONS) ASSOCIATED WITH TRANSPLANTATION

General Considerations

Transplantation is a science that is still in its infancy. There are many problems associated with organ transplantation, and complications of transplant procedures are common. Several of these complications can occur with any type of transplant, and we shall discuss these, and the care necessary to prevent and treat them, in this section. We will discuss specific problems with lung or liver transplantation separately.

One problem that many people with CF wonder about is whether their transplanted lungs or liver will develop CF. They will not. CF is a part of the cells that make up the actual tissue of each organ, and if you get a new organ, that organ will not develop CF. There are many other problems that can develop, some of which are related to the fact that the patient still has CF, even though the transplanted organ does not. Patients with CF who receive a new lung or liver will still have to be seen regularly by their CF doctor in addition to their transplant doctor. Many other problems are complications of the transplant itself, and we will discuss these problems now.

Immunosuppression: Too Much or Too Little (Infection or Rejection)

The saying, "each one of us is unique," has special importance in relation to transplantation. Each of us has built-in systems designed to protect our body from attack from bacteria, viruses, and fungi. These complex defense systems, known as our immune system, work together to kill invading germs and keep them from harming us.

But our immune system can do more than protect us from germs that may try to invade our bodies: it can recognize and destroy cells or organs from another person. When a new organ is transplanted into someone, the immune cells of the recipient will know that the new organ is from someone else, and they will set about to destroy it. This destruction of the transplanted organ is known as *rejection.*

Rejection is one of the major problems following transplantation, and medical researchers have struggled for years to understand it and try to prevent it from destroying transplanted organs. There are a couple of ways to do this. The first way is to transplant an organ or tissue that is not foreign. That can be done if the organ comes from oneself (as can be done with bone marrow transplants in some cases of cancer treatment: a person donates some of his or her own bone marrow for storage, and then that same bone marrow is transplanted back into the person after the cancer treatment). It can also be done if the organ comes from the recipient's identical twin, since these two people are immunologically identical. Such transplants have been done very successfully; but of course this option is open to very few people, because most of us don't have an identical twin, and the bone marrow, a kidney, or a single lobe of a lung is about the only tissue or organs that a living donor can safely contribute.

For people who don't have an identical twin to donate an organ or who need an organ (like lungs or liver) that a living twin can't do without, we must interfere with the immune system's ability to recognize and attack foreign tissue. In other words, we must suppress the immune system. The most common way of doing this is by giving the recipient medicines that weaken the immune system, making it incapable of rejecting the transplant. Such drugs are known as *immunosuppressive agents* (or immunosuppressive drugs or *immunosuppressants*) (Table 8.1).

Few immunosuppressive drugs were available at the time of the first transplants. Steroids, such as prednisone, were used to decrease the function of certain white blood cells known as lymphocytes. An anticancer drug known as azathioprine (Imuran®), which interferes with the ability of any cell to divide, was also used. Unfortunately, it decreases the production of good cells as well as potentially harmful cells. Steroids and anticancer drugs like Imuran® were somewhat effective, but they could not prevent rejection completely without causing severe side effects.

With an improvement in our understanding of the mechanisms involved in rejection came the development of new immunosuppressants that were more powerful in their actions on the immune system, yet didn't have as many side effects. Table 8.1 describes the major types of immunosuppressive medications now in use at most transplant centers, how they work, and what major side effects they have. We discuss them in the next several paragraphs.

A revolution in transplantation occurred in the early 1980s with the development of a drug called cyclosporine, which was the first of these more specific and powerful agents. The improved success of liver and lung transplantation is a direct result of the development of new antirejection drugs like cyclosporine. Cyclosporine and other modern immunosuppressive drugs (including FK506, which is now known as tacrolimus, or Prograf®) are more effective than earlier drugs, and have fewer side effects. Unfortunately, fewer side effects does not mean *no* side effects, for all drugs have side effects. We'll discuss several of the more important side effects of each class of immunosuppressive drugs in the next section (see also Appendix B, *Medications*).

Probably the most important "side effect" of the immunosuppressive drugs is that they might work too well. Remember, the immune system's primary job is to protect us from infections, and weakening it too much with immunosuppressants will result in an increased risk of developing infections. As we might expect, transplant recipients who take immunosuppressive agents are at increased risk for developing infections, in either the transplanted organ or elsewhere. Some of these infections may be life threatening. Infections can be caused by bacteria, such as *Pseudomonas* species, or by viruses or fungi. Viral infections can be particularly difficult to treat and may have further complications, which we will discuss later.

Two particular viral infections deserve special mention here. These are *cyto-megalovirus*, known as *CMV*, and *Epstein–Barr virus*, called *EBV*. CMV is a common virus, which many of us have been exposed to (often without realizing it) by the time we are adults. If we've been exposed to CMV, we have built up immunity to it and don't usually get sick if we are reexposed to it, even if we take immunosuppressive drugs. CMV is a very clever virus, however, and seems to be able to hide in lungs, liver, or blood of people who have had the virus. It can stay there, not causing any trouble as long as the person's immune function is normal. If the lungs of a donor who had CMV in the past are transplanted into someone who has never had CMV (and therefore doesn't have any immunity to CMV), and the recipient has to get immunosuppressive drugs, the CMV can cause serious disease in the transplanted lung as well as in other sites such as the eye, the intestines, or the liver. Another situation can lead to CMV disease in a transplant recipient: if neither the recipient nor the donor has ever had CMV, the recipient can still be exposed to CMV after the transplantation. This can happen simply by coming into contact with someone who has CMV (remember, a lot of healthy people have CMV and don't know it) or—as was common up until recently—through blood transfusions from someone who has had CMV. Transplant recipients now get blood only from people who have no evidence of ever having had CMV. Children may not have had CMV disease (and therefore have no CMV immunity), and if they undergo transplantation and are exposed to CMV while they receive immunosuppressive medicines, they may become quite ill. Fortunately, there are new medicines to treat CMV, but it is still a major problem, particularly in lung transplant recipients, and we shall discuss this a little more, below.

EBV is the virus associated with mononucleosis ("mono"). Like CMV, it seems to have the ability to "hide" in the tissues (and possibly blood) and cause severe problems in people who receive immunosuppressive drugs. Also like CMV, many adults have had EBV, even though they may not have had an illness like mononucleosis. Children, however, are less likely to have had EBV. They may become infected with EBV after transplantation and become ill with a disease that is similar to mononucleosis. Of more concern, however, is the association of EBV

TABLE 8.1

Immunosuppressive Medications

Type of Drug	Brand Name	Generic Name	How Given	How it Works
Corticosteroids *Decrease inflammation and can treat or prevent acute rejection. The exact mechanism of action of corticosteroids is not understood. They are able to decrease lymphocytes (the cells that are involved in rejection) directly. Corticosteroids attach to proteins called receptors; the steroid–receptor combination then goes into the nucleus (control center) of cells, where it affects the activities of the cell. Corticosteroids also interfere with the activation of lymphocytes by other cells.*	Deltasone (and others)	Prednisone	Oral	See Column 1
	Medrol, Solumedro	Methylprednisolone	Oral; IV	See Column 1
	Prelone	Prednisolone	Oral	See Column 1
Lymphocyte-specific drugs *Decrease the ability of lymphocytes known as T-helper cells to function properly. These T-helper lymphocytes are central to the immune system's ability to reject foreign tissue such as a transplanted lung or liver.*	Sandimmune	Cyclosporine	Oral/IV	Attaches to a protein called cyclophilin inside lymphocytes. This inhibits the ability of the lymphocyte to make proteins called interleukins, which stimulate other cells to attack the graft.
	Neoral	Cyclosporine/microemulsion	Oral	Works like cyclosporine, but may be absorbed better from the gastrointestinal tract.
	Prograf	Tacrolimus	Oral/IV	Similar to cyclosporine, except that it has a different binding protein and is more potent in its action.

Antimetabolites
Interfere with the ability of cells to manufacture normal DNA, which is essential for cell division.

Rapamune	Sirolimus	Oral	Similar to cyclosporine and tacrolimus, but with a different binding protein and acts on a different part of the lymphocyte cell cycle.
Imuran	Azothioprine	Oral/IV	Metabolized in the body to a compound called 6-mercaptopurine, which interferes with DNA production.

This decreases the number of cells available to reject foreign tissue.

CellCept Oral	Mycophenolate mofetil	Oral	Metabolized in the body to a mycophenolic acid, which interferes with DNA production.

Antilymphocyte antibodies
Preparations of antibodies that can bind to and attack proteins on the surface of lymphocytes. This will inactivate or destroy those lymphocytes.

Atgam	Antithymocyte globulin	IV	See Column 1. This antibody preparation is derived from horse serum. The horses are "immunized" with human cells.
Orthoclone OKT3	Muromonab-CD3	IV	See Column 1. This antibody preparation is "bioengineered." It is produced by mouse cells in cultures.
Zenapax	Daclizumab	IV	"Bioengineered" antibodies directed against a specific protein on the surface of lymphocytes.
Simulect	Basiliximab	IV	"Bioengineered" antibodies directed against a specific protein on the surface of lymphocytes.

IV, intravenous.

infection in transplant recipients with a special complication, which is a tumor of lymphatic tissue (lymphoma). This lymphoma is called *post*transplantation *lym*-phoproliferative *d*isease, or PTLD. If PTLD occurs after transplantation, it is usually treated by decreasing the immunosuppressive medications. On rare occasions, PTLD may require other special forms of therapy. Although PTLD often responds to treatment, it doesn't always, and can be fatal.

Another problem with immunosuppressive drugs is that they may not work well enough. When this happens, the immune system recognizes the transplanted organ as being foreign and tries to destroy it, leading to rejection. There are two major "types" of rejection: acute and chronic. Rejection, along with infection, remains a major problem for transplant recipients, and is discussed later in this chapter.

In summary, transplant doctors try to use immunosuppressive drugs in just the right amount. Too little immunosuppression leads to the threat of rejection; too much immunosuppression leads to the risk of infection or PTLD. Transplant physicians and scientists are constantly trying to widen the distance between the extremes of rejection and infection that can cause severe illness in the recipient. As more research is done, it is likely that safer yet more powerful immunosuppressive drugs will be discovered, allowing for better control of both rejection and infection.

Side Effects of Immunosuppressive Drugs

As we've already said, the major "side effect" of immunosuppressive drugs is either having too much immunosuppression, which leads to infection or PTLD, or too little, which leads to organ rejection. Immunosuppressives are medicines that can have other true side effects, that is, effects that are unrelated to the main reason you take them in the first place.

The main side effects of cyclosporine, tacrolimus, and similar drugs are kidney damage, high blood pressure, diabetes, seizures, increased growth of the gums in the mouth, and excessive body hair. Despite this long list of possible side effects, many of the most serious ones can be minimized by measuring the blood levels of the immunosuppressive drugs and adjusting the dosage as required. In some cases, however, where the immunosuppressives are harming the kidneys, it may not be possible to lower the drug without causing or worsening lung rejection. In those few cases, it comes down to a choice between saving the lungs and saving the kidneys. The lungs always win, because you can live (with treatments several times a week from a kidney dialysis machine) without kidneys, but you cannot live without lungs. Some patients have even received kidney transplants after a heart or lung transplantation because of the kidney damage caused by the immunosuppressive drugs. Some of the recipients who develop diabetes from the immunosuppressive medications may need to receive insulin shots.

The other immunosuppressants that have been used for the prevention of rejection also have side effects. Azathioprine (Imuran®), as we've already discussed, interferes with the development of blood cells. Because of this, anemia and a low white blood cell count, which can increase the risk of infection, are the main side effects of Imuran®. In addition, nausea and diarrhea are fairly common with the use of this drug. Because of the side effects of Imuran®, many transplant centers have switched to something called mycophenolate mofetil (Cellcept®). Of course Cellcept® comes with its own set of side effects such as stomach upset and disruption of the development of blood cells, but it seems to be better tolerated in some people than Imuran®. Steroids such as prednisone may lead to high blood pressure, diabetes, obesity, cataracts, ulcers of the stomach and bowel, excessive bruising, and some decrease in the ability to fight off infections. Our body normally makes its own steroids similar to prednisone, and these naturally occurring steroids are important in helping us withstand stresses like infection, surgery, or exposure to cold temperature. Taking prednisone for a long time can decrease the body's ability to make these natural steroids and lead to an increased risk if we encounter any of these stresses.

Surgical Complications

Transplantation—as we've seen—involves very complex surgery. During any such procedure, it is possible that something (a blood vessel, nerves, the organ itself, etc.) could get cut that shouldn't get cut. This can cause problems after surgery. Despite their significant complexity, the surgical techniques of lung transplantation have improved significantly since the first lung transplantation. For the most part, the improvement in the survival of patients who have undergone lung transplantation has come from improvements in surgical techniques.

Complications of Lung Transplantation

Aside from the general complications of transplantation that we've mentioned already as "side effects" of the immunosuppressive drugs, most important, infection and rejection, there are several complications specific to lung transplantation. These complications include organ failure, bleeding in the chest, damage to nerves in the chest, blood clots in the veins going from the lung to the heart, and narrowing of the airway where the donor lung is attached to the recipient. Some of these complications happen soon after transplantation (early complications), while others happen later (late complications).

Early Complications of Lung Transplantation (Hours-to-days After Transplant)

Organ Failure

Any organ that does not have a healthy blood supply can be damaged. This can happen to a donor lung when it is removed from the donor or when it is still in the donor, if the donor's illness or injury has interfered with the blood supply to the lung (or harmed it in any other way). Once the organ has been removed from the donor, it is washed free of blood with a special solution designed to keep it healthy for the trip to the operating room, where it will be put into the recipient. If the trip takes too long, or if the preservative solution doesn't work perfectly, there can be damage to the organ. Any one factor or combination of these factors can damage the transplanted organ badly enough that it may not be able to function. This kind of problem shows up in the early hours or days after transplant, and is referred to as "preservation injury." This injury is believed to be the result of either inadequate blood supply to the lung for too long a time, poor preservation of the lung, or both. A severe form of this injury results in damage to the air sacs throughout the lung and can lead to respiratory failure soon after transplantation. While this injury may resolve, it may leave scarring in the lung that will limit the amount of healthy lung the patient will have after recovery.

Bleeding in the Chest

The surgery for lung transplantation involves opening the chest by making an incision across the front of the chest wall (the "clamshell incision"). As we've already mentioned, one of the important reasons this incision was developed was because of the problem of bleeding from the lining of the chest wall (pleura) following surgery, bleeding that is common in patients with CF because of frequent scarring of the pleural space that has resulted from chronic lung infections. This can be a problem when a surgeon tries to remove the lungs from a patient with CF to put new lungs in. The clamshell incision, by allowing better access to the lungs, helps the surgeon find and stop the bleeding, but bleeding after surgery (after the chest is closed again) is still a problem in patients with CF following transplantation, particularly in those patients who had to go on heart–lung bypass during their surgery.

Blood Clots

Blood clots can form in the veins leading from the transplanted lungs to the left side of the heart, and can greatly interfere with heart and lung functions right after a transplant procedure. To find such clots, the physicians usually use a technique known as *transesophageal echocardiography*. In this technique, a plastic probe about as big around as a finger is passed through the mouth, down the back of the throat, and into the esophagus. The probe contains a miniature echocardiograph machine, similar to the machines used for ultrasound. Because the esophagus is behind the heart and because the veins from the lungs enter the backside of the heart, the physicians can see them better with this approach. Transesophageal echocardiography is usually done with the patient heavily sedated.

Nerve Damage

When lungs are transplanted, the nerves that usually accompany them are cut and not reattached. Although this might seem to be quite dangerous, it usually has a relatively small effect on recovery and this will be discussed later in this chapter. There are, however, several other important nerves that run through the chest rather than into the lungs, and these may be damaged accidentally during surgery. The most important of these nerves are the *phrenic nerves.* These nerves go to the diaphragm, which is the main muscle involved in breathing; damage to these nerves may decrease the ability of the diaphragm to contract, which limits the ability to breathe. Damage to one of these nerves may lead to the diaphragm on that side being too high in the chest. Although the nerve may regrow, this can take a very long time. Treatment of this injury involves surgically "pulling down" ("*plicating*") the affected diaphragm. The other nerves that can get damaged are the ones that control the vocal cords. If the vocal cords do not move appropriately, there can be problems with a weak voice or choking during swallowing (aspirating food). Like the phrenic nerve, the nerves that supply the vocal cords usually recover from injury. If not, treatment involves "retraining" the vocal cords (something that speech therapists do).

Narrowing (Stenosis) of the Airway

It sometimes happens that one or both of the main bronchi become narrowed following transplantation. This is most often right where the donor and recipient airways are joined (the bronchial anastomosis). If the narrowing is severe, it can be hard to breathe and move mucus past the narrowed area, setting the stage for hard-to-control infection. The narrowing can be caused by the surgeon's having sewn the bronchi too tightly, by the bronchi simply being too small, or (and this is by far the most common) by the formation of scar tissue at the anastomosis.

Rejection

Despite the use of immunosuppressive drugs, rejection remains a major problem following lung transplantation. Rejection, which is the result of the recipient's cells trying to destroy the "foreign" lung tissue from the donor, takes two major forms, called *acute* and *chronic* rejection.

Acute rejection is especially common in the first weeks to months following transplantation, but may occur years after transplant. Episodes of acute rejection tend to occur abruptly and cause breathing difficulties, cough, lowered blood oxygen levels, and changes in the chest radiograph. If acute rejection is diagnosed and treated promptly and aggressively, it usually responds well to treatment, and the patient improves. The usual treatment of acute rejection is with high doses of steroids given through an intravenous (IV) line for several days. The other immunosuppressive drugs, such as cyclosporine or tacrolimus, are often given in higher doses to prevent acute rejection from coming back. If the steroids don't work (they usually do), some other treatments may be used and are often effective. These more specialized treatments are designed to attack the specific kind of blood cells (lymphocytes) that are causing the acute rejection. The two major treatments are known as OKT3 and ATG (which stands for *anti*t*hymocyte g*lobulin). Both of these must be given, in the hospital, by IV over several days.

Chronic rejection is less well understood than acute rejection and is more difficult to treat. It tends to have a slower onset, and last longer, with more subtle symptoms of shortness of breath with exercise, cough, or a fall in PFTs. We will discuss chronic rejection in more detail under the section that deals with the late complications of lung transplantation.

The diagnosis of rejection is made with certainty only by examining a piece of lung tissue under the microscope. The piece of tissue, known as a *biopsy* specimen, is usually obtained during a procedure called *bronchoscopy*, which will be discussed later in this chapter. Acute rejection is easier to diagnose than is chronic rejection with this type of biopsy. At times, the biopsy specimen must be fairly big to diagnose chronic rejection, and this may lead the transplant physicians to recommend an "open" biopsy, in which the chest is opened surgically and a piece of lung removed by a surgeon.

Infection

As we've seen, immunosuppressive medicines increase the risk of infection in transplant recipients. This risk is greatly increased in the lungs of patients with CF. In fact, the major cause of death following lung transplantation in patients with CF is infection. The windpipe (trachea) and sinuses of the patient with CF still "have" CF, even though the new lungs don't. Bacteria such as *Pseudomonas* or *Staphylococcus* organisms will remain in the airways (sinuses, trachea, and bronchi) of these patients and can cause infection in the transplanted lung. The combination of immunosuppression and *Pseudomonas* organisms, particularly if the *Pseudomonas* organisms are resistant to antibiotics, can prove deadly for the recipient. Because of this risk, some centers decrease the immunosuppression as much as possible in CF lung transplant recipients. More important, virtually all transplant centers look closely at the bacteria in their patients with CF before transplantation. As we've already discussed, organisms that are resistant to all antibiotics are considered by many centers to be a contraindication to transplantation. Infections can be an early or late complication of lung transplantation. Infections can occur in the transplanted lungs, or elsewhere.

The new lungs are the most common targets for infections after transplantation, for several reasons. First, the lungs are the only major transplanted organs in direct contact with the outside world after transplantation. Every time we breathe, air enters our lungs; the very air we breathe is often contaminated with materials that can harm us. Bacteria, viruses, small particles of dust or dirt, or certain toxic gases may be in that air. Our lungs normally have a set of barriers or ways to deal with many of these dangerous materials. Scientists and physicians refer to these as the lung defenses. Transplanting lungs directly affects lung defenses, and this makes the lungs more susceptible to infection. Some of these have been discussed in Chapter 3, *The Respiratory System*, but we'll review the affected lung defenses in the next few paragraphs.

Since the nerves supplying the lungs are cut and not reattached during transplantation, the new lungs do not have any sensation. One important sensation that we all normally have in our lungs is what we call the *cough reflex,* which is the stimulation to cough that is brought about when any material like increased mucus builds up in the airways. This urge to cough is lost at least for the first months after transplant, meaning that mucus can build up in the new lung without the recipient's feeling the need to cough. Of course, some people—who have coughed all of their lives up to the time of the transplant—might think that the lack of cough is wonderful. But, we must remember that cough is one of the lung's most effective ways of getting rid of bacteria and excess mucus. Thus, this loss of the cough reflex adds to the risk of developing infections in the lung. Lung transplant recipients can still cough, but they must actually *decide* to cough because, without the cough reflex, coughing won't happen on its own.

Another of the lung's usual defenses that is altered by a transplant is *mucociliary clearance.* Normally, secretions such as mucus help to trap unwanted small particles such as bacteria and keep them from damaging the lung. Because the airway cells are continuously making mucus, a way to move the mucus out of the lung is needed. This movement is the responsibility of the cilia, which are very small, hairlike tufts that project out from airway cells and are in contact with the mucus. Normally, these cilia move in a regular way that slowly but surely moves the mucus up the airways to the trachea, from which it can be coughed out, or to the back of the throat, where it can be swallowed. For unknown reasons, even though the cilia are still present on the airway cells following transplantation, they just don't move as well, allowing mucus to build up in the lung.

Finally, for reasons that we don't yet understand, the white blood cells that fight infection in the lungs do not seem to be able to get into the lung as well as they should following lung transplantation. All of these defenses and their status following lung transplantation are the subject of intense scientific study. It's likely that we'll have better ideas on how to improve the lung defenses and decrease the risk of infection following lung transplantation as we learn more about the way the lungs defend themselves normally.

Late Complications of Lung Transplantation (Weeks-to-Months After Transplant)

Infection

As we just mentioned, infection can be an early or late complication of lung transplantation. Infection can be caused by bacteria like *Staphylococcus* and *Pseudomonas* organisms that the patient with CF has had in the sinuses and trachea for months or years before transplantation. These bacteria can infect the new lungs at any time.

Although we discussed it earlier, the problem of CMV infection deserves special mention when discussing the late complications of lung transplantation. Once CMV has infected a person, that individual will make antibodies to CMV, which is one of the body's ways to try to fight off infection: antibodies attack specific targets; antibody to CMV fights CMV. The virus is a clever one, however, and it may not be eliminated from the body, and instead may lie dormant in the lung, intestines, kidney, or liver, temporarily not causing trouble. We can determine whether antibodies to CMV are present in the blood of a lung donor and a lung recipient. If the donor is positive for the antibodies (meaning the donor at one time had a CMV infection), then CMV may be lying dormant in the donated lung. The immunosuppression given to the recipient will allow the CMV that has been lurking in the donor lung to become free to cause a new infection, particularly if the recipient is negative for the antibodies (meaning that the recipient has probably not ever been infected with CMV and has no antibodies to help fight CMV). CMV infection in this setting can be especially bad, causing fever, sore throat, or other symptoms. In addition, it now seems that CMV disease in the lung recipient may increase the risk for the development of chronic rejection, which we mentioned briefly before and will discuss further below.

Several approaches have been used to try to prevent and/or treat CMV disease and chronic rejection in lung transplant recipients. In some transplant centers, recipients and donors are now "matched" whenever possible, so that lungs from CMV-positive donors are transplanted into CMV-positive recipients, while lungs from CMV-negative donors are reserved for CMV-negative recipients. Another approach is to treat CMV-positive and CMV-negative recipients who have received CMV-positive lungs with an anti-CMV medication known as ganciclovir. A third approach is to give CMV-negative recipients a special antibody preparation that is high in antibodies directed against CMV. These approaches are not all always feasible (particularly the method of "matching" donors and recipients) or completely effective. Physicians and scientists are working on new approaches to try to minimize the effects of CMV in transplant recipients.

Chronic (long-lasting) *rejection*, which was mentioned earlier, is a poorly understood form of lung rejection. Rejection is the recipient's body's way of attempting to attack and destroy the new lung. In chronic rejection, the part of the lung that is attacked is usually the small airways. This leads to a very serious form of airway damage known as *bronchiolitis obliterans*, which is characterized by scarring of the small airways. We don't yet know the reason for this pattern or the exact cause of chronic rejection. Chronic lung rejection is sometimes associated with CMV infection. Several other factors, including recurrent episodes of acute rejection, especially severe episodes of acute rejection, and stenosis of the airway anastomosis, have also been associated with chronic rejection. Approximately 25% to 35% of all lung recipients develop some form of chronic rejection, and it remains a major cause of death in transplant recipients. Of those lung recipients who develop chronic rejection, approximately 35% to 50% will die, and most of the remaining 50% to 65% of patients will have some degree of compromise of their airway function. As is the case for acute rejection, steroids as well as medications such as OKT3 and ATG have been suggested for the treatment of chronic rejection. In chronic rejection, attention is focused on making sure that the immune-suppressing medications are optimized. In some cases, more immune-suppressing medications are added. One such medication is sirolimus (rapamycin or Rapamune®) which, in combination with Prograf®, can provide very potent immune suppression. Several experimental treatments are being tested for the treatment of chronic rejection. One such treatment is the early initiation of azithromycin (Zithromax®) when chronic rejection is suspected. It is thought that the anti-inflammatory effects of this antibiotic can help prevent further damage and chronic rejection. Another recent discovery is the link between gastroesophageal reflux (see Chapter 4, *The Gastrointestinal System*) and chronic rejection. Because of this, many transplant centers are aggressive about identifying and treating reflux in patients who have received lung transplantation. Sometimes even surgical procedures to prevent reflux are done to give the best chance of preventing chronic rejection of the transplanted lung. We hope that as more is learned about chronic rejection, we will get better at preventing and treating it in lung transplant recipients.

Other Late Complications of Lung Transplantation

Although infection and rejection are the most common and usually most serious complications of transplantation, there are some others.

Narrowing (stenosis) of the airway was discussed under the section *Early Complications . . .* above, but actually is more likely to be a problem weeks to months after the transplant. A little bit of narrowing of the airway usually causes no problems. More severe narrowing can cause difficulty in breathing, difficulty moving mucus, and therefore worse problems with infection beyond the narrowed area. Sometimes the physician can open the stenosis with bronchoscopy (we'll describe bronchoscopy later in this chapter). This can happen in several ways: sometimes just pushing the bronchoscope through the narrowed area can stretch it open. Instead of a bronchoscope, surgeons or radiologists may be able to pass a special deflated balloon to the narrowed anastomosis, inflate the balloon with a lot of pressure, making the now-rigid balloon stretch open the stenosis. Sometimes the extra scar tissue that is blocking the airway can be cut away during bronchoscopy. A third way of dealing with stenosis is to use a special laser beam (again during bronchoscopy) to "burn off" some of the scar tissue. Finally, in very severe cases, a surgeon or radiologist may be able to place a plastic or metal *stent* in the airway. This device is stiffer than the airway and props it open. This is a difficult procedure, and is used only when there seems to be no other choice. If the length of narrowed bronchus is short and the stenosis is severe, in rare cases the surgeon may reopen the chest and cut out (resect) the narrowed portion, sewing the open ends of the normal-sized bronchus back to each other.

Psychological, Social, and Financial "Complications" of Transplantation

Transplantation is very expensive. Figures from one major transplant center for 1995 show that pretransplant care for a patient with CF averaged $80,000 per year. These costs have not changed very much since. The transplantation itself (and the hospital stay afterward) cost $200,000 to $250,000, and the costs for the first year after transplantation were about $100,000. Most, but not all, insurance companies will pay for transplantation, but some still consider the procedure (and some of the medications used afterward) experimental and therefore not covered.

A lot of care is required after transplantation and, in addition to costing money, this adds to the inconvenience and discomfort of the process. Many patients will have one or more of the complications of transplantation and will require further testing and care. All this may increase the time spent in the hospital and away from work, school, family, and friends. Often these hospitalizations are at the transplant center, which may be hundreds (even thousands) of miles away from home.

Transplantation is stressful for patients, their parents, and their physicians and nurses. Even for someone who does very well, there can be emotional challenges: it is often not easy for someone who has had trouble breathing for months or years to adjust to not needing oxygen, and to trust in his or her newly gained energy.

As in any new field of medicine, difficult lessons about transplantation are learned all the time. Unfortunately, many of these lessons are taught by the patients who develop problems related to the transplantation or to the medications given to prevent rejection. The history of transplantation (particularly for lung transplants) is short, and the length of survival following a new lung or liver is impossible to predict. The uncertainty of the course someone will take after transplantation adds to the stress of the procedure. Transplantation is probably not a good treatment for someone who needs assurance that "everything will be fine." We'll discuss this further in the section entitled "Making the Decision."

CARE AFTER TRANSPLANTATION

General Considerations

During any transplantation, the patient is unconscious, under general anesthesia, with his or her breathing being done by a machine (a ventilator) through a tube that goes in the nose or mouth into the trachea (endotracheal tube). The patient will have other tubes in as well: drainage tubes from the chest, a urine tube in the bladder, and several different catheters in blood vessels, including IVs, sometimes a tube in an artery (an "a-line") for easy measurement of the oxygen and carbon dioxide levels in the blood, and sometimes an IV that goes into the heart to be able to measure blood pressure very accurately. Immediately after the transplant surgery, the patient is cared for in the intensive care unit (ICU) until he or she is strong and healthy enough to breathe on his or her own, and to withstand the removal of the various tubes. During this time in the ICU, tests will be done to make sure that the new organs are working satisfactorily and that there haven't been any immediate problems associated with the surgery, like bleeding or formation of large blood clots. Once it seems that there are no major postoperative problems, and the patient is ready to breathe on his or her own, the endotracheal tube can be removed (we say the patient is "extubated"). Getting to this point usually takes a few days, but can take longer. There are a couple of different approaches to extubation of a patient after surgery: one approach is to get the tube out absolutely as soon as possible, since the tubes are very uncomfortable, and the patient cannot talk while the tubes are in place. The other approach is more conservative, and delays extubation until it is absolutely clear that the patient is ready because an extubation that is done too early can fail (if the patient isn't strong enough yet, he or she could tire and must then be reintubated). Reintubation may be harder for patients than a slightly longer single intubation.

In the ICU, the patient will usually need a lot of pain medication and sedatives. While a patient is on the ventilator, medications are often given that paralyze the patient, to make it easier for the ventilator to "breathe" for him or her. Once the patient is breathing on his or her own, is relatively alert and not requiring large amounts of sedatives and pain medication, and all organ systems are working satisfactorily, he or she can be moved to a regular hospital room. This usually takes several days to a week or so, but in some cases can take weeks or even months.

After transplantation of any organ, that organ requires a lot of care and close monitoring to be sure that it continues to function well. Rejection of the organ and infection (in the transplanted organ and in other parts of the body) remain dangers forever after transplantation. The posttransplantation care is at least as time consuming, bothersome, and important as regular CF care is. Because of the health risks, and because of the care required after transplantation, we often say that getting a transplant is like trading one disease for another (the new lungs or liver don't have CF anymore, but they will have other problems that need to be treated). And of course, someone with CF who has new lungs or a new liver still has CF, even if the new organs don't. So digestive enzymes, vitamins, and so on, continue to be important. Care of the lungs remains essential after transplantation of any organ in a patient with CF.

Testing a patient for rejection is necessary on a regular basis following transplantation of any organ. PFTs can give early hints that there might be a problem with the transplanted lung, but any kind of problem, not just rejection, can make these tests abnormal. The most accurate way to see if rejection is present in a transplanted organ is to examine a small piece of it under the microscope. The technique of taking a small piece of an organ is known as a *biopsy* procedure, and the small piece itself is referred to as a biopsy specimen, or sometimes just a "biopsy." For liver or lung transplant recipients, it is not uncommon for 5 to 10 biopsy procedures to be done in the first year after transplantation.

Tests After Lung Transplantation

After lung transplantation, several kinds of tests are done in the ICU, in the regular hospital room, and afterward when the patient has gone home.

The most common tests that help to monitor the health of transplanted lungs are PFTs and chest radiographs. PFTs are described more in Chapter 3, *The Respiratory System*, and are no different from the PFTs used for most people with CF who have not undergone transplantation. In addition to regular PFTs at the clinic, most patients are given small electronic PFT machines to take home with them, which they are asked to use two or three times per week. If the results of these home PFTs get worse, the patient notifies the doctor for further testing. The radiographs are no different from the usual chest x-rays that CF patients have had for years. The types of problems that might show up on PFTs or radiographs can be different from the pretransplantation CF lung problems, and might prompt the physicians to recommend specific treatment or further testing, which will almost always mean a special test known as *bronchoscopy*, **bronchoalveolar lavage** (called BAL for short), and *transbronchial biopsy*. We'll describe this test, which is commonly done for lung recipients, in the next several paragraphs.

Bronchoscopy is a way of looking into the trachea and bronchi of the lung, using a tube called a *bronchoscope*. There are different kinds and sizes of bronchoscopes. In most cases, the kind used for patients who have had lung transplants is flexible, so it can be passed through the nose or (more commonly) an endotracheal tube or laryngeal mask airway (LMA), bend around curves down the back of the throat, through the vocal cords, and into the trachea and bronchi. It has a light and lens at the end, so the physician doing the procedure can see into the dark bronchial tubes. In most transplant centers, the bronchoscope is connected to a video camera, and the physician doing the bronchoscopy (the "bronchoscopist") moves the bronchoscope while watching the television image. (The patient can watch the procedure "live" on the television, too, if she or he likes, or afterward on a video playback.) There is also a hollow suction channel running the length of the bronchoscope through which liquids can be squirted in or sucked out, and through which thin, flexible wire instruments can be passed.

BAL means, quite simply, that a liquid, usually saline (salt water) like that used for an IV solution, is washed ("lavaged") into an area of the lung through the thin channel of the bronchoscope and then sucked back out into a sterile container. The total amount of fluid used is often several ounces, given a small amount at a time, with suctioning after each individual amount of fluid. As the saline washes into the airways, it mixes with the cells and fluid in the airways and alveoli. When it is sucked back, it carries with it some of those cells and fluid. In addition, if there are bacteria or viruses in the airway, some of them will be in the suctioned fluid as well and can be cultured in the laboratory. Cultures of the fluid for bacteria, viruses, or fungi take several days to weeks to give definite answers. The laboratory can determine the number of cells taken out of the airway and the type of cells removed. These tests will help tell the physicians if there is evidence of an infection in the lung or if there might be rejection. To diagnose rejection most accurately, the physician will also want to do a biopsy through the bronchoscope (see below).

Within the first day or so after lung transplantation, one of the physicians might perform a bronchoscopy for a quick look at the bronchial anastomoses (the places where the donor bronchi are sewed to the recipient bronchi). For this procedure, the bronchoscope can simply be passed through the endotracheal tube into the trachea and bronchi, and the procedure should not be much of a big deal for the patient.

Beyond the first days, bronchoscopies with BAL and biopsy are performed every few weeks at first, then every few months if things are going well. Bronchoscopies will also be performed if there is any hint that there is a problem. These "hints" might come from symptoms, such as increased cough or sputum production or laboratory test results, like lower oxygen level, worsened PFTs, or some new findings on the chest x-ray.

A biopsy done through the bronchoscope is known as a *transbronchial biopsy*. There are other types of lung biopsies, and we'll describe those later in this section. For a transbronchial biopsy, the physician using the bronchoscope will pass small forceps through the bronchoscope. These forceps are at the end of a long thin wire and are a tool that has small jaws with tiny teeth. The jaws of the forceps can be opened and then closed to take biopsy specimens ("bites") of the small bronchi and surrounding lung tissue. These samples are also sent to the laboratory for examination under the microscope. It usually takes a day or so for the biopsies to be prepared and examined. The biopsies can give some information about possible infection, but their main use is to tell if there is rejection. The more pieces of tissue the physician obtains, the better the chances that they will give a true representation of the situation in the lungs. However, the more pieces taken, the greater the chances of a complication of the procedure, too (see below).

Complications of Bronchoscopy

There are several important possible complications of bronchoscopy, but fortunately, complications are relatively rare. The most important of these complications are oversedation, nosebleed, cough, bleeding within the bronchi, and pneumothorax (collapsed lung). These will be discussed in the next several paragraphs.

The usual bronchoscopy procedure is done by passing the bronchoscope through the patient's nose, down the back of the throat, through the vocal cords, and into the trachea and bronchi. The procedure sounds brutal, but is surprisingly easy to tolerate. The bronchoscope itself is soft and flexible, and the procedure, while a bit uncomfortable, is not painful. To minimize the discomfort, several things are done. Most patients are given sedatives through an IV. This will help the patient relax and make it easier for the physician to do the bronchoscopy. Notice, we didn't say the patient had general anesthesia: most flexible bronchoscopies are done with the patient sedated and breathing on his own. This is important, because the patient has to breathe around the bronchoscope. The usual bronchoscope is about as big around as a pencil, and most patients breathe around it without any difficulty. Occasional patients don't want any IV medications, and actually watch the procedure being done on the same TV screen that the bronchoscopist watches. Others prefer to see the video afterward, while others want nothing to do with the bronchoscopy, preferring to be asleep for it. As much or as little sedation as the individual patient needs can be given.

The other option for sedation is to have an anesthesiologist deliver gas anesthesia by facemask so that the patient falls asleep and then place either an endotracheal tube into the trachea through the vocal cords (the patient is "intubated") or an LMA. The LMA is a tube that is passed through the mouth to the back of the throat where it sits just above the voice box (the larynx). The LMA for delivery of gas anesthesia and sedation has recently become popular for performing bronchoscopy because it does not require deep sedation to place an endotracheal tube, it is more comfortable, and it allows the person doing the bronchoscopy to advance the bronchoscope through the LMA and see the vocal cords and upper trachea well, which is not possible if the procedure is performed through an endotracheal tube.

Whenever sedative (or any other) medicines are used, there is a small chance that the patient can get too much. In this case, that could cause the patient to be oversedated and fall so deeply asleep that he or she doesn't breathe. To prevent this complication, sedative doses are checked carefully and are usually given in relatively small amounts, with extra being given as needed. Furthermore, the patient is monitored carefully for any signs of not breathing enough (a pulse oximeter, or "pulseox," is attached to the finger to give a continuous reading of blood oxygen levels). Finally, medicines are readily at hand to reverse the effects of the sedative medicines. The sedatives are usually very effective in keeping patients comfortable, without their needing general anesthesia as they would for painful surgical procedures. The sedatives used most often have the added benefit of causing what is known as retrograde amnesia, which means the patients forget what happened while they were sedated.

As soon as the patient is comfortable, if the bronchoscopy is being done through the nose, the nose and back of the throat are numbed with Xylocaine® drops (like the dentist uses, but not injected with a needle), Xylocaine® jelly on the end of a cotton swab, or even Xylocaine® aerosols. As the bronchoscope is passed through the nose or through the LMA or endotracheal tube, the vocal cords are also numbed with Xylocaine® dripped through the suction channel of the bronchoscope. The nose is the narrowest part of the patient's body that the bronchoscope has to pass through, and it can sometimes bleed from the rubbing. These nosebleeds are not serious and not common (about 1 of every 20 or 30 patients).

The bronchoscope is then passed through the patient's vocal cords into the trachea. The trachea also gets some Xylocaine®, not really to prevent pain (it doesn't hurt), but to prevent cough (the body's natural reaction to an "invader" like a pencil-sized tube at the vocal cords or in the trachea is to try to expel it with cough). In some patients with CF, it is difficult to numb the vocal cords and trachea completely, and they do cough a bit during the procedure. Once the bronchoscope reaches the bronchi of the new lungs, the need for anesthetizing the airways has lessened, since the new lungs do not have nerves connected to them. The new bronchi do not have any feeling or cough reflex.

Once the bronchoscope is in the small bronchi, it is pushed gently so that it temporarily blocks the airway (this is known as "wedging" the bronchoscope). When the bronchoscope is wedged into place, blocking off the bronchus, the physician performs the BAL (that is, she or he washes in the saline, and sucks it back out again, saving it for culture and microscopic examination). Sometimes, just pushing the bronchoscope down bronchi, especially bronchi that are inflamed because of infection or rejection, can cause bleeding. Usually this bleeding is not serious, but occasionally it can be.

After doing the BAL, the physician repositions the tip of the bronchoscope so that it's well placed to obtain biopsies. Most often, the physician uses a radiograph screen (fluoroscopy or just "fluoro") to show the exact position of the bronchoscope and the forceps. The physician then passes the forceps through the suction channel and takes a few "bites" of tissue for the biopsies. One might think that the taking of biopsies would be painful, but it is not–remember that the transplanted lungs do not have nerve connections any more. Taking bites from the lung (or any living tissue) usually causes some bleeding, as you might expect. Usually the bleeding stops very quickly, but on occasion, particularly if the lungs are inflamed (infection or rejection), the bleeding can be difficult to control and can be dangerous. In extremely rare cases, it has even been fatal.

Taking a bite of tissue can also cause a hole in the outside of the lung, allowing air to leak outside the lungs. The air that escapes through a hole in the lung is still trapped within the chest, and can accumulate around the lung, press in on the lung, and cause it to collapse. This condition is called a *pneumothorax*, and is discussed a bit more in Chapter 3, *The Respiratory System*. A pneumothorax is much more likely to occur in a patient who is breathing with the help of a ventilator, since the ventilator works by blowing air into the lungs under pressure. This added air pressure can open up a small hole and prop it open, preventing it from sealing itself shut, and allowing air to escape with each breath in. If someone develops a pneumothorax, he or she will usually need to have a tube placed through the skin, between the ribs, and into the chest to let the air escape and allow the lung to reexpand. These tubes are called chest tubes, for obvious reasons. A pneumothorax is usually painful, and chest tubes are always painful, so pain medications are given if this problem develops.

There are some situations where a biopsy with the flexible bronchoscope (a transbronchial biopsy) might not be possible, but a biopsy of the lung is needed. For example, the patient may be too small to breathe around the flexible bronchoscope, the patient may be too sick to have flexible bronchoscopy, or the physicians believe that the bites taken with biopsy forceps are likely to be too small to give an accurate diagnosis. In these cases, an *open* lung *biopsy* might be necessary. An open biopsy is done in the operating room, under general anesthesia. The surgeon makes an incision into the chest to expose part of the lung under his or her direct vision, and cuts out a small piece of the lung, sews the hole, and closes the chest. This procedure is more involved, requires general anesthesia, and takes more time to recover from, but, in a very sick patient, is probably safer than the transbronchial biopsy, and guarantees a bigger piece of tissue, which is more likely to allow for a correct diagnosis.

Ongoing Care

After transplantation, as you've heard many times already, continuing care is absolutely essential and never-ending. Treatment with immunosuppressant (anti-rejection) medications is essential. Other CF treatments, such as enzymes and nutritional supplements, are also important. Many patients will still need to do airway clearance for clearing mucus from their new lungs. Some patients may have to have special treatment for their sinuses, if their physicians feel that infected sinuses have been causing problems in their new lungs. In most cases, care can take place at your regular CF center, but with periodic visits back to the transplant center. Your physician and the transplant team will work together to make sure your overall care is as good as it can be.

RESULTS OF LUNG TRANSPLANTATION (PROGNOSIS AFTER TRANSPLANTATION)

Lung transplantation for patients with CF is still a relatively young science and art. The first procedure, you'll recall, was in 1983, and for the first several years of lung transplantation, patients did not live more than a few weeks. Although we have improved a great deal since then, we are certainly not at the point where it's simply a matter of ordering a set of new lungs, getting them hooked up, and going on about our business. Now, and for the foreseeable future, lung transplantation, perhaps especially for patients with CF, will be a very difficult procedure, with many deaths and with much suffering for many of those who survive. In fact, as of 2008, "transplant complications" was in second place on the list of reasons for death of patients with CF (CF pulmonary disease accounted for 68% of the deaths of patients with CF and transplant complications accounted for 13%).

Nonetheless, many patients have done spectacularly well, with full resumption of work, school, recreation, and family life, some of them 9 or 10 years after transplantation. As transplant centers gain more experience, and as scientists develop better ways to preserve lungs outside the body and devolop better and safer immunosuppressive drugs, we can expect the results to improve. It is worth keeping in mind that the first kidney transplant recipients did not survive long, and liver transplantation had no long-term survivors for the first several years when the procedure was performed. Now, both of these procedures are accepted as standard care for many conditions, and the outcome is excellent. As experience with lung transplantation increases, the results will almost certainly improve.

At the writing of this book, most centers report approximately 75% two-year survival after lung transplantation for patients with CF. That means that if 100 patients get a transplant, 75 will be alive 2 years later; 25 will be dead. Let's look at some other numbers that don't have anything to do with transplants: patients with CF with the worst PFTs have approximately a 50% two-year survival (without transplant). So, of 100 of these patients, 50 will be alive and 50 dead in 2 years. Transplantation may allow up to 25 more out of a hundred of these sickest patients to survive for 2 years than would have survived without transplantation. Other factors need to be considered too: of those who survive, about half will develop bronchiolitis obliterans, a severe condition seen in transplanted lungs. Bronchiolitis obliterans causes progressive difficulty breathing and is ultimately fatal in about one third to one half of the patients who develop it.

In one recent report from UK, 76 patients with CF were referred for lung transplantation. Of those 76 patients, 36 died waiting on the transplant list, and 15 were alive (still waiting for transplant) at the time of the report; 25 patients received their transplants, and of those, 10 died and 15 were still alive. So, of the original 76 patients put on the transplant list, 46 died (10 after transplant, 36 waiting for organs) and 30 were alive, 15 of them still waiting for transplant and 15 of them after getting their new lungs. Of the 15 alive after the new lungs, we can assume that 7 or 8 will likely develop bronchiolitis obliterans, and become sick. The seven or eight others are likely to be doing well. Although such numbers make lung transplantation appear too risky for many people, we should stress that scientists and physicians continue to improve the outlook for lung transplant recipients, and we have reason to expect that more and more patients will do well after the procedure in the future.

MAKING THE DECISION

The decision to proceed with transplantation is always a difficult one. Most patients express disbelief when told that they should consider a transplant; often they just don't feel sick enough to require a transplant. This is especially true for lung transplant candidates. Because there can be a long wait for lungs, patients must get on the list early. In addition, the idea of transplantation can be frightening. It is, after all, an unknown procedure to the patient, and this can be especially difficult for patients (and families) who are used to a routine of treatment for CF. Deciding to undergo a transplantation often means the patient and family will have to get used to a whole new set of physicians and nurses (the transplant team); adding this new care team may interfere with the patient's ways of dealing with his or her original CF team. Finally, a patient who is very sick with CF may be able to accept his or her illness and decide to be comfortable and in control of his or her destiny. Such a patient may not want the uncertainty of transplantation, and may feel it is better to die peacefully rather than be expected to fight to stay alive long enough to receive lungs that may never come.

This last point is one of the most difficult aspects of a family's decision in "going for" transplant.

When your CF doctor suggests that a transplant may be the best thing to do, you must first find out why he or she feels that way. Is it because your PFTs are very bad? Have you gotten worse quickly over the preceding year? Ask your own CF physicians; they will tell you.

Your family can often help you with your decision. For a major procedure like transplantation, particularly one that will surely require lots of care afterwards, you will need help and support. Any form of transplantation is something that should be viewed with both eyes open. The more you and your family understand the procedure and the risks involved, the better you and your physicians will be able to deal with the consequences of transplantation.

Finally, remember that no one can really make your decision about transplantation for you. In addition, *there is no right or wrong decision when and if you are asked to consider having a transplant.* Many patients are eager to have a transplant, many others don't want to consider one under any circumstances. Both groups of patients (and all of those patients whose feelings are in between the two) are right. You must be comfortable with your decision, for you will have to live with the results of your decision.

Deciding to be considered for transplantation, however, does not mean you have to actually undergo transplantation. This is an extremely important point. It is possible, in other words, to be evaluated for a lung transplant, to get on the list for the transplant, be on the top of the list, and *then* decide that you really don't want a transplant. Obviously, if you do this, you will have to have the tests needed for evaluation, and you may have to go on the "inactive" transplant list if you decide not to have a transplant. On the other hand, if you decide *not* to have an evaluation for a lung transplant and change your mind a year later, you may become more sick and possibly too sick to have a transplant safely. Unless you are definitely opposed to a transplant, you should at least discuss it with your physician when it is suggested to you. After you have all the information available, it will be possible for you to make an informed and responsible decision about proceeding or not proceeding with the process of transplantation.

LIVER TRANSPLANTATION

Who Should Be Considered for a New Liver?

Liver transplantation is usually considered in two situations (see Chapter 4, *The Gastrointestinal Tract*, for more details): (a) when there is liver failure, with buildup of toxic chemicals that the liver normally clears from the body, and low levels of chemicals (including protein and factors that help blood clot properly) that the liver normally makes; and (b) when there is uncontrollable bleeding from esophageal varices (the details of this problem are spelled out in Chapter 4).

Who Should Not Be Considered for a New Liver?

Just as there are some people who feel that they don't want any part of the high-tech world of lung transplantation, with its many unknowns and its possible complications, some people make the same decision about liver transplantation. There also are some situations in which there are medical contraindications to (reasons not to do) liver transplantation. A widespread bloodstream infection carries such a high risk of death after transplantation that it is considered an absolute contraindication for any transplant, including liver, by most transplant centers. *Very severe* lung disease is also believed by many to be a contraindication to liver transplantation alone. Perhaps surprisingly, there have been many patients with CF with mildly or even moderately affected lungs whose PFTs have stayed the same or even improved after liver transplantation (see below). There have even been a couple of patients with CF who have received lung and liver transplants during the same surgery.

Transplant List for Liver Transplants

The system for determining your spot on the liver transplant list takes into account the time on the list and how sick you are. Each patient is assigned a score and "patient status" that affects where you are on the list. The score (much like in lung transplantation) is dependent on the severity of the liver disease. For adults (older than 18 years) the score is referred to as a MELD (Model for End-stage Liver Disease). For children (younger than 18 years) the score is referred to as a PELD (Pediatric End-stage Liver Disease). The MELD and PELD help determine how sick people's livers are and set a priority for who should get a liver transplant first. The MELD takes into account bloodwork that includes liver function, kidney function, and blood clotting factors. The PELD takes into account the bloodwork used for the MELD, but also takes into account growth and nutrition. Aside from the MELD and PELD, a patient that is really, really sick from their liver can be assigned a "status 1" classification. Status 1 is given to patients who are in the ICU and not expected to live more than 7 days because of their liver disease. This new system was adopted in 2002. Prior to this, patients with liver disease were given a status based on the severity of their disease (1, 2a, 2b, or 3) and were offered liver transplantations based on their status and the amount of time they had been on the list. The current system with the MELD and PELD allows patients to be prioritized on the list by a severity score. In the event that two patients have the same score, time on the list breaks the tie and the patient with more time on the list will be offered a liver transplantation first.

The wait for a liver is not as long as for lungs, partly because livers can be preserved longer than lungs and therefore can be brought from farther away, and partly because the liver is less delicate than the lung and more likely to have acceptable function despite the injury or illness that has killed the donor or the treatment the donor has received in attempting to save his or her life.

Technique of Liver Transplantation

The liver is located in the upper portion of the right side of the abdomen, just below the diaphragm. Its blood supply comes from an artery (the hepatic artery), and a vein (the portal vein). Blood leaves the liver in a vein known as the hepatic vein. The liver is also connected to the gallbladder, which releases bile into the small intestine through the bile duct. To transplant a liver, the surgeons must make a very large incision across the upper part of the abdomen of the recipient, carefully remove the liver, and then attach the blood vessels to the blood vessels going to and coming from the transplanted liver. The bile duct from the new liver may not be reattached at the time of surgery, and instead is often allowed to drain directly into the small intestine. Because of the difficulty in taking out the damaged liver and replacing it with the transplanted liver, it is not unusual for a liver transplant operation to take more than 9 hours. Because of the many blood vessels that must be attached and because the liver contains a large amount of blood, many transfusions are often needed during the surgery. In addition, some patients have their blood diverted away from the abdomen using an artificial pump to take blood from the lower part of the body and return it directly to the heart while the liver is being replaced.

Because bleeding in the abdomen is fairly common after the surgery, several drainage tubes are placed in the abdomen at the time of surgery. These tubes go out through the skin into small plastic reservoirs, which can hold blood or other secretions that come out of the abdomen. This will allow the surgeons to see if there is a large amount of bleeding in the abdomen following surgery. The drainage tubes will also help with the healing process by removing excess blood from the abdomen. They are usually removed within the first 2 weeks after surgery.

Complications of Liver Transplantation

The most worrisome complications specific to liver transplantation are organ failure, bleeding, and blood clots in the artery or vein to the liver. As with any organ transplantation, rejection of the transplanted organ and infection (of the new organ or elsewhere in the body) are also major concerns, and necessitate very careful dosing of the immunosuppressive medications.

As is the case with any transplanted organ, the liver must be obtained from a donor, and then must be kept alive long enough for the surgeon to place it into the abdomen of the recipient. Over the years, the technique of organ preservation has improved, but it is still not perfect. The liver, once removed from the donor, has its blood washed out to prevent the donor's blood from clotting within the vessels and to prevent the donor's white blood cells from damaging it. The blood is washed out of the liver through the blood vessels, by rinsing a large amount of a special solution that contains minerals and special sugars that will allow the liver to remain alive even though the blood is gone. Sometimes, despite the best efforts to preserve the function of the liver, it is injured, either while it is still in the donor, or after it has been removed (this might be or because the preservation process is inadequate). If this occurs, then the liver will not work after transplantation, and the patient will have liver failure. In some instances, the liver damage may be so severe that the patient dies. In other cases, the liver may recover enough function to allow the patient to survive and ultimately do well.

As mentioned before, bleeding is a fairly common problem during the liver transplantation procedure itself. Bleeding can also be a dangerous problem in the hours and days following transplantation. The drainage tubes placed into the abdomen at the time of surgery can alert the surgeons to bleeding after surgery. Although blood and clotting factors given to the recipient after surgery may stop the bleeding, there are instances in which the only way to stop the bleeding is for the surgeon to reopen the abdomen and find the blood vessels that are bleeding and stop the bleeding directly.

Blood clots can form and block the blood vessels to the transplanted liver. In some cases, these clots can decrease blood flow to the liver, leading to liver damage. At times, such clots must be removed surgically, by opening the abdomen, locating the clot in the blood vessel, opening the blood vessel, removing the clot, and then surgically closing the blood vessel. Clotting within major blood vessels to the liver, unfortunately, does not always resolve, or may lead to irreversible liver damage before the clots can be removed.

Care After Liver Transplantation

Tests After Liver Transplantation

As with lung transplant recipients, liver recipients must undergo regular tests to make sure the new liver is functioning well. Blood tests of liver function (usually abbreviated as LFTs) are followed on a frequent basis, but if rejection is thought to be likely, biopsies are necessary.

A liver biopsy is done by cleaning and numbing the skin over the liver and then inserting a special needle directly into the liver. This needle is designed to cut into the liver and hold a small piece of the liver inside the needle as the needle is removed. The biopsy can then be sent to the laboratory and examined. As with the lung biopsies, liver biopsies are usually performed after the patient has been given some IV sedative medication.

Complications of Liver Biopsy

Most liver biopsies are performed with no ill effects. But, as with any procedure, there is a small chance of problems. The biggest risk of liver biopsy is bleeding. The liver has a rich supply of blood vessels, and it is possible to tear one of these and cause bleeding. In most cases, the bleeding isn't serious, but, particularly if the liver isn't working well and not making blood clotting factors normally, it can be difficult to control.

Ongoing Care

After liver transplantation, as with lung transplantation, continuing care is absolutely essential and never-ending. Treatment with immunosuppressant (antirejection) medications is very important. Other CF treatments, such as enzymes and nutritional supplements, are also necessary. Patients will still need to do airway clearance. In most cases, care can take place at your regular CF center, with periodic visits back to the transplant center. As in the case of lung transplantation, it is important that your CF physician and the transplant team work together to deliver the best care possible to maintain good liver function as well as to preserve lung function.

Results of Liver Transplantation

The results for liver transplantation for people with CF are a little harder to know for certain than those for lung transplantation, because there have been far fewer liver transplantation procedures done in patients with CF. In 2008, out of the more than 25,000 people with CF in the United States, only 8 had liver transplantations. In one large CF and transplant center, approximately 92% of the patients with CF who received liver transplants survived 1 year after the procedure, and 75% survived 5 years.

One surprising result has been that patients with CF who have received liver transplants do not have an immediate worsening of their lung infection, as many people worried they would. The reason for the worry, of course, was that these patients have to take immunosuppressive medications to prevent liver rejection. Immunosuppressive medicines decrease the body's ability to fight infection, and there already is infection in the lungs of people with CF. So most physicians assumed that lung infection would worsen as soon as someone with CF was started on immunosuppressive medicines. Instead, what happens is that in most cases the lung function of patients with CF either doesn't change or actually gets a bit better in the weeks to months after liver transplantation. The reasons for this are not completely clear, but one possible explanation is that the immunosuppressive medicines cut down on the inflammation within the airways. As you've seen in Chapter 3, anti-inflammatory medicines, such as steroids, can sometimes be helpful in patients with CF. It may be that this anti-inflammatory action of the immunosuppressives helps more than the increased risk of infection hurts.

LUNG AND LIVER TRANSPLANTATION

At this point you may be asking yourself, "If you can transplant both lungs and livers for CF, and if CF affects both lungs and livers, can you transplant both a lung and a liver at the same time if someone needs both?" The short answer is "yes." But, this is not a very common thing to have done.

It is not very common that someone would have very sick lungs and a very sick liver that would need to be transplanted at the same time. Because of this, not many people have had a combination lung–liver transplantation. But it has been done.

The difficulty with doing a combination lung–liver transplantation is that both surgeries are difficult surgeries on their own. To combine the two surgeries significantly increases the risks. Also, just as there are not a whole lot of lungs and livers available for donation, getting a combination lung–liver for transplantation is pretty rare. Nevertheless, there are situations in which the patient would need to have both organs transplanted at the same time mostly because each organ is too sick to survive a significant surgery like a transplantation. That is, someone with sick lungs would not be able to survive a liver transplantation. Conversely, someone with a sick liver would not be able to survive a lung transplantation.

Fortunately, the medications used to prevent rejection after lung and liver transplantation are the same. Because the lungs require more antirejection medications after transplantation, the medications used to prevent rejection of the lungs can be used (and are actually more than enough) to prevent rejection of the liver.

THE FUTURE OF TRANSPLANTATION

Transplantation is a young science, and many physicians and research scientists are working to unravel its secrets and solve its many problems. With the development of newer antirejection medications and an improved understanding of the ways to prevent and treat the complications of transplantation, the future of transplantation is bright. It remains, however, a major medical and surgical commitment for any patient who wishes to pursue this avenue of treatment. Confidence in the transplant physicians, a willingness to undergo special tests, an ability to cooperate with the transplant team, and a firm commitment to taking on a difficult posttransplant care program will increase the chances for any one patient to undergo transplantation successfully. It is clear that there is much to learn about transplantation, but the many patients with CF who are alive following liver or lung transplantation are a testimony of the promise inherent in this form of therapy.

Daily Life

9

Jonathan E. Spahr, David M. Orenstein, and
Daniel J. Weiner

THE BASICS

1. Most patients with cystic fibrosis (CF) should be expected to live a very normal daily life (except for treatments): They go to school, do homework, have friends, play sports, grow up, many marry, and so on.

2. Children with CF should have the same expectations and responsibilities as other children.

There are many aspects of daily life that are altered very little by having CF: Babies cry and laugh, and children still sleep through the night, wake up, go to the bathroom, have breakfast, go to school, play with friends, play sports, do homework and chores, watch television, and go to parties. They may go on trips with or without their families. They grow up and finish school and take up jobs; many marry and may decide to raise a family. It is very important for a child's emotional well-being, and that of the family, that daily life be approached with these expectations. The emotional aspect of living with CF is discussed in Chapter 12 (*The Family*), and the issues that relate specifically to teens and adults are addressed in Chapters 13 (*The Teenage Years*) and 14 (*Cystic Fibrosis and Adulthood*), respectively. This chapter addresses the few areas in which CF does have an effect on the patient's (or his/her family's) daily life.

In most stages of life, patients with CF require some form of airway clearance therapy, anywhere from one to four times a day. Approximately 90% of people with CF must remember, or be reminded, to take digestive enzymes with each meal and usually with snacks. Most patients will also have to take vitamins each day, and many will need to take antibiotics by mouth fairly frequently.

Clinic visits for checkups will be required anywhere from one to eight times a year, depending on your physician's approach and your health. These visits are very important for health maintenance(see Chapter 3, *The Respiratory System*).

During periods of pulmonary exacerbation (see Chapter 3), it may be necessary to pay visits to the hospital for 1 to 3 weeks or to receive intravenous antibiotics at home (see Chapter 7, *Hospitalization and Other Special Treatments*). This treatment may be necessary one to three times a year for as many as one in every three or four patients.

Patients who have more severe lung disease may need to lessen the intensity of their physical exertion, and a very few may even need to wear oxygen tubing while they sleep, and perhaps when they are up and around.

Meal times should not be too different for people with CF than they would be if they did not have CF, except for remembering to take enzymes. Individuals with CF-related diabetes may need to check their blood sugar levels and give themselves insulin. If someone has had trouble putting (or keeping) weight on, they may need meals with added fats and calories, or even nighttime tube feedings, (see Chapter 6, *Nutrition*).

MEDICATIONS AND TREATMENTS: WHO IS IN CHARGE?

During a child's the early years, the parents are responsible for medications and must know which medicines should be taken when, why they are needed, and what additional treatments are required. By the time a young adult leaves home, he or she must be in charge. Most experts believe that a good time for the transition of this responsibility from the parents to the young patient is early in the teenage years, but you need to start early promoting responsibility and decision making. This which takes practice. Both the parent and child need to practice together.

You may have noticed that children, at times, can be defiant and will "push back" when asked to follow certain rules. Getting children to "follow the rules" can be difficult for any parent. With CF care added to daily life, this can be more challenging.

Rules may fall into different categories that deal with things such as safety, behavior, personal business, etc. "Don't play in traffic" is a rule that most children will not struggle with because if the reason behind the rule is explained ("we don't want you to be hit by a car"), most children will understand and obey the rule. This is a rule about personal safety. "Put your coat on, it's cold out" is a little bit more difficult. While the parent may be able to explain that they don't want their child to be cold, the child may counter with "So what if I'm cold, it's my decision." And, the child has a point. Unless you live in North Dakota and it's February, there is probably not a life-threatening situation that would arise from your child not wearing a coat. This is a rule about personal business. This category of rules can be very difficult to negotiate between the parent and child. Other situations that fall into this category include personal hygiene, child chooses to hang out with, curfews, and the list goes on and on.

Depending upon one's perspective, CF care can fall into both categories of rules (safety or personal business). From the parent's perspective, CF care is a matter of health and safety. Parents know that if consistent, good care is given to children and adults with CF, they have a much greater chance of living a long and healthy life. From the child's perspective, CF care may be a matter of personal business ("It's my life and my body. I get to choose whether I take care of myself or not.") Get ready for this and know that it will only get worse before it gets better (see Chapter 13, *The Teenage Years*).

What is a Parent to do? What are the Options?

It is important to prepare yourself and your child for these situations that will inevitably arise. The parent needs to be prepared and practiced in the art of providing situations that allow the child to accept responsibility, and the child needs to be prepared and practiced in accepting that responsibility. One of the best ways to prepare a child to accept responsibility is to give them responsibility. Giving a child a set of tasks (ugh, chores) for which they are responsible builds their confidence and organizational skills. Children can accept this responsibility early (3 to 7 years of age). Parents should be prepared to reward for successful completion of these tasks. Start with hugs or stickers. If you start with money, things can get out of control quickly—trust us. The responsibility/reward interaction can be great preparation and practice for CF care.

Another way to promote responsibility in children is to give them the sense of control. A lot of this can be accomplished by how a request is phrased. Give options that allow your child to make decisions for themselves. "It seems to be pretty cold out, would you like to wear your new blue coat or your Steelers sweatshirt?" "Would you like to take all of your enzymes at the beginning of the meal or would you like to take half now and then half midway through the meal?" "Would you like me to do chest clapping or would you rather use your vest and watch a show?" The option that your child chooses may not be your ideal option, but remember, the treatment/medication that gets at least partially done is much better than one that is not done at all.

There will be times when certain treatments or medications are non-negotiable. These non-negotiable tasks are life lessons that are important for all of us to learn. Allowing some responsibility or personal choice for certain tasks that are negotiable will make the non-negotiable tasks easier for your child to take. If you really hit a roadblock, *gasp* . . . talk with your child. Find out why there is such resistance to doing a treatment. This conversation may open up an opportunity to decide together what tasks are negotiable and, in return, what tasks they just have to do.

Exerting your dominance and using fear as motivators may be effective in the short-term, but are not effective long-term motivators. Saying "Because I said so," "As long as you live under my roof . . .," and "I brought you into this world and I can take you out," is easy and may work, but who is benefitting from this type of interaction? Showing patience and treating your child with respect teaches them that they also can respond to difficult situations with patience and respect for others. This can be really, really hard. Again, practice is necessary. Don't give up.

Of course, this is all very easy to say and much harder (for us, anyway) to do. No one is perfect and no one has received extensive training in how to be a parent, much less how to be a parent to a child with CF. Talk to those who have done it before you, read books, talk to your CF doctor/nurse/social worker/dietician, practice how you might respond to situations that you can predict, and admit to yourself that you will make mistakes. This is another important lesson that your child will learn from you.

Again, if it seems challenging now, it can get worse once your child becomes a teenager. Therefore, the sooner you can establish a mutually respectful means for transferring responsibility over to your child, the better. Allowing a teen to take day care on responsibility without practice can set them up for failure during a particularly fragile time with regard to their emotional and physical health. Eighteen is just an age. Don't expect your child to all of the sudden become an adult and take on adult responsibilities at 18. They, as we did, need a lot of preparation.

Even when children are properly prepared, adolescence is both a good and a bad time for accomplishing the transition in responsibility for medical care. It is a good time because the teenager wants very much to become independent of the parent and is looking for ways to assert that independence. Teenagers welcome the trust that accompanies responsibility as well as the absence of nagging that results when they have learned all their medications and take them faithfully. Adolescence can be a difficult time, however, for the transition in responsibility, because in normal teenage rebellion against authority there is a strong urge to ignore what the parents want. More discussion on this will follow later (see Chapter 13).

DAYCARE

Daycare has become very common for many families with babies, especially if both parents work. Babies in day care get more colds than those kept at home. Babies with CF will get neither more nor fewer colds than the other babies, but some of these colds may develop into bronchial infections (*pulmonary exacerbations*). This fact has made some families avoid day care. For the first months of an infant's life, when the bronchi are very tiny and when infants with CF may have more trouble keeping the bronchi clear, it may be advisable to delay day care. However, if this is financially difficult, it should not be considered a major setback. Remember that the goal of avoiding all colds is impossible to achieve, especially if there are other children in the family, and that careful attention to an infant's health, with quick treatment for any pulmonary infections, is likely to result in very good maintenance of health.

Occasionally, a misguided day care supervisor, parent, or even physician may be concerned that the presence of an infant with CF will pose a danger to the other children in daycare. *CF is not contagious.* Even if a baby with CF is coughing a lot, the bacteria in its lungs are not dangerous to children without CF. Of course, a baby with CF can get a regular cold, just like any other baby, and pass that cold on to anyone else, but babies with CF should not be excluded from day care just because of having CF or cough.

SCHOOL

School is very important for all children, and virtually all children with CF should be able to go to school and carry a full load, including homework and extracurricular activities. When a child has a lung infection, he or she may not feel as well as usual, but in most cases this should not interfere with education. Children should be encouraged to go to school, even if they are coughing more than usual, as long as they are receiving the appropriate treatment (antibiotics and increased airway clearance treatments).

Teachers may need to be educated about CF to make a very few special considerations for the child with CF. They need to be aware that the child with CF is likely to have more cough than other children and should never be discouraged from coughing. The child with CF may also need to have more frequent bathroom privileges. Most CF centers have a very good booklet designed for teachers (see Appendix F, *Bibliography*).

Homework should be required from the child with CF, just as from his or her peers. There should be almost no exceptions to this rule. Even if a child has to be hospitalized, he or she should keep up with schoolwork. If a child is hospitalized, the school district should provide tutoring to enable the child to keep up with the class.

Physical education class is as important (or even more important) for children with CF as for other children. Physical education class should not be graded on the basis of athletic performance for any child, especially those who might have a physical reason for lower than average performance, as a child with CF and lung disease might have.

COLLEGE

See Chapter 13 (*The Teenage Years*) for a discussion of going to college—going away or staying home.

SPORTS AND EXERCISE

In general, there is no reason for children, adolescents, or adults with CF to avoid exercise. Exercise is good for most people, including people with CF. Everyone, with CF or without it, needs to adjust the amount and intensity of exercise to his or her own abilities and needs, but this can be done fairly easily. (Exercise and sports are discussed more in Chapter 10, *Exercise*.)

VISITS WITH FRIENDS

Visiting with friends, either at their houses or your own, is an important part of growing up, learning to get along with others, and learning to become independent away from home. Children and adolescents with CF should have these same opportunities as anyone else. In most cases, special arrangements will have to be made to ensure that medications are being taken and that treatments are being done. In some cases, for a single overnighter for a grade-school child, it might not be a problem to skip a single day's treatment, but this should not become a habit. Adolescents who give themselves their own treatments (especially if they do their airway clearance with a portable device like the acapella® should be able to do this anywhere. If either part of the visiting pair is sick, changes may have to be made, but this is no different from what would be done if neither child had CF. All experts now advise against close contacts (like overnights) between patients with CF, to avoid the possibility of their sharing potentially harmful lung bacteria. Although the bacteria that patients with CF may cough out or have on their hands present absolutely no danger to people without CF, there is a small but real risk of harm to someone with CF (see Chapter 3 for more discussion of the issue of *person-to-person transmission* of CF bacteria).

SMOKING

People with any form of lung disease should not smoke, nor should they inhale other people's smoke. This is certainly true for people with CF. Smoke is harmful to children's lungs, even if the lungs are normal. Someone who has abnormal lungs, especially if asthma is part of the condition, has a greatly increased risk of complications if he or she must breathe cigarette smoke. Smoke from cigarettes can be harmful to a child's lungs even if the person smoking the cigarette loves the child very much. Parents whose child has CF should stop smoking immediately, and smoking should not be allowed in their homes. Most people, including smokers, know that smoking is very harmful to the smoker; not everyone realizes that it is also harmful to the lungs of children who are forced to breathe in the second-hand smoke. *It has been shown unequivocally that being exposed to parents' cigarette smoke causes worsened lung function in children with CF.*

Many parents who have been unsuccessful at stopping smoking are able to stop when they realize that it is not just for their own health but for the children's as well. If you cannot stop right away, it is essential that you stop smoking in the house. If you are smoking in the same house, the child will get the fumes. You must especially never smoke in the car, even with the windows down, since it is a space where smoke can get very thick and irritating. If you need help stopping, your physician may be able to help. For someone who is truly addicted to cigarettes, the addiction is every bit as serious as—and *harder to break* than—a heroin addiction. (Some people feel it's even worse than heroin, since with heroin it's mostly the person directly taking the drug whose health is impaired, while with cigarettes, it's also the "innocent bystanders.") Nicotine chewing gum and patches have been helpful for people who are dedicated to stopping smoking but cannot do it on their own.

TRAVEL

Patients with CF can travel, just as people without CF can travel. There are a few practical considerations for the traveling CF patient.

Remember to Take Your Medicines

Some medications used for patients with CF (especially enzymes) may not be carried in every pharmacy, so it may be difficult to replace medications while you are away from your regular pharmacy. For longer trips, it may be advisable to speak with your CF doctor about providing a prescription for antibiotics "just in case" you run into problems while away and need to start treatment for a CF exacerbation. If you travel out of state, you may find that a pharmacy will not accept your doctor's prescription if he or she is not licensed in the state you are visiting. In most cases, pharmacists are very helpful and will do what they can to provide you with the service you need, but it is better to be prepared for an emergency.

Remember to Take Any Equipment You Might Need for Aerosols or Airway Clearance Treatments

If you are going on a short trip, it may be possible to bring less bulky equipment than you use at home. For example, if you use the vest for airway clearance, your doctor might approve the Flutter® or acapella® device for your trip; you might be able to user inhalers instead of nebulizer treatments for a short time (see Chapter 3 for more details). If you are traveling to a different country, you may need to bring special electrical outlet adapters for whatever electrical equipment you use, because different countries use different power sources. Adapters are available to enable you to convert the power source to fit your own equipment.

High Altitude

If you live at or near sea level and travel to higher altitudes, you may experience difficulty because of the lower oxygen pressures at altitude. The air in Denver, for example, has only 80% as much oxygen as that in San Diego or Boston. Someone whose lungs are in excellent condition should have no trouble in these places, but someone who has serious lung involvement may be comfortable and safe at sea level but may develop problems in the mountains. It is a good idea to discuss travel plans with your doctor before embarking on a journey.

Low Altitude (Scuba Diving)

Most scuba diving outfitters will not allow people with chronic lung disease (asthma, CF, emphysema) to participate in scuba diving. The risk is that the pressure changes that occur while scuba diving can cause harmful and even life-threatening complications in lungs that are not completely healthy. This is a risk even in people who do not have chronic lung disease. This risk is not worth taking for people with CF and so scuba diving should be discouraged. Snorkeling is a different story. In snorkeling, there are no significant pressure differences that can cause lung damage. So, snorkel to your heart's content.

Airplane Travel

Commercial airlines pressurize their cabins from 5,000 to 8,000 feet. That means that the oxygen level inside the cabin is comparable to Denver's or a place even higher. The majority of patients with CF and with mild or even moderate lung disease can fly in commercial airliners without any problem. If you need oxygen at sea level, you will need more in an airplane, and if you are close to needing it at home, you may need it while you fly. The major airlines are used to dealing with requests for oxygen during flights, and usually are very helpful, but *most insist that you contact them well in advance* to let them know about your plans and needs (usually there is a special medical department to contact at the airline).

SUMMER CAMP

Summer camps can provide valuable experience for children and adolescents, and most children and adolescents with CF should be able to attend camps if they want to. Most children whose lungs are in good shape and whose digestion is fairly well controlled with enzymes should be able to attend any kind of camp, as long as arrangements for medications and treatments can be made with the camp physicians and nurses. Many areas used to have CF camps, especially for kids with CF. These have now all disappeared, because of the risk of infection (see Chapter 3).

WHERE TO LIVE

People often wonder whether there are areas of the country that are better than others for children (and adults) with CF. From what is known now, the answer is no. In individual patients, it is possible that they might do better in one geographic location than another, but so many factors influence how a person will do and patients are so different from each other, so that no one place has the perfect combination of factors that make for good health for all people with CF.

Cities and states differ in the amount of pollution, cold, wetness, allergens, and in the availability of good medical care. While one might think that the cold, wet, polluted, industrial, northeastern cities (Cleveland, Pittsburgh, Boston, Toronto, etc.) would be the worst places for CF patients to live, national survival statistics, which measure how long people live, previously showed that it was exactly these cities that had the best CF survival. The explanation almost certainly lies in the fact that these cities have had excellent CF centers for the longest time. Excellent CF centers now exist in most regions of the United States, Canada, Europe, and Australia, and the survival statistics now reflect this change. Most CF physicians believe that ready access to a good CF center is very important, but other than this criterion, there is very little basis for recommending one geographic area over another for a person with CF.

Exercise 10

David M. Orenstein and Daniel J. Weiner

THE BASICS

1. Exercise is good for virtually all people with CF.

2. People with CF lose more salt and drink less fluid than normal when they exercise in the heat.

3. Physically fit CF patients live longer than those who are not fit.

4. Children with CF should be encouraged to be active from a very young age, and that active lifestyle should continue throughout their lives.

Everyone is interested in exercise these days. People with cystic fibrosis (CF) are no exception. Exercise done properly, in the right amount, the right intensity, and with the proper safety precautions, can be fun and beneficial for nearly everyone and may enable you to live longer as well!

EFFECTS OF EXERCISE ON PEOPLE WITHOUT CF

Single Sessions of Exercise

When someone begins muscular exercise, the body has to make some fast adaptations, most of which relate to supplying the exercising muscles with considerably more oxygen than is needed at rest. These adaptations help the muscles remove excess carbon dioxide, which is produced when they are active. Muscles are able to contract and move the body without oxygen, but this is much more difficult than muscular work performed with adequate oxygen. Work that is performed without adequate oxygen being supplied to the muscles is called *anaerobic* work, and work that is performed with enough oxygen is called *aerobic* work. Anaerobic exercise can be carried out only for a period of seconds or minutes, whereas aerobic exercise can be sustained for many minutes or even hours. Anaerobic exercise is not only more difficult and less efficient than aerobic exercise but also results in the production of lactic acid in the muscles and in the production of considerably more carbon dioxide, which then has to be removed.

Since oxygen is supplied to the exercising muscles (and carbon dioxide is removed) by circulating blood, one of the first changes at the beginning of exercise is an increase in blood flow to the active muscle. Since the heart has to pump more blood, it has to pump faster, and the heart rate (pulse) increases. The heart rate reaches a maximum which can be predicted fairly accurately from a person's age: maximum heart rate $= 220 -$ age (in years). Thus, a 20-year-old person would have a predicted maximum heart rate of $220 - 20 = 200$ beats per minute. It is also necessary to increase the amount of oxygen available to the blood, and, especially with anaerobic exercise, to increase the disposal of carbon dioxide. The increase in oxygen supply and carbon dioxide removal are both accomplished by increasing the amount of air that is breathed each minute. The accuracy of these adjustments is astounding, as you've already seen in Chapter 3. During heavy exercise, the heart may increase its output five- or sixfold, and the lungs may bring in (and exhale) 5 to 10 times as much air as they do during naps, and, yet, the level of oxygen and carbon dioxide in the bloodstream remain nearly constant.

It takes anywhere from a few seconds to $1\frac{1}{2}$ minutes to adjust the amount of blood the heart pumps to the exercising muscles. Therefore, during the first seconds of exercise, the muscles are undersupplied with oxygen. In other words, the first seconds of any form of exercise are anaerobic exercise. Exercise that is strictly "stop-and-go," in which you exercise, rest, then exercise again (for example racquet sports) is anaerobic exercise. Exercise is also anaerobic if it is very heavy work and the muscles demand more oxygen than can be supplied (like heavy weightlifting, hard running, or riding a bike up a steep hill). In contrast, aerobic exercise is a low-intensity, rhythmic type of activity, such as walking, swimming, easy jogging, and bike riding.

Exercise in the Heat

The more someone exercises, especially in hot weather, the more heat the body produces. If the body temperature becomes too high, it can be dangerous; so there has to be a way for body temperature to be regulated and for excess heat to be lost. This is accomplished through several mechanisms. The first is that a greater amount of blood than usual is sent to the skin, especially to the scalp and hands. This is a way of bringing the warmth of the body close to the surface, where it can be given off to the surrounding air (unless the air is hotter than body temperature). If all of the blood stayed in the heart and other internal organs, it would be insulated by the skin, muscles, and fat, and the heat would build up. The other way of giving off excess heat is through sweating. As sweat evaporates, it cools the surface of the body. This is why you sweat when you exercise, especially in the heat.

Exercise Tolerance

When someone is given a test on an exercise cycle, it becomes progressively more difficult to pedal and, eventually, *everyone* will arrive at a point where he or she can no longer pedal. In most healthy people, the point at which this occurs is determined by two factors. The first is that the heart reaches a point at which it can no longer increase the amount of blood it pumps to the muscles, so the muscles become relatively undersupplied with blood and oxygen and become fatigued. This usually happens when the heart has reached the maximum rate of beating. If a 20-year-old person is exercising so hard that the heart rate is 200 beats per minute, it will not be able to go any faster, so the amount of blood being pumped out will not be able to increase any further.

The second limiting factor may be the muscles themselves: there is a limit to how much oxygen the muscles can process, so they may become fatigued even though enough oxygen has been delivered. In someone with normal lungs, the lungs are never the limiting factor in exercise. Even at total exhaustion, the lungs have considerable reserve. Recall from Chapter 3 that the maximum voluntary ventilation (MVV) is the measurement that estimates the largest amount of air a person can move in and out of the lungs in a minute. During exercise, even at the point of total exhaustion, most people don't use any more than 70% of their MVV; that is, their lungs could still deliver another 30% effort. But this wouldn't help, since other factors would have impeded the exercise before the extra breathing reserves were needed.

Repeated Sessions of Exercise (Exercise Programs)

If you exercise each day, or at least 3 days a week, for a certain minimum time (10 to 30 minutes a day) and at a certain minimum intensity (hard enough to raise your heart rate to approximately 75% of its maximum, which is around 150 beats per minute for adolescents and young adults), after a few weeks (6 to 12 weeks), you will become more fit; that is, you will be able to do more of the same kind of exercise with less stress on your body. If the type of exercise you were doing each day was aerobic, then you will increase your *aerobic fitness*. If it was anaerobic exercise, then your *anaerobic fitness* will increase. Jogging 30 minutes each day will make it much easier for you to jog, but it will not make you able to lift 200 pounds, whereas lifting weights every day will make your muscles stronger (and bigger) for weightlifting tasks, but will not improve your endurance or your ability to carry out prolonged walks or bike rides.

With repeated aerobic exercise sessions, involving walking or jogging, one of the ways in which you become more fit is that your heart becomes stronger and can pump more blood with each beat; therefore, you need fewer heart beats to deliver the same amount of blood to the muscles. You can see this change by checking your heart rate for a certain workload before you start an exercise program, then rechecking it after a few months of exercise. The easiest "workload" to check is no work at all, that is, measure your heart rate while you're resting. The more fit someone is, the lower his or her resting heart rate. You may know runners who brag about having a resting heart rate of 45 or 50 beats per minute. Please don't make fun of them; just let them brag.

Another change that occurs with a training program and increased fitness is in the muscles themselves: They become able to process much more oxygen and to put that oxygen to use in performing work.

One change that does not occur with an exercise training program is in lung function. Most scientific studies have shown no important changes in lung function in healthy people after they train and become very fit. Since lung function doesn't have much to do with one's exercise ability if the lungs are normal, this doesn't make much difference to most people.

There is increasing evidence that people who engage in lifelong exercise live longer than sedentary people and have lower risks for various diseases, especially heart disease and some kinds of cancer.

Exercise training programs have long been felt to be valuable to the emotional health of the people as well as their physical health, with decreased depression and stress levels and increased work productivity. Many big corporations have installed impressive gym facilities for their employees because they have felt that fit employees were happier, healthier, and more productive.

Heat Training

Another change that comes with an exercise program, especially if it's been carried out in the heat, is that you become heat-acclimatized; that is, you can withstand exercise and heat stress better than you could before you got in shape. Several changes account for this improved heat tolerance. The first is just that exercise itself is easier because of your being more fit (lower heart rate, etc.), without regard to the heat. But additional changes occur that are related specifically to increased heat tolerance. People who train in the heat begin to sweat earlier during an exercise session, thus cooling themselves earlier, through evaporation. In addition, and quite remarkably, when someone without CF trains in the heat for several weeks, the sweat that is produced contains less salt. This may be the body's way of preserving salt, since a lot salt can be lost when someone sweats excessively. (People running a marathon can easily lose 5 to 10 pounds of sweat in 3 or 4 hours.)

EFFECTS OF EXERCISE IN PEOPLE WITH CF

Single Sessions of Exercise

The responses to exercise of people with CF are generally similar to those of people who don't have CF. To meet the increased needs of exercising muscles for oxygen supply and carbon dioxide removal, both the heart's output and the amount of breathing are considerably increased. If a person's lung function is normal or nearly normal, he or she will have exactly the same responses to exercise as anyone else. However, there are some differences in the response to exercise in someone with CF whose pulmonary function is not normal. One difference is that people with CF frequently stop exercising before their heart rate has reached the maximum predicted based upon age. In these cases, the minute ventilation (the amount of air being breathed each minute) may be very large in comparison with the person's capacity or reserve. Remember that people with normal lungs seldom breathe more than 70% of their MVV (where MVV is an *estimate* of their maximum capacity), even during strenuous exercise. People with CF often use more than 80% of their MVV (in some cases, more than 100% of their "maximum" capacity is used!). Even as you can't expect a person with a normal heart to make the heart beat faster than its maximum, you can't expect *anyone*—with or without healthy lungs—to be able to use more than 100% of the predicted capacity of the lungs.

Most patients with CF maintain their blood levels of oxygen and carbon dioxide during exercise. In some patients, the blood oxygen level actually increases with exercise. However, in people with severe lung disease, the blood oxygen level may fall during exercise, and in some of these patients, the carbon dioxide level may increase. [This decrease in oxygen level does not occur in anyone whose forced expired volume (FEV1) is greater than 50% of their forced vital capacity (FVC; see Chapter 3), and it doesn't occur even in most people whose FEV_1 is that low.] If someone's whose oxygen level does fall, and/or carbon dioxide level increases, this means that for the amount of oxygen being used and the amount of carbon dioxide being produced by the exercising muscles, the person is not breathing enough. It is not known if this is harmful, but most CF physicians recommend that patients avoid this situation. That does not mean to avoid exercise altogether. Specific exercise guidelines are discussed later in this chapter.

Some people with CF also have asthma, particularly in response to exercise (*exercise-induced asthma,* or EIA). This is a common condition and one that need not curtail your exercise program—about 10% of the athletes on the United States Olympic team in several different recent Olympics have had EIA! We mention this not to guarantee you a spot on the team, but just to let you know that people with EIA may still be able to exercise and compete at a very high level. People with EIA will experience cough, wheeze, chest tightness, chest pain, or a combination of these symptoms when they exercise—typically, it's a few minutes *after* they exercise. The exercise that is most likely to bring on these symptoms is vigorous exercise—especially running—lasting 6 to 8 minutes and especially in cold air. The problem can be prevented in the majority of people with a couple of puffs from a bronchodilator (like albuterol) metered-dose inhaler about 15 minutes before exercise.

Many people with CF (whether or not they have asthma as well) cough during or after exercise. This may be distressing to someone who is watching, if they don't know about CF, and may be somewhat uncomfortable to the person coughing, but it is not dangerous. In fact, it is probably helpful in bringing mucus up out of the lungs.

Exercise in the Heat

Having CF should not prevent someone from exercising in the heat. People with CF have the same ability as those without CF to keep their body temperature down while exercising in hot weather. However, since they have the same mechanisms for doing this, including sweating, and since CF sweat is so much saltier than any other sweat, athletes with CF lose much more salt than their non-CF teammates. They may lose so much that the blood levels of sodium and chloride drop. In most cases this does not cause a problem. Young people with CF also have a very accurate salt "thermostat" that enables them to know how much salt they need to take after exercise to replace what they've lost during exercise. Replacing salt is something that can be done over a period of hours and does not have to be done immediately after it's lost.

Replacing lost fluid is quite another matter, though, for anyone with or without CF. It is very important for all people who exercise in the heat to drink plenty of fluid, but it is particularly important for children and adults with CF to drink while they exercise in hot weather, because while their salt "thermostat" works well, their fluid "thermostat" is a little sluggish. *All* children tend to drink less fluid than they lose during exercise in the heat, but children with CF are especially bad at drinking as much as they need.

Exercise Tolerance

Many children and adults with CF who have good lung function are limited in their exercise capacity by the same factors that limit their classmates; namely, the heart reaches a limit to how much blood it can pump, and/or the muscles reach a limit to how much oxygen they can process. These factors will be especially limiting if someone has not exercised much and is out of shape. But those whose lungs are affected more extensively by CF are likely to be limited by the lungs before the heart and muscles are pushed to their limits. This does not necessarily mean that their blood oxygen levels will fall, but rather that the work of breathing may just become too uncomfortable and they will need to stop because of that discomfort. Even in people whose oxygen level does fall, it is probably the discomfort of hard breathing and not the lowered oxygen level that forces them to stop running or pedaling. Even so, there are some people who benefit from using oxygen during exercise and are able to do considerably more exercise if they use extra oxygen when they are active.

Although coughing may be severe, it seldom limits exercise.

Exercise Programs for People with CF

Exercise programs have the same benefit for people with CF that they have for people without CF, namely, increasing their fitness and sense of well-being and probably improving their overall outlook on life. "Increased fitness" is defined as being able to do more physical work and having a lower heart rate for the same workload. Some studies have shown better lung function after a CF exercise training program, and other studies have shown no change in lung function. A very important study showed that CF patients' fitness level corresponded more closely with their survival (how likely they were to be alive 8 years later) than any other factor. So, although it hasn't yet been proved that becoming more fit means you'll live longer, it's tempting to think so and act as if that's so by working to get and stay in shape!

For people with normal lungs, strenuous aerobic exercise programs should raise the heart rate to 75% of its maximum, or about 150 beats per minute. A number of people with CF will not be able to exercise this hard, because their breathing will stop them before their heart rate has risen that high. This does not mean that someone with CF cannot become more fit. In fact, it seems that CF patients can become more fit by exercising hard enough to raise their heart rates to 75% of *their own* maximum and not the maximum that you'd predict on the basis of their age. Thus, if someone with CF has a maximum heart rate of 150 beats per minute (that is the pulse goes up to 150 during the most strenuous exercise he or she can tolerate), that person will be able to benefit from regular exercise sessions with the heart beating around 115 beats a minute (roughly 75% of 150).

Fortunately, it's not necessary to measure the heart rate precisely during all exercise sessions to know if you're working hard enough to bring about improvements; instead, you can strive for a *pleasantly tired* feeling. If you're not at all tired, you are not working hard enough. On the other hand, if you're so tired that you don't feel at all good, you're pushing yourself harder than you need. That becomes important in planning a long-term exercise program, because human nature is such that no one wants to do unpleasant things, and exercise is no exception: if your exercise sessions leave you exhausted and feeling bad, you will be much more likely to find excuses to skip them than if they are enjoyable. In the section after the next, there will be an introduction to the nitty-gritty of carrying out an exercise program.

Heat Training in CF

Like everyone else, people with CF can become adapted to exercise in the heat. If you exercise in the heat every day for a week or more, at the end of that period, your heart rate and body temperature will be lower when you do that same exercise in the heat than they were on the first day.

When you have CF, you are likely to lose large amounts of sodium and chloride (in your sweat) during each exercise session in the heat. This is very important, because a major difference between the normal response to heat training and the CF response is that CF sweat glands cannot decrease the salt content of sweat. This means that even though you have greater tolerance for exercise and heat stress, you still lose much more salt than is normal. In addition, after you've trained for a while, you will begin to sweat earlier in the exercise session (this change occurs in everyone during heat training) and you will also be able to exercise for a longer period, thus losing even more salt after you've become adapted to the heat.

In between exercise sessions, if you allow yourself to eat and drink without restriction, you will find that you automatically select items that will completely replace the lost salt, but you should be careful to make sure you drink more than you think you need *during* the exercise sessions. Consuming sports drinks like Gatorade® can help.

GUIDELINES FOR AN EXERCISE PROGRAM

General

Most CF physicians now feel that exercise is beneficial for all CF patients and that an active lifestyle should begin early in childhood, well before a formal "program" is prescribed. In most cases, more activity is better than less, and parents should encourage activity from very early on. As with any child, parental encouragement is good; aggressive parental pushing is probably not. Parents can often help establish the exercise habit in their children by example: if they exercise, their children are likely to. And the family that exercises together is more likely to maintain the exercise longer than those who don't. As children get older, they may want to participate in sports, and this is fine. There are virtually no limits to what sports or activities they can engage in. Patients' bodies will usually give them the indication when they need to stop, so they need not be limited by parents or coaches. However, for patients with some degree of lung disease, their coaches must be aware of their condition and must allow the patients to limit themselves: the patients should not be pushed beyond their comfort/tolerance. Teenagers and adults may want to have some guidelines for setting up their own exercise program. Read on.

Medical Advice

Check with your doctor before you start. If your lungs are severely affected by CF, your doctor may recommend an exercise test first to check your oxygen level. If your FEV_1 is less than 50% of your FVC (or 50% of the predicted normal level— for a lot of people that's about the same as 50% of FVC), it's a particularly good idea to see if your oxygen level falls during exercise and, if so, at what intensity of exercise: If your oxygen level is good until your heart rate reaches 150 beats per minute, it's relatively easy to keep your exercise program light enough that your heart rate stays below 145. Your doctor might even want to prescribe some oxygen for you to use while you exercise. For most people with CF, this will not be necessary.

Time Allotment

Set aside a time to exercise. This should amount to about 30 minutes a day, three to five times a week for the exercise itself, in addition whatever time you need to shower and dress. You should guard this exercise time jealously and keep it for yourself. It doesn't matter what time of day you exercise. Some people prefer to exercise in the morning, whereas others prefer to wait until they've been awake and active for several hours. Of course, if your exercise is in gym class or with a team, you won't have much choice as to timing.

Type of Activity

Pick an activity that is a good aerobic conditioner. These activities are ones that are continuous, not stop-and-go; they are light enough that they can be carried out for a long duration at a time, without causing total exhaustion. Typical aerobic activities that are discussed below in greater detail include running, swimming, and biking. Others include rowing, skating, stair-stepping, "elliptical trainers," aerobic dance, cross-country skiing, indoor "skiing" on a NordicTrack® or similar equipment, and vigorous walking. Brisk walking (including race-walking) is excellent and has recently become one of the most widely practiced forms of regular exercise. Activities that require you to support your body weight (walking, running, skating) have the additional advantage of helping to keep your bones strong.

Activities that are *an*aerobic include weight training, most racquet sports, and volleyball. These activities are also beneficial, and many are fun; some may make you stronger and build your muscles, including the chest muscles that you use for breathing. Anaerobic activities will probably not help your endurance. For most CF patients, it's probably ideal to include a hefty dose of aerobic exercise, whether or not you do anaerobic exercise also.

Regular daily activities should not be overlooked in planning a more active lifestyle. If you usually walk the dog around a short block, try going around a long block instead; walk or ride a bike to the corner store when you run out of milk instead of getting a ride; take the stairs instead of the elevator whenever possible; and so on. Try cutting down on TV time in favor of exercising time. It does you a lot more good to walk or run around the block than to watch someone else doing it on TV.

PACING YOURSELF

Getting Going

Whatever activity you pick, remember not to overdo it, especially when you first begin to train. Listen carefully to what your body is telling you about how hard or fast or far you're going. It's much better to take a few days, weeks, or even months, to work your way up to the desired amount of exercise than to get injured or discouraged by trying too much too soon. If you haven't been particularly active, limit your first exercise session to no more than 10 minutes. Continue to exercise for 10 minutes each day for the first week. With each successive week, try adding

2 minutes to each session. By the time several months have passed, you'll find that you're exercising for as long as 30 minutes.

Listen to Your Body

If you're getting winded, go slower until you've caught your breath, and then continue at an easier pace. If you feel as though you've hardly exerted yourself after 10 minutes, you can push a little harder for a little longer.

Injuries

Minor injuries can occur with most forms of exercise. Don't ignore them. While you can continue to exercise with some discomfort, real pain is a signal to stop. Let a few days pass without exercising, and if your pain persists, inform your doctor.

Medications, Food, and Drink

If you have asthma or if you take any inhaled bronchodilators, it is advisable to take an inhalation before you exercise. It is not wise to exercise after a heavy meal; in fact, waiting a while after a meal before you run or swim will make your exercise more pleasant.

Exercise in the Heat

If you're exercising in warm weather, you should drink *while you exercise—even more than you think you need.* You do not need to take salt pills, but sports drinks, like Gatorade®, are especially helpful for people with CF, as they help replace the sodium and chloride that you lose.

RUNNING

Equipment

The only special equipment you need for running is a good pair of running shoes. Gym shoes or tennis shoes are not appropriate for regular running. A long-term running program involves a lot of pounding of your feet on the pavement. If you don't have the proper shoes, this pounding travels from your feet to your shins, knees, and hips and can cause an injury. It is advisable to buy your shoes in a store that specializes in runners' supplies. When shopping for running shoes, pick a shoe that feels good on your foot. Do not expect an uncomfortable shoe to "break in" after a while the way a leather shoe might (most running shoes are made of synthetic materials that do not change their shape with time and wear).

Clothes

You can run in clothes that you probably already have. For summer running, dress as lightly as possible. Nylon shorts and shirts are light and dry out quickly, but cotton is more absorbent. Some newer synthetic materials like "polypro" help wick sweat away from the skin for better evaporation and cooling. For running in colder weather, you are more likely to overdress than underdress. When the temperature is below freezing, cotton socks and sweat pants or stretch tights are the best. Cover your chest with several light layers rather than one heavy layer. On the coldest days, a T-shirt, cotton turtleneck, and hooded cotton sweat shirt should be enough. If it is very windy, a thin nylon shell suit over your running clothes will insulate you and keep the wind out. GoreTex® and similar high-technology fibers are expensive, but are impressive in their ability to keep you dry: they don't let rain or snow in, but they do let sweat out. Be sure to cover your head with a wool cap or the hood from your sweat shirt or jacket, because much of the body's heat is lost from the head. A scarf or mask over your nose and mouth may make breathing easier, particularly if you have EIA. Your feet are working hard, so they won't get very cold, but your hands will. To keep your hands warm, mittens or socks are better than gloves, since they let your fingers keep each other warm. Some petroleum jelly on your lips and cheeks will reduce the sting of the cold.

Starting to Run

Remember not to push yourself too hard, especially in the beginning. You should be exercising to make yourself feel good; if you push so hard that you feel bad, you've missed the point. Start with a 10-minute run/walk session. Run slowly, and when you get tired, start walking. When you are ready, run again. Continue this for three or four sessions during your first week, trying to run for most of the 10 minutes. As the weeks go by, you should gradually add time to your run/walk sessions. Add 2 or 3 minutes each week, so that, after 7 to 10 weeks, you are running for most of each 30-minute session. If it takes longer to add the extra minutes, don't worry, there's no rush. It doesn't matter how far you go or how long it takes you to work up to 30 minutes of running.

Safety

You should be able to avoid injury to your muscles if you warm up properly before running, stretch and cool down afterward, and build up gradually to a regular exercise program. However, if you feel pain after running, be sure to have it checked. Other safety factors to consider include not running in traffic or other polluted areas and not running in dark clothes at night. You can avoid these problems by running on an athletic field, golf course, track, or jogging trail rather than on the sidewalk or street.

If you start your running program in the spring, summer, or fall, you may become discouraged when the weather turns bad in the winter months. There is really no reason you shouldn't run in the winter, as long as you dress properly. Running on icy or slippery surfaces is dangerous, so be careful and sensible about running in the winter; a broken leg or sprained ankle will not promote your general conditioning. Running in cold weather may be hard for people with EIA. Two easy steps can make it much easier: take two puffs of albuterol or other bronchodilator before you go out and wear a mask or scarf around your nose and mouth, so the air you breathe in will be warm and a bit moist. Many athletic clubs or "Y"s have treadmills you can use for comfortable indoor running.

SWIMMING

Where to Swim

You will need a pool, lake, river, or ocean. Unless you live in a part of the country where the weather is good and you can swim outside all year round, you will want to swim in a pool that is convenient to get to and affordable to use. A summer swimming program at a beach or lake won't give you any long-term benefit if you only swim for 2 or 3 months out of the year. Additionally, rivers and oceans have currents, waves, and tides that may interfere with a regular, sustained swimming program. If you don't have a pool or ocean in your backyard, there are a lot of places where you should be able to swim for free or at a moderate cost. Many high schools and colleges have pools that are open to the public during certain hours. Many people swim at municipal or community pools. Most YMCAs and many health clubs and hotels have swimming pools that can be joined for a reasonable fee.

Equipment

Once you have found a place to swim, the only equipment or special clothing you really need is a bathing suit. For a regular exercise program, a one-piece nylon or lycra tank suit is best. Both nylon and lycra suits wear well and dry out quickly. Goggles are useful if you are swimming in a pool or in salt water, since both chlorine and salt can be very irritating to the eyes. If you wear glasses or contact lenses you can purchase goggles with corrective lenses for very reasonable cost (ask your eye doctor or swim shop for details; if you don't have a local swim shop, there are several excellent ones online). If you have long hair, a bathing cap will keep your hair out of your face, as well as out of a pool's filter system. Caps also protect hair and scalp from the drying effects of chlorine.

Safety

Never swim alone! There should always be a lifeguard at the pool or beach. While you are probably less likely to drown in a swimming pool than in a lake, river, or ocean, always make sure that there is a lifeguard present. Failing that, use the "buddy system": swimming with a friend who can pull you out of the water or run for help if you need it. You should also learn some basic water safety techniques. The risk of pulling muscles or tendons while swimming is much less than while running or bicycling. If you are swimming smoothly, your muscles should get an even workout. Most swimming-related injuries occur from diving into shallow water, swimming into the side of the pool, or sustaining cuts from rocks or trash on the bottom of a river or lake.

Learning to Swim

Swimming is most enjoyable when you have a smooth, comfortable stroke. If you do not know how to swim well or if you want to improve your stroke, swimming lessons will be helpful. This does not mean that you have to start training to make it to the Olympic team, but you should be able to execute the various strokes properly. As in running and bicycling, the goal is not speed, but rather sustained, even exercise over time. There are many places where you can learn to swim. The Red Cross and the YMCA are probably best known for their swimming programs, but any reputable class will do. Many places offer swimming lessons designed especially for adults.

Starting to Swim

As with running, don't push yourself too hard or too fast in the beginning. A 10-minute session that alternates a strenuous stroke like the crawl (free-style) with a more restful stroke (breast stroke or side stroke) should get you off to a good start. Try to schedule your swimming sessions three or four times each week for the first few weeks. Gradually work up to longer sessions by adding a few minutes to each session after the first week or two. Your goal should be to swim for at least 30 minutes during each session. Again, remember that you can take as many weeks as you need to reach this goal. It doesn't matter how many laps you swim or how fast you swim them.

BICYCLING

Equipment

If you plan to cycle out-of-doors, a sturdy bike with 3 to 12 speeds is your basic piece of equipment. You can get a touring bike, with relatively skinny tires, or a fat-tired bike, which can be used for off-road cycling or for handling rough or wet roads more readily than the skinny tired bikes. If you want to go really fast on a smooth road, the skinny-tire bikes are the ones for you; if you're more into riding on rough surfaces, for feeling more secure, look into fat-tired models. A cycling helmet is also essential to prevent head injuries if you fall or are thrown from your bike. You should always wear a helmet, even if you don't *plan* to fall! If you plan to cycle indoors, there are many good models of stationary exercise bikes. However, before you buy one, remember that riding a stationary bike can be extremely boring. Some people set the bike up in front of the TV and pedal as they watch. Some health clubs have snazzy computer systems hooked up to the exercise bike, which make you feel like you're riding in the country, and can even set different paces, and make you feel like you're going up and down hills, etc. Most people who just cycle in a bare cellar don't stay with it very long.

Preparing Your Bicycle

Your bicycle should be in good condition each time you begin a ride. Make sure that the seat is properly adjusted, because this will increase the efficiency and comfort with which you ride. Raise or lower the saddle so that your leg is fully extended when your heel is placed on the pedal at the bottom of its cycle. This will cause your leg to be slightly bent while pedaling with the ball of your foot on the pedal. Before each ride, briefly inspect the tires, brakes, and wheels of your bike to make sure that they are in good order. If any part is not working properly, have it fixed. Proper maintenance of your bike will help to ensure safe riding.

Safety

Wear a bike helmet! Bike paths and lightly trafficked roads are recommended over city streets and highways. *Wear a bike helmet!* Familiarize yourself with the traffic laws regarding bicycling and obey them. *Wear a bike helmet!* If you plan to ride in the evenings, be sure that you have the proper lights and reflectors on your bike and wear light-colored clothes so that motorists and other riders can see you. There are wonderful little battery-powered blinking lights available to attach to your belt or bike seat, which are visible from a long way away. And, did we mention? *Wear a bike helmet!*

Clothes

The clothes needed for bicycling are similar to those for running, except that you will build up less heat and give off more heat on a bike than on foot, so you'll have to dress more warmly (and with more wind protection) on the bike. Be sure that your pant legs fit snugly so that they won't get caught in the gear sprockets or chain. Be sure that your shoe laces are tucked in so that they don't get caught in the sprockets or chain. And on your head? *Wear a bike helmet!*

Starting to Cycle

As with running and swimming, start out slowly and build up to longer periods of exercise. A 10- to 15-minute ride three or four times a week is a good way to start out, adding extra minutes to each session after the first week or two. Alternate slow, easy riding with fast, hard riding until you are riding for 30 minutes, three to five times a week. Strive toward a continuous, comfortable ride of increasing duration, rather than a ride that covers a certain distance.

SUMMARY

Patients with CF can and should exercise, at virtually every stage (and age) of life. They reap the same benefits from exercise programs and an active lifestyle that other people do (and perhaps even more): they can become more physically fit and can do more exercise than if they are sedentary. Exercise helps CF patients keep their lungs clear of mucus. Exercise helps a lot of people emotionally, too, by reducing stress. Exercise may even enable CF patients to live longer.

Genetics

11

Barbara Karczeski, Garry R. Cutting, and
David M. Orenstein

THE BASICS

1. Cystic fibrosis (CF) is inherited. In order to be born with CF, you have to get two nonworking CF genes (one from each parent).

2. People with just one nonworking CF gene are called "carriers," and do not have CF.

3. Each time two carriers have a baby, the chances are one in four that that baby will have CF, even if the couple has already had one or more babies with CF.

4. All states now screen newborns for CF.

5. It is possible to test during a pregnancy whether the baby will have CF.

6. It is possible to test to see whether someone is a CF carrier, but the test will miss some carriers.

7. Gene therapy may some day cure CF.

Cystic fibrosis (CF) is a genetic disorder, which means that it is determined by the genes a person has inherited. Our genetic material is called DNA. DNA is a blueprint for building and growing a human being, and there's a complete copy of our DNA in almost every cell we have. DNA is made up of thousands of genes. Genes are individual instructions for how to make a protein our body needs. The genes are packaged into chromosomes. We have 23 pairs of chromosomes: 22 numbered pairs and the sex chromosomes (XX in girls and XY in boys). If your genetic material was a set of encyclopedias, the volumes would be the chromosomes, the entries would be the genes and the letters would be DNA. Genes come in pairs, and we get one copy of each gene from each of our parents. When parents make sex cells (eggs and sperm), they split their full set of genetic information into half sets. In this way, half a set of genetic information from the mother and half a set from the father make a full genetic information set in each child. Our genes are the blueprint to make us, so they determine many of our physical characteristics, from the shape of our ears to the color of our hair. What makes each of us unique physically is the combination of genes that make up our cells.

Different traits are caused by different gene combinations. In some cases, a trait is *dominant*, meaning that it is caused by one of the two genes that person has, regardless of what other gene accompanies it. A gene for a dominant trait completely determines the outcome. An example of this (although it's a bit oversimplified) is brown hair. If a baby gets one brown hair gene, he or she will have brown hair, no matter what the other hair color gene is. In other cases, a trait is *recessive*, meaning that the trait will show up only if both of the genes for that trait are the same. Red hair is a recessive trait, so most redheads have received two red hair genes—one from each parent. A baby with one red hair gene and one brown hair gene will usually have brown hair. Finally, there is the gene interaction in which each gene contributes something so that the resulting trait is a combination of what each would have determined by itself. An example of this is blood type. When a parent with Type A blood and a parent with Type B blood have a child, that child could have Type AB blood. We all have two copies of the CF gene (called CFTR)—the gene that determines whether or not we have CF—and for most people both copies are working. CF is a recessive disorder, which means that a baby who gets a nonworking CF gene from only one parent will not have CF and will have no sign of CF. CF occurs *only* if a person has received a nonworking CF gene from each parent. For a parent to pass on a nonworking CF gene to a child, she or he obviously must have one of those genes. In almost every case, the parent carries one nonworking CF gene and one working CF gene in each of his or her cells. Yet there is no evidence at all that they carry the nonworking CF gene until they have a child with CF. People who have one nonworking CF gene and one working CF gene are called *carriers* because they are not affected by the gene but carry it and can pass it along to their children. Whether their children will have CF depends on what gene the other parent contributes. In the unusual case in which a parent has CF, he or she has two nonworking CF genes in each cell and *must* pass on one of those to each child. As with carriers, whether their children will have CF depends on what gene the other parent contributes.

Some readers may be asking: Why don't carriers have any symptoms? Isn't there any effect on their health? Those are great questions, so let's stop for a little detour. A carrier does not have and will not develop symptoms of CF. Carriers have about one half (50%) of the CFTR protein that they should (since they have half the number of working *CFTR* genes); however, this is actually enough protein to control the movement of charged particles (ions like sodium and chloride) in and out of cells. Carriers of *CFTR* mutations may have an increased risk for pancreatitis (inflammation of the pancreas), sinusitis (infection or inflammation of the sinus cavities), or bronchiectasis (overstretching of airways in the lungs), but most carriers will not develop any symptoms related to CF. OK—back to the possible combination of CF genes from two parents who are carriers of *CFTR* mutations.

Figure 11.1 shows the possible combinations if two parents who are each carriers have children. For each parent, half of his or her eggs or sperm will have the nonworking CF gene and half will have the working CF gene. The chances of a

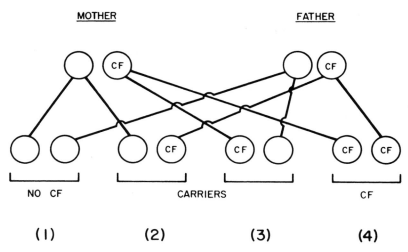

FIGURE 11.1 The inheritance of cystic fibrosis (CF). Each parent of a child with CF has one abnormal CF gene (*circle* labeled "*CF*") (*1*). The abnormal CF gene causes no problems if it is paired with a normal CF gene (*empty circle*). When two parents who each carry an abnormal CF gene have children, each parent passes on either the abnormal or the normal CF gene. The figure shows the possible combinations of genes that children of carriers can have: (*1*) A normal CF gene from both father and mother; (*2*) a normal CF gene from the mother and an abnormal gene from the father; (*3*) an abnormal CF gene from the mother and a normal gene from the father; and (*4*) an abnormal CF gene from each parent. Each of these four combinations is just as likely to occur as the others, meaning that the chances of two carrier parents having a child with CF is one in four each time they have a child.

sperm that carries the nonworking CF gene fertilizing an egg with a nonworking CF gene are exactly the same as the chance it fertilizes an egg with a working CF gene. This means that there are only four possible combinations of genes from these parents, and each is just as likely to occur as the others. *Each time this couple has a child*, the chances are one in four that the baby will get two nonworking CF genes and will have CF; two in four that the baby will get one nonworking CF gene, and therefore will not have CF but will be a carrier; and a one in four chance that the baby will not get any nonworking CF gene at all.

Chance and statistics can be confusing to understand at first. People may assume, mistakenly, that if their chances are one in four that a baby will have CF, and they've already had a baby with CF, then the next three children can't have CF. This is not so—*each* time they have a child, there is one chance in four that the child will have CF. There are families with three children, *all* of whom have CF, and others in which both parents are carriers, yet *none* of their children have CF. With statistical chance, the numbers work out over hundreds or thousands of cases, which doesn't help make predictions for a specific family.

Consider the example of a deck of cards. There are four suits: hearts, diamonds, spades, and clubs. If the cards are shuffled well and are not marked and you pick a card, hoping for a diamond, your chances will be one in four. Now, put that card back, shuffle again, and pick another card. Once again, your chances of getting a diamond are still one in four. But you know that you might repeat this process of picking and replacing cards, and that you might pick 10 times before you get a diamond, and another time you might pick four diamonds in a row. If you picked cards all morning, by the time you'd picked 1,000 cards you'd have come pretty close to 250 diamonds, but those first few may follow almost any pattern.

So, in families trying to decide on their family's future, they can consider their statistical chances. If they have had a child with CF, it means that the parents are both carriers, and the chances for each pregnancy resulting in a child with CF are one in four. Some people consider one chance in four to be great odds, whereas others think that they're dreadful. Great chances or dreadful, brothers and sisters of patients with CF should all be tested to see whether they have CF, even if they have been perfectly healthy, because each child born to the parents of someone with CF does have a one in four chance of having received the two nonworking CF genes, and many people with CF can be healthy for a long time before symptoms appear.

What about the chances of having a child with CF if there is CF in the family of one parent (or parent-to-be) or the other? What if you have a nephew, niece, brother, sister, or cousin with CF? Table 11.1 shows the chances in different situations, depending on the parents' family background.

TABLE 11.1

Risks for Individuals of North European White Background of Having a Child with Cystic Fibrosis[a]

One parent	Other parent	Risk with each pregnancy
No CF history	No CF history	1 in 3000
No CF history	First cousin has CF	1 in 400
No CF history	Aunt or uncle has CF	1 in 300
No CF history	Nephew or niece has CF	1 in 200
No CF history	Sibling has CF	1 in 150
No CF history	Has CF	1 in 50
Sibling has CF	Sibling has CF	1 in 9
Sibling has CF	Has CF	1 in 3
Sibling has CF	Known carrier	1 in 6
Known carrier	Known carrier	1 in 4
Known carrier	Has CF	1 in 2

CF, cystic fibrosis.
[a]Risks are actually slightly higher than listed because the list assumes that (excluding siblings of patients with CF) someone who is a carrier has one parent who is also a carrier. It is actually possible that both of this person's parents are carriers, and that means that each of this person's siblings has greater than a 50:50 chance of being a carrier. Risks to other ethnic groups will generally be different (see Table 11.2).

HOW COMMON IS A NONWORKING CYSTIC FIBROSIS GENE?

Sometimes it can seem to new parents of a child with CF that it was just unbelievably bad luck that both were carriers of the same nonworking gene. But, carrying a nonworking gene is very common: Geneticists estimate that every healthy person carries between 10 and 20 different nonworking genes. And the nonworking CF gene is not unusual. In fact, it is quite common, occurring in about 1 in every 25 white people in North America. It's less common in other ethnic groups (1 in 60 black people; 1 in 375 Asian people) but has been reported in individuals on every continent (except, perhaps, Antarctica!) and from virtually every racial and ethnic background. Table 11.2 shows how common CF is in different countries.

Not only is the CF gene common, it's also old: CF has been with us for somewhere between 3,000 and 53,000 years. People sometimes wonder how an altered gene that causes disease can persist for so long. Getting two copies of the altered gene clearly gives a person big disadvantages, so why should the gene still be around? For some other genes that cause recessive disorders (remember, those are problems where you need to get one nonworking gene from each parent), we think that there might be an advantage of being a carrier, meaning that carriers of the gene have some benefit over those who do not carry the gene. Many different guesses

TABLE 11.2

Incidence of Cystic Fibrosis in Different Countries

Country (or group)	One baby with CF per live births[a]
Alberta (Canada) Hutterites	313
Afrikaners (Southwest Africa)	622
Ireland	2,000
Australia	2,500
United Kingdom (England)	2,500
North America	2,500
France	3,000
The Netherlands	3,500
Germany	4,000
Denmark	4,500
Ashkenazi Jews in Israel	5,000
Sweden	8,000
Italy	15,000
Finland	40,000

CF, cystic fibrosis.
[a]Numbers listed are patients with CF per live births (so, for Ireland, of every 2,000 babies born alive, one has CF).

have been made about what the "carrier advantage" might be for CF carriers. Things like increased fertility of the carriers, less asthma, or increased resistance to intestinal infections have all been suggested, but none has been proven.

Recent advances in molecular genetics enabled researchers to zero in on the CF gene to determine that CF is caused by a single gene (and not a series of genes) and to discover and analyze the gene itself in 1989. That gene is located on the seventh of the 23 chromosome pairs. The discovery of the gene has led to a virtual explosion in our knowledge about CF and has expanded our ability to identify CF carriers and diagnose CF in living patients, in unborn fetuses, and even sometimes in patients who have already died. The discovery of the gene has even enabled people to hope that the day may be approaching when CF will be cured with gene therapy or treated very effectively with new medications.

To understand the importance of this discovery, let's take a little detour to a crash course in basic genetics.

WHAT IS A GENE?

A gene is a pattern for building a protein. It carries a code to tell the body what amino acids to put into the protein and in what order. It "codes" through DNA. DNA is made of pairs of chemicals called *nucleotides*. The chemicals or *bases* that make up these nucleotides are adenine, guanine, thymine, and cytosine (abbreviated A, G, T, and C). These nucleotides form long double chains, wound around each other in a "helix." The strands are held together by specific pairing of the nucleotides. Adenine always pairs with thymine, and cytosine with guanine. These chains of pairs of nucleotides ("base pairs") are the DNA. The average gene is made up of about 30,000 DNA base pairs. To get an idea of the dimensions we're dealing with here, take a look at Table 11.3. This table compares our genetic information to time and distance to give you an idea of how much genetic information our cells carry.

TABLE 11.3

The Relative Dimensions of the Components of Human Genetic Material, Expressed as if They Were Time or Distance

Unit	Time	Distance
Nucleotide	1 second	1 inch
Gene	8½ hours	700 yards
Chromosome	4⅓ years	1,900 miles
Genome	1 century	2 equators

Courtesy of Dr. John Mulvihill, formerly of the University of Pittsburgh.

The way genes dictate what our body's cells do is by directing ("coding") the production of proteins; it's the proteins that really do the work. These proteins are made of building blocks called *amino acids,* and it takes three nucleotides to "code" for an amino acid. All together, the particular amino acids and the order in which they are placed determine what the resulting protein looks like and does. It turns out that not all of the gene is involved in coding for protein production; relatively short portions, called *exons,* carry the protein code. These exons are separated along the length of the gene by long stretches of noncoding DNA that are called *introns.* When the cell is ready to make a protein, it makes a template from the DNA and then cuts and pastes all of the coding sections (exons) together.

Changes in genes are called "mutations." A mutation can replace one DNA base with another which can cause the code to be wrong and the protein to have a mistake in the amino acid order. A mutation can also cause the code to be cut and pasted together incorrectly, leaving some introns in the mix or cutting out part of the exons. Sometimes all or part of the gene is missing. However, not all mutations in a gene cause it to malfunction. Sometimes, mutations create a slightly different version of the gene that still works fine. One way to think of this relates to different spellings of the same word; for example, let's look at the word "doughnut." Some changes to this word don't make any real difference. If you delete some letters—ugh—and change "doughnut" into "donut," you can still communicate your meaning. But if you delete other letters—ghn—the new word "douut" doesn't mean anything, and the person you're writing to won't know what you mean. Mutations are the same way—not all of them lead to nonworking proteins. Some of them make proteins that work just fine, whereas others make proteins that work, but not as well as the original spelling, or don't work at all. Thus, it is very important to verify whether a mutation causes a loss of gene or protein function or not.

THE CYSTIC FIBROSIS GENE

The CF gene is very large, containing about 250,000 base pairs (about eight times the average gene). The protein made from the CF gene contains 1,480 amino acids. (For those of you who've been following the complicated math here, you would have noted that if it takes three base pairs for one amino acid, 250,000 base pairs could have resulted in more than 80,000 amino acids, instead of a measly 1,480; this shows how much of the CF gene—like most genes—is made up of introns, that is, noncoding DNA.) This 1,480 amino acid protein has the unwieldy (but accurate) name *CFTR,* for *c*ystic *f*ibrosis *t*ransmembrane conductance *r*egulator protein. The main function of this protein is to direct traffic across cell membranes, especially traffic of salt (sodium and chloride). Abnormal movement of chloride and sodium (and water) across cells seems to explain many of the health problems seen in people with CF. This is discussed more in Chapter 1. Since the CF gene is responsible for producing the CFTR protein, the gene is sometimes referred to as

CFTR. To make things even more complicated, *everyone*, not just people with CF, has two *CFTR* genes that make CFTR protein. The difference between patients with CF and people without CF is in the structure (and therefore also the function) of the CFTR protein: whether it works or not. When the CFTR protein is working, sodium, chloride, and water all travel normally in and out of cells. Cell secretions are not extra thick and no disease results.

When the CF gene makes nonworking CFTR protein, it will not do its job properly. If both copies of the CF gene make nonworking protein, sodium, chloride, and water will not travel properly. This causes the problems that make up CF. Far and away the most common *CFTR* gene mutation occurs in exon 10 and is the loss of three (out of a total of 250,000!) base pairs, leading to a protein that is missing one amino acid (out of 1,480). The missing amino acid is called "phenylalanine" (we abbreviate it using "F"), and it is missing from position 508. The name of this mutation is Δ*F508*. Here's why: Δ (delta–for deletion) F (for phenylalanine) 508 (the position in the protein). It has also been called "F508del," *deltaF508*, or *508delF*. About 70% of CF chromosomes (in North America) have the Δ*F508* mutation. About 50% of North American patients with CF have two copies of Δ*F508* (one from each parent), whereas 40% have one Δ*F508* gene and one of the other *CFTR* mutations. (After Δ*F508* was discovered, it was originally thought that there would probably be five or six other mutations that would account for the other 30% of CF mutations. By the time of the writing of this book, 22 years later, we know about more than 1,800 different CF mutations! Most of these mutations are very rare, occurring in only a very few patients, sometimes in only one patient. There are a few mutations that are not so rare, and the frequency of different mutations varies, depending on a population's ethnic and geographic background. For example, W1282X is uncommon in non-Jewish people but found in nearly 50% of the chromosomes of all Jewish patients with CF. G551D is relatively common in people of Celtic origin, occurring in 5% of abnormal CF genes in Ireland and England. See Table 11.4 for other examples. Taken all together, the known mutations explain about 98% of all CF chromosomes. In a few specific ethnic groups, a very few of the known mutations account for almost all of the patients with CF (Table 11.5).

DIFFERENT MUTATIONS: DIFFERENT DISEASES?

Whenever several different variations of a gene can cause problems, people wonder whether the kind of genetic variation a patient has will affect the kind of symptoms that patient has. Geneticists talk about the *genotype–phenotype relationship*. Genotype means the combination of gene changes that one has. "Phenotype" comes from the Greek word that means appearance, and it refers to what you see in a person. In this case, it means the outward evidence of a genetic disease. We know that some people with CF seem to have a worse form of the disease, with severe lung disease and lots of hospital admissions, whereas others are pretty healthy.

TABLE 11.4

Some of the More Common Cystic Fibrosis Gene Mutations and Their Characteristics

Mutation	Geographic/ethnic incidence	Characteristics
ΔF508	70%–75% in North America	Pancreatic insufficiency
W1282X[a]	50%–60% in Ashkenazi Jews; 2.1% worldwide	Pancreatic insufficiency
G542X[a]	3.4% worldwide	Pancreatic insufficiency; more meconium ileus
G551D[a]	2.4% worldwide	Pancreatic insufficiency
3905insT[a]	2.1% worldwide	Pancreatic insufficiency
N1303K[a]	1.8% worldwide	Pancreatic insufficiency
R553X[a]	1.3% worldwide	Pancreatic insufficiency
621 + 1G → T[a]	1.3% worldwide	Pancreatic insufficiency
1717–1G → A[a]	1.3% worldwide	Pancreatic insufficiency
A455E[a]	3%–7% in The Netherlands 0%–0.2% in North America	Pancreatic sufficiency[b]; mild lung disease
3849 + 10 kb C → T[a]	1.4% worldwide; 4% in Israel	Pancreatic sufficiency[b]; normal sweat chloride; most males not sterile; lung disease varies from mild to severe
R117H[a]	0.8% worldwide	Pancreatic sufficiency[b]; slightly lower sweat chloride; older age at diagnosis
R334W[a]		Pancreatic sufficiency[b]; older age at diagnosis
R347P[a]		Pancreatic sufficiency[b]
P574H[a]		Pancreatic sufficiency[b]
Y563N[a]		Pancreatic sufficiency[b]

[a]"Compound heterozygotes," in most cases, meaning these patients had one copy of the particular mutation noted and one other cystic fibrosis mutation (usually ΔF508).
[b]Pancreatic sufficiency in most, but not all, cases.

Whether someone needs to take pancreatic enzymes and how healthy his or her lungs are make up his or her phenotype. So when people wonder about the genotype–phenotype relationship in CF, they wonder whether different CF mutations cause any of the variations we see in how CF affects different patients.

As with so many things, the answer seems to be "yes and no." The "yes" part has mostly to do with pancreatic function and whether someone needs to take enzymes or not. Almost everyone with two copies (one from each parent) of the most common CF mutation, *ΔF508*, needs to take enzymes (they have "pancreatic

TABLE 11.5

Ethnic Groups in Which a Few Mutations Account for Most of the Cystic Fibrosis Chromosomes

Group	Mutations, No.	Cystic fibrosis chromosomes, %
Alberta (Canada) Hutterites	2	100
Welsh	29	99.5
Brittany Celts	19	98
Ashkenazi Jews	5	97
Belgian	17	94.3

Courtesy of Dr. Garry Cutting, Johns Hopkins University.

insufficiency"). There have now been several different CF mutations discovered that are associated with pancreatic sufficiency, that is, you don't need to take enzymes, even if that mutation is paired with one $\Delta F508$ gene. Table 11.4 lists some of these genes. Some geneticists have referred to the genes associated with pancreatic insufficiency as "severe," whereas those associated with pancreatic sufficiency are called "mild." The "mild" versus "severe" distinction holds true only for how the pancreas is affected (the need to take enzymes or not), not the overall phenotype or the overall health of the patient, so this can be confusing to patients and families.

The more important question is harder to answer: Are variations in the severity of lung disease related to different CF mutations? With few exceptions, the answer seems to be "no." The differences in the severity of lung disease among people with the exact same *CFTR* mutations is great, so we know that factors other than the specific type of mutation are very important in determining how bad someone's lungs are.

Factors that are known to influence lung health in patients with CF more than their particular mutations include things in the environment (like cigarette smoke and viruses) and how aggressive treatment is. In a way, this is good news, since things over which patients and families have some control (treatment and avoiding cigarette smoke) are more important to their survival than some things over which families have no control (the family mutations).

We also know that other genes and proteins can influence someone's CF phenotype. For example, if the protein set that responds to infection is stronger in a person with CF, that person will be less likely to have multiple and severe lung infections. If it is weaker in another person, that person may have more severe lung disease. Scientists are just now starting to unravel the complicated gene and protein networks that determine a patient's CF phenotype.

REPRODUCTIVE TESTING

For nearly every couple who already has a child with CF, it is now possible to tell reasonably early in pregnancy whether an expected child will have CF. This is called "prenatal testing" and can be done in one of two ways. The first is called "amniocentesis," and it can be performed after 16 weeks of pregnancy. In an amniocentesis, a small amount of the fluid surrounding the developing fetus is collected through a needle into the uterus through the mother's abdomen. The second prenatal test method is called "chorionic villus sampling," and it can be performed even earlier in the pregnancy (10 to 13 weeks). Chorionic villus sampling involves inserting a thin tube through the vagina and cervix into the mother's uterus. Once the tube is in the uterus, a small sample of cells from the placenta is taken. These tests do involve some risks to the pregnancy, but they have been used safely for many years.

Both the amniotic fluid cells and the placenta contain the complete genetic information set of the fetus, so they can be analyzed for *CFTR* gene mutations. Most of the time, this DNA analysis involves looking for the specific mutations known to cause CF in the family, but sometimes the testing will include a handful of the most common of more than 1,800 known CF mutations. If the fetal cells have the CF mutations from both parents, we would predict that the fetus will have CF. If only one or none of the mutations is inherited, we would predict that the fetus would not have CF.

Many families have used these new methods to decide to continue a pregnancy if the fetus is shown not to have CF, or to stop the pregnancy (with an abortion) if the fetus has CF. For people who would not consider having an abortion, these tests may still be useful for preparing for the new child with CF, or providing peace of mind if the test shows the baby will not have CF. It is up to each family to decide whether prenatal testing is the best option for them. Another option for families who want to decrease the chance that they have an affected pregnancy is preimplantation genetic diagnosis (PGD). Couples having PGD go through in vitro fertilization (IVF; where egg and sperm are brought together in the lab and early embryos start growing outside of the mother). One or a few cells from these embryos are taken and genetic analysis for CF can be performed. Only the embryos predicted not to have CF are transferred back to the mother's uterus. PGD does not guarantee a healthy baby, and prenatal testing is often recommended, but PGD greatly improves the chance of having a baby without CF. Because PGD for CF involves IVF and is done in only a few labs, it needs to be highly coordinated and can be very expensive for the family. The main use of reproductive testing is for couples who already have a child with CF. But there are a few other instances in which it might be used. For instance, if the cousin of a patient with CF wants to get pregnant and she and her husband are found to be carriers, they would be able to use reproductive testing. In fact, in any couple where both partners are carriers, testing could be done to see whether their baby would be born with CF. Of course, if carrier testing (see later) shows that one spouse is not a carrier, then the risk of having a child with CF is very low (but not zero, see later) for the couple.

Newborn screening for CF is now performed in every state in the United States. Most states use a combination of testing for a pancreatic protein called immuno-reactive trypsinogen (IRT) and a genetic test for common *CFTR* mutations (see Chapter 2, *Making the Diagnosis*). Newborn screening is most helpful for identifying children with CF in families who do not know that they are at risk (they have no family history of CF). It is also a way for families who know that they are at risk, but don't want to have reproductive testing, to find out about CF in their children very early in life. Most newborn screening programs will not be able to identify children with the mild or unusual forms of CF we've discussed earlier in this chapter.

CARRIERS

If a brother or a sister of someone with CF does not have CF, there are two chances in three that this sibling is a carrier. Here's why: As illustrated in Figure 11.1, if both parents are carriers, there are only four possible combinations of CF and non-CF mutations that their children could have. One combination gives CF (two mutated CF genes), two combinations result in carriers, and one combination has no CF mutation. Once you know that a brother or a sister does not have CF (and you'll know that after a properly performed sweat test), there are only three possible combinations, two of which result in carriers. Table 11.6 shows the chances of various people being CF carriers. Genetic testing can tell whether a relative of a patient with CF is a carrier.

When a person is at risk to be a carrier of CF because of his or her family history, his or her health care provider can draw some blood or collect some cells by

TABLE 11.6

Risks of Being a Cystic Fibrosis Carrier[a]

Relationship to patient with CF	Risk of being a carrier
Parent of a patient with CF	1 in 1 (100%)
Unaffected sibling of a patient with CF	2 in 3
Aunt or uncle of a patient with CF	1 in 2
Nephew or niece of a patient with CF	1 in 3
Cousin of a patient with CF	1 in 4
None known (northern European)	1 in 25

CF, cystic fibrosis.
[a]Risks are actually slightly higher than listed, because the list assumes that (excluding siblings of patients with CF) someone who is a carrier has one parent who is also a carrier. It is actually possible that both of this person's parents are carriers, which means that each of this person's siblings has greater than a 50:50 chance of being a carrier.

gently swirling a cotton swab inside the person's cheek. The genetic laboratory can analyze the DNA in the blood or cheek cells, specifically the *CFTR* gene, for the known disease-causing mutations in the family. If a brother or a sister of the patient with CF does not have one of the same CF mutations that the patient has, he or she is not a carrier–Period. If cousins, aunts, or uncles are being tested, and they don't have one of their relative's known CF mutations, they probably are not carriers either.

But what if you don't have a family history of CF? What if you are married to a carrier or are just concerned about what your risk might be? You can still have carrier testing. In fact, many couples without a family history will be offered carrier screening for CF when they are early in pregnancy or contemplating becoming pregnant. Instead of looking for one or two known mutations (already seen in relatives) the carrier screening test looks at a small panel (23 or more) of the most common CF mutations. Carrier *screening* is a little different from carrier *testing*. In carrier screening, there's not a specific mutation to rule in or out, and since the test doesn't include all known CF mutations (just the most common ones), a negative carrier screening test will decrease the chance that someone is a CF carrier but will not take it away completely. The left over chance (called residual risk) depends on your ethnic background, your family history, and the set of mutations that were tested. As Table 11.5 shows, in a few ethnic groups just a few mutations account for virtually all cases of CF, whereas 2 to 3 dozen most common mutations account for about 85% to 90% of CF chromosomes.

GENETIC DIAGNOSIS OF CYSTIC FIBROSIS

In some cases, gene testing can be used to help make the diagnosis of CF itself. This issue is discussed at greater length in Chapter 2. The procedure for obtaining cells for testing is the same as for carriers: either a blood sample or a gentle brushing from the inside of the cheek can be used. If two of the known CF gene mutations are found, almost certainly the person has CF. If one or none is found, it is less likely, but not impossible, that the person has CF.

Even though DNA analysis seems to be state-of-the-art, the sweat test remains the "gold standard" for diagnosing CF in most patients. But there are some cases in which gene testing may be very useful in making the diagnosis of CF. The first and most common is in someone who has signs, symptoms, and perhaps even family history that suggest CF, yet the sweat test does not give a definitive answer. Sometimes there is not enough sweat to perform the test. In other patients the sweat test result is in the "gray zone": not definitely positive, not definitely negative. Finding two CF genes in someone like this will make the diagnosis of CF much more likely.

Some families may not be able to get to a center with the skill and experience to perform the sweat test correctly. Genetic testing can usually be arranged over a long distance with a local doctor. Lastly, DNA testing can help make or confirm the diagnosis of CF in someone who has died. This situation arises more often than you might think: A baby gets very sick and dies before testing can be done (or before CF is considered) or someone has a relative who died a long time ago, and only now is the possibility of CF being considered. If blood or a small piece of tissue is available from that relative in the hospital's pathology department, those cells may still be enough for testing.

Rarely, a person with two *CFTR* mutations does not have CF in its classic or usual form. This may be particularly true for men who are otherwise healthy but are being evaluated for infertility: You'll recall from Chapter 5 (*Other Systems*) that most men with CF are sterile because they have a complete blockage, or even absence, of both the right and left *vas deferens*, the tubes that normally carry sperm from the testicles to the penis. There is an uncommon form of male infertility not associated with any other symptoms of CF, called "congenital bilateral absence of the *vas deferens*," usually abbreviated CBAVD (congenital: you're born with it; bilateral: both sides). It turns out that a lot of these men have one or two nonworking CF genes. In this case, finding two *CFTR* mutations does not make the diagnosis of CF.

GENE THERAPY

Gene therapy is discussed at greater length in Chapter 16. Gene therapy is placing a healthy gene into cells affected by an abnormal gene and having that healthy gene take over the function of those cells. In CF, this would be getting a healthy *CFTR* gene into cells to correct the abnormalities in salt (sodium and chloride) and water traffic across the cell membranes. This would be most important in the lungs. Big strides have been made toward developing successful (safe and effective) gene therapy since the discovery of the CF gene in 1989: Gene therapy has worked in the test tube, in individual CF cells, and it seems to have worked in mice with CF. But there is still much work to do before it is widely available for treating CF.

The Family

David M. Orenstein and Daniel J. Weiner

12

THE BASICS

1. Hearing that a child has cystic fibrosis (CF) is very stressful for parents.

2. As parents learn more about CF and see their children doing well, the stress lessens.

3. CF center staff expect you to have a lot of questions and want you to ask them. They know that it takes a long time (years) to learn all there is to know about CF.

4. Children with CF should be treated normally: they need to do homework and chores and should be allowed to participate in all normal childhood activities. Children treated this way grow up healthier emotionally and physically.

As a chronic disease that requires a vigorous schedule of daily treatments, cystic fibrosis (CF) imposes significant stress on the affected child, the parents, and any brothers and sisters (whether or not they also have CF). Understanding the reactions to this stress and learning about effective methods to cope with them are important to the care of the child with CF and to the functioning of the family.

In this chapter, we discuss the variety of reactions that parents have to the diagnosis and management of CF, the methods for dealing with the daily stresses, and suggestions for how the family and the medical team can work together most effectively.

YOUR CHILD HAS CYSTIC FIBROSIS

Parents and other family members experience various emotions when they are told that a child has CF. Family members may say to themselves, "I can't believe this. This can't be happening to my child and my family. I don't know what to

235

do. What does the future hold? Is there anything I can do for my child? Could I have prevented this?" All of these reactions—anger, denial, shock, grief, helplessness, confusion, despair, sadness, and fear—are very normal responses. These emotions are part of a *grieving* response. Just as a person experiences many of these feelings when a loved one dies, parents feel many of the same emotions when they learn that a child has a serious health problem. The parents "mourn" the loss of the perfect, healthy child that they had expected. Another very common response upon learning the diagnosis of CF is one of relief—if a family has taken their child to many doctors over a long period, they may be *relieved* finally to have been given a reason for their child's health problems. This sensation of relief may be very puzzling, and the parent may even feel guilty about it. With more babies being diagnosed through newborn screening (see Chapter 2), the opposite may be true: a perfectly healthy-seeming baby and a blind-side "hit"— often in the form of a call from the pediatrician's office: "your baby has CF," or "you need to schedule an appointment at the CF clinic." This can certainly come as a shock.

No matter what the reaction, it's important that each family member has someone to confide in—a trusted, understanding friend, health professional, member of the clergy, or other person with whom he or she can share feelings. It may be difficult for parents to talk about CF with one another, especially immediately after the diagnosis is made. Strong emotions may make it too hard to listen and understand another person's pain, grief, or anger—even if it is a spouse. A husband and wife may find that they react very differently to the diagnosis ("how could he feel *that* way?"), making discussion even more difficult. Since they are two individual people, they may experience varying reactions at different times. And it is hard to *give* support and understanding to anyone—even your spouse— when *you* may be hurting badly yourself. This can put a strain on the relationship unless both parents try to remember that it is normal and that the spouse's reaction does not reflect a lack of caring. It is important to try to be open and nonjudgmental about each other's reactions. A third person may be able to help a couple get through this difficult time.

At the time of diagnosis, the family will be given extensive information about CF and its management. The flood of emotions may make it hard to concentrate on what the doctor is saying and to remember this information. Despite an initial lengthy discussion with the doctor, it is not uncommon for parents to retain very little of what they have been told; they may feel that they have a poor understanding of CF and have many unanswered questions.

The team at the CF center is aware that it is difficult to comprehend all this information at such a stressful time. They know that it is important to review the information many times and they plan to spend ample time with the family for this purpose. Learning about CF is a continuous process that goes on over many months and years. The CF center staff *expect* this, view education as a very important part of their jobs, and *want* you to ask your questions, big or small.

Many parents find it helpful to write down their questions and discuss them with the doctor, nurse, or social worker, in person or by phone. Typical questions that many parents ask are the following:

- Will CF affect my child's brain function?
- Will my child look any different from other children?
- How will CF affect my child's daily life?
- How long will my child live?
- Is there something I did during the pregnancy to cause my child to have CF?
- Could I have prevented this?
- Should I limit my child's activity?
- Can my child go to daycare and school?
- Do my other children have CF?

Some families are reluctant to ask these questions out of fear of what the answers might be, or fear that they may appear insignificant or too simple. Your physician and the team members at the CF center understand and encourage families to ask all their questions—no question is too insignificant to be considered, and even answers that are hard to hear are seldom as horrible as people's imaginations.

Because the manifestations of CF are so different in each child, it is often difficult for the doctor to be specific in answering many of the parents' questions. No one can predict the exact effect of CF on a child's lung function, growth, activity, or life span. The uncertainty is very frustrating and frightening, for it means that the family must live with the unknown from day to day. Even though the doctor cannot make any predictions for a specific child, he or she can explain to the parents the range of disease in CF and perhaps where the child falls in this range. On the whole, most children with CF should be expected to attend school regularly, to be able to participate in sports, and to play with other children without restriction, that is, in general, to carry out the work and play of normal children.

It can be very helpful if you are aware of the different normal stages of development that your child will go through and how these might influence CF care. For example, it helps to be prepared for the wonderfully challenging time when a toddler begins to express her or his own preferences ("NO!!"), which you'll notice we didn't call "the terrible twos." Social workers and others in your CF center can help you anticipate these times and how to work in important treatments *and* enjoy your toddler. Similarly, teen years can bring their own challenges and anticipating them can help both you and your child.

BEGINNING HOME CARE

In addition to obtaining information about CF, it is important that parents learn techniques for caring for their child with CF—particularly the methods for respiratory treatments and enzyme administration. In the past, many physicians recommended that the newly diagnosed infant or child be admitted to the hospital for thorough evaluation of respiratory function and growth and for education of the parents. While this idea was frightening to the family (and disapproved by short-sighted "bottom-line" oriented insurance clerks), it often helps if they realize that an admission to the hospital provides the valuable opportunity for the parents to have daily contact with the CF team and lays the groundwork for a lifetime of successful health care—perhaps preventing or minimizing the need for future hospitalizations. The doctors, nurses, social worker, respiratory therapists, and dieticians used this time to teach the family about home management of CF and begin to develop an important working relationship with the family.

In recent years, hospital admission for initial CF education has become much less common. Instead, many centers schedule several clinic visits back-to-back (e.g., every week for several weeks in a row) to try to accomplish the same goals of initiating the learning process and helping families through the difficult time that follows their hearing the diagnosis. Families may be invited to bring other important people (most often grandparents; sometimes older siblings, aunts or uncles, etc.) to these sessions.

No matter how thorough are the instructions and how skillful are the parents, most families are nervous about beginning therapy at home. At the same time they are beginning enzyme administration and respiratory treatments, they may be facing an already busy child-care schedule, work schedule, or both. With the help of a nurse or social worker, the parents may benefit from sketching out a daily schedule, which takes into consideration *their* family's needs. The doctor, nurse, or social worker may be able to arrange for a meeting with a family more experienced with CF who can serve as an important source of information and support.

In addition to the confusion of a new schedule and nervousness about new treatments, parents may find themselves faced with a cranky baby who is hard to comfort. Some babies with CF are fussy eaters and before diagnosis have been irritable because of lung infection, hunger or chronic abdominal discomfort, and diarrhea. Because they have been hard to feed, hard to soothe, and haven't grown well, their parents may feel helpless and incapable.

Many parents say that although they *love* their infant, they find it difficult to *like* him (or her) because he or she is so irritable and is frustrating to care for—and they feel guilty about resenting their own child. It may be hard for the parents to talk about these feelings or even to admit them to themselves. These feelings, while very troublesome to the mother and father, are very common, normal reactions.

Gradually, as babies become accustomed to their new medications and treatments, the chronic digestive symptoms will be relieved and they will begin to gain weight. As babies feel better, they become more contented, and their parents can draw much satisfaction from their daily efforts and the successful "settling in" at home.

EXPLAINING CYSTIC FIBROSIS TO OTHERS

Once the diagnosis of CF has been confirmed and the parents have begun to learn about CF, they must begin to explain CF to grandparents, other family members, and friends. This may be difficult to do. However, an honest, simple explanation is essential—it will set the tone for how others react to their child for many years to come. Although CF is a chronic progressive disease that may result in a shortened life span, many patients live to middle age, or even beyond. In fact, CF used to be only a disease of childhood (patients died before they became adults), and now in many CF centers, there are more adult patients than children! As the prognosis for CF improves, it is important that children and teenagers be raised with the idea that they should look forward to being active, productive adults. To promote independence and goals for the child with CF, the parents and others with whom the child lives and works must share an outlook of hope and encouragement for the child. Many questions are difficult to answer, but each successful encounter makes the next one easier to handle.

Following are some of the important points that parents may want to share with others:

- CF does not affect the brain or intelligence.
- No part of CF, including the cough and loose stools, is contagious.
- CF is a genetic disease caused by inheriting a gene mutation from each parent; it is no one's *fault* (some grandparents have difficulty accepting the idea that an abnormal gene came from *their* side of the family).
- CF is not curable, but it is treatable.
- The treatment for CF must be carried out each day and consists primarily of respiratory care and enzyme administration, both of which must be made non-negotiable and normal parts of every day.
- There are currently exciting treatments in clinical studies directed at the basic underlying cellular defect in CF, and the prognosis is constantly improving.

YOU AND YOUR CHILD

One of the most valuable gifts you can give your child with CF (and yourself) is to treat him or her as a *normal* child *who happens to have CF*, and *not* as a *case of CF*, nor as a poor, sickly weakling who should not be expected to do normal things. First of all, the large majority of children and adolescents with CF *are not limited* in their physical or mental capacities by their disease. Many play sports, some even excel at sports; many excel in school. But as surely as day turns into night, children whose parents *expect* them to fail and to be unable to take care of themselves *will* fail and will grow up thinking poorly of themselves. Children should know that they have CF, and that having CF means certain things are different from other kids (need to do chest treatments, need to take enzymes with meals). Many children who feel unfairly singled out because of having to do special things because of their CF take some comfort in knowing that *many* kids have to do different things: some children may have diet restrictions that the CF child doesn't; some may need a wheelchair, as the child with CF doesn't; some may need braces, and so forth.

But they should also know that they have the same rights, privileges, and responsibilities as anyone else in the family or school. They go to school, have friends over, play sports, and so on. They need to do homework, help with the dishes, and so on. Treated normally, they will think of themselves as normal and will *be* normal. In reviewing this book, several teenagers and young adults with CF urged us to stress that children with CF should never be allowed to use CF as an excuse for getting out of unappealing chores or responsibilities.

In fact, most parents and children with CF are able to adopt this very positive outlook, which in turn not only makes the children wonderful to be around but also has a very positive influence on their health.

YOU AND YOUR OTHER CHILDREN

In many ways, having two children is more than twice as hard as having one. Although the bond between siblings in most cases ends up being among the strongest on earth, sibling rivalries and jealousies exist at one level or another in most families. Most parents are able to keep these rivalries and jealousies from erupting into outright armed conflict, but at times the peacekeeping role can be challenging. If one child has CF, this can add a dimension to the challenge. The child with CF may resent the other child for *not* having it ("Why me? It's not fair!"), whereas the child without CF may resent the extra attention the child with CF gets (treatments, trips to the clinic, perhaps even visits and gifts in the hospital). It's a balancing act—that most parents end up doing very well—to make absolutely certain that the child or children with CF get all the needed treatments, while the other child or children realize that they too are cherished.

YOU AND YOUR SPOUSE

In conjunction with the treatment of CF, parents find themselves faced with new stresses on their marriage: care of the child takes up more time—how should they divide the responsibilities? Medicines and doctor visits are expensive—how can their budget accommodate this? There is a risk of subsequent children having CF—how can they work out their sexual relationship and family planning? The child with CF needs discipline as any other child—how should they handle discipline for a "sick" child? The other children need attention or one parent's job may be in jeopardy—how can they cope with preexisting family problems in the midst of this new stress?

An important starting point for handling each of these stresses is for the couple to be open and honest in sharing their feelings with one another. Good communication will help to define the problems from each partner's perspective, starting them on the path to developing mutually acceptable solutions. As the parents work *together* to resolve conflict, many couples report that their relationship is strengthened and they are better prepared to face future challenges together. Many experts in family relationships stress the need for couples to make some time alone with each other, whether it's an evening out to dinner and a movie or just a walk together in a local park. These times can reinforce the couple's relationship with each other and make it easier for them to face any stresses, including those brought by CF. The child benefits from parents having some time for themselves, too: parents leaving a child with a trusted babysitter, be that a relative, friend, or professional, gives the child an important lesson in security and teaches the child that (a) the parents *will* return and (b) the world is safe place, even without the constant presence of the parents.

If one parent is employed outside the home and the other is responsible for child care, the employed parent will probably have a limited amount of time to administer treatment. However, it is important that parents share responsibility for the child's care, even if it can be only to a limited extent. This shared responsibility demonstrates to children that their parents are unified in their approach to their care; it may also help to avoid resentment that can arise when one spouse is solely responsible for treatments.

Financial worries can cause much strain within a family. Insurance coverage may be inadequate or nonexistent. State-aid programs may be helpful in some situations. Many clinics have a "patient representative" or a social worker who can put parents in contact with appropriate financial resources.

As the parents cope differently with their reactions to the diagnosis of CF, their desire for sexual intimacy may be altered. These differing needs may serve to create further conflict and misunderstanding. Overshadowing these differences may be fear of another pregnancy and the birth of another child with CF. An atmosphere of open, honest communication is essential for the resolution of these differences.

Sometimes the stresses associated with a diagnosis of CF are too much for a couple to handle without outside help and guidance. The CF center team can be a valuable resource in assisting the family; they may recommend further assistance from a psychologist, counselor, or clergy. The family's pediatrician or family doctor may also be of great assistance. Although these professionals are not CF experts, they may have known the family for a long time and often are very willing to provide support. It is essential that a family seek help promptly if difficulties arise in coping with the diagnosis of CF or with related issues. Such problems do not "just go away," and must be handled directly and aggressively. Unless properly managed, problems with stress and communication within the family may persist, having an impact on CF management and adversely affecting the child's health.

GOING TO THE CYSTIC FIBROSIS CLINIC

Most patients with CF will have clinic visits scheduled for between four and eight times a year, more just after diagnosis and when someone is sick. These visits are very important in maintaining the patients' good health, but for many people they are not easy. Depending on the distance you live from the center, the number of tests to be done, and how busy or organized the clinic happens to be that day, a variable amount of time (often a whole day) is lost to other activities. This may mean losing a day's work (and wages), spoiling a perfect school attendance record, missing a team or chorus practice, and so on. It may be expensive to drive and park.

Beyond the financial and logistical nuisance of clinic visits, they may be difficult emotionally, too. For some young patients, there is the fear of shots (despite experience and assurances that there are unlikely to *be* shots, except for a yearly "flu" shot, and yearly blood work) or the fear of hospital admission. For some patients and families, it may be less focused, but scarier than that: going to CF clinic is a rude reminder that the child *has* CF. Many families—including many who do absolutely every treatment, every day—are able to put CF aside and not think of it or its long-term implications most of the time. But a clinic appointment brings CF back into the center of the family's existence for a brief time.

There are some things that may help ease the emotional burden of a trip to clinic. The first is the realization that most clinic visits are actually quite pleasant, with a number of people who are truly glad to see you and your child, and with a minimum of unpleasant tests or treatments. At most visits, there's a positive report from the physician or an optimistic and realistic plan arrived at to attack a problem you knew about before you came: it's relatively unusual for a bad problem to be discovered at the clinic visit that is a big surprise. Parents can help nervous children prepare by stressing the positives: "You'll get to see_____" (fill in the blank with a favorite nurse or doctor or waiting room toy), and we'll go out to eat afterward (or to the museum, zoo, mall, etc.). It is *not* helpful to say over and over to a frightened toddler, "They're not going to *HURT* you; I won't let them *HURT* you," as that can even plant the idea of hurting in the child's mind.

GOING TO THE HOSPITAL

Occasionally, hospitalization may be necessary. Admission to the hospital upsets the daily routine of a family and, in effect, creates a crisis. This topic is dealt with at length in Chapter 7.

SUMMARY

Having a child with CF adds stress to a family, particularly when the diagnosis is made. With time and education, if parents make an effort to work together, the stress eases, and the family can even be made stronger by this stress. Parents can work together with CF center staff to learn about CF. CF center staff expect (and want) parents to ask many questions, since learning about CF is very important and takes years. Children with CF should be brought up normally, with the same plans, expectations, and responsibilities as other children. The large majority of children with CF grow up with healthy positive attitudes they've gotten from their parents, and this positive outlook helps their physical health as well.

The Teenage Years

Jonathan E. Spahr, David M. Orenstein, and
Daniel J. Weiner

13

THE BASICS

1. The teenage years can be wonderful and healthy for people with cystic fibrosis (CF).

2. The teen years are a crucial time for CF patients' health. If the lungs are neglected, they can easily be damaged and scarred; with good care, they can often remain very healthy.

3. Teens with CF can do virtually everything that their friends without CF do: school, college, date, plan careers, and so forth.

HOW DO TEENAGERS RATE THEIR OWN CHAPTER?

If you read the *Preface* to this book, you saw that teenagers with cystic fibrosis (CF) are one of the main reasons for this book's having been written. There are a few reasons for that and a few reasons why you deserve your own special chapter. Teenagers are caught between two extremes: adults—out on their own, totally *independent*, and with their own chapter in this book—and children—totally *dependent* on parents for everything, and with a lot of the rest of the book focused on their needs. There are special questions that are of more concern to teenagers than other people (education, deciding on a career direction, establishing relationships—including intimate relationships, and even deciding who you are and who you are going to be). And, there are a lot of you: In 2008, there were 25,651 patients with CF aged from 0 to 82 years (that's right, 82!) seen in CF centers in the United States, and over 20% of those people were between the ages of 13 and 20. Finally, perhaps more than any other 7-year period, the teenage years determine what will happen to your health for the rest of your life, based in large part on what you yourself decide to do about it.

Unfortunately, many teens with CF have made what they later realize have been *bad* decisions about their health, and have paid a big price for those decisions, for the rest of their lives. We all make bad decisions at times. It's part of growing up.

245

Fortunately, during the teenage years, you have that little voice, that constant reminder that it is important to take care of yourself. We're not talking about your conscience. We're talking about your family, friends, and CF care team. It's your support team that is important during this time period that can help you make *good* decisions and to be able to reap the benefits of them, for the rest of your longer, healthier lives. Sure, at times it may seem like nagging. There is definitely a language barrier that can exist between adults and teens. In addition to the problems that everyone always talks about with the teen years, these years can be wonderful, and your CF does not need to change that.

You will find some of the information in this chapter in other chapters of the book as well, particularly Chapter 14 (that's the one about adults). Also, check out www.cfvoice.com for more information about CF and tools to help you learn to take care of CF.

MEDICAL ISSUES

This section will address the various organ systems of the body that are affected by CF and how either the effects or the treatment might be different for teenagers. You'll find more details about each organ system in its own chapter (for example, lungs are discussed at great length in Chapter 3). You probably know a lot of this stuff already, since you've had CF all your life, but most likely you haven't had the opportunity just to sit down and learn about CF. If you are like most teens with CF, up until now, you have been kept out of the conversation regarding your health. That is, when you were diagnosed with CF as a baby, the CF care team spoke with your parents about CF. Then when you were a toddler and had trouble gaining weight or your enzymes needed to be adjusted, the CF care team spoke with your parents about that. Then, when you were in elementary school and you had a cough, the CF care team spoke to your parents about that. You may have been in the clinic, and even in the same room, but it just made sense to speak with your parents. Now, we're speaking to you. It's your time to learn about CF and how to take care of your health. And it's a perfect time since you have the experts on your health, your parents, by your side (commence eye-rolling . . . now).

Lungs

Far more than any other part of the body, it's the lungs that determine the health of people with CF and how long they live. The lungs account for 95% of the deaths from CF. Fortunately, there's a lot you can do to influence the health of your lungs.

First, you need to know what happens in the lungs of people with CF. For the full story, you can go back to Chapter 3 but for the brief version, here we go: Thick mucus blocks the bronchi (air tubes, sometimes called *airways*) of people with CF. It doesn't *totally* block them, but it blocks them enough so that infection and inflammation can take hold. Infection you understand: Germs (mostly bacteria, but also viruses, and occasionally fungi) can grow in the bronchi and cause damage. *Inflammation* is what happens when the body responds to these invading germs: White blood cells are sent to fight the infection, and—in a kind of chemical warfare—they release toxic chemicals that attack the bacteria. Unfortunately, these chemicals can also damage the cells that line the airways, causing swelling and cell damage. Some of the bacteria themselves release the same kinds of chemicals and cause the same kind of damage. If the infection and inflammation go on too long or too often (and nobody knows exactly how long "too long" is, or how often "too often" is), airway cells are killed, and scar tissue is formed. For each little infection, it's probably only a little bit of scar tissue that's formed, but once scar tissue forms, it can never become normal, and over months and years that "little bit" of scar tissue for each little infection adds up, so that eventually, virtually the whole lung becomes a mass of infected *cysts* (fluid-filled sacs) and scar tissue. In fact, since scar tissue is called *fibrosis*, you can see where the name *cystic fibrosis* comes from.

So, the idea in treating the lungs of someone with CF is to prevent this progression of airway blockage, infection, inflammation, and scar tissue formation. Since there are three ingredients in the recipe for scar formation, there are three targets for treatment, namely: (a) reducing or preventing airway obstruction, (b) treating or preventing infection, and (c) treating or preventing inflammation.

Minimizing Bronchial Blockage

Airway-clearance techniques are used to minimize bronchial blockage. These techniques include CPT (for *chest physical therapy*), the Flutter, the Acapella, the Quake, percussion vests, *huffing, autogenic drainage, PEP* (positive expiratory pressure) masks, and several others. There is even a device called The Frequencer that sends thumping bass into your lungs to break up mucus (no lie, google it). You've probably heard of one or more of these, and have probably had countless treatments with at least one of these techniques. You *may* even have realized how effective they can be in keeping your airways unblocked, and you never miss a one. But, there's a reasonable chance that you've thought they don't make any difference, or perhaps part of you realizes they help, but you skip a lot of treatments because they're a bother.

The thing is, they *do work*. Studies have shown a significant deterioration in lung function after 3 weeks of missed treatments, even in people whose lungs are in pretty good shape. But a big catch is that if your lungs are in pretty good shape, you will probably not *feel* a difference after getting (or missing) an individual treatment. Our lungs—all of us, CF or no—are notoriously insensitive. We cannot tell when our bronchi are blocked. In a famous experiment, people breathe through a small plastic tube, with their eyes closed. Then the doctor conducting the experiment gradually blocks the end of the tube until the person doing the breathing feels a blockage. Most people can't tell those tubes are blocked until they're more than 50% blocked! The same is true if the breathing tube is your own airways and not a plastic tube you hold in your lips. So, you can't go only on the basis of how you feel: "My breathing feels good, so there must not be any blockage." There can be substantial blockage before you feel it. This is true if the blockage happens quickly (as you just saw, with that tube-blocking experiment); it's 10 times truer if the blockage develops slowly. As with so many other things, gradual changes are very hard to notice: You don't see a kid brother or sister (or the grass) grow taller from day to day, but let a few months go by and they don't fit their jeans anymore (and the grass now looks like a wild field). The difference between those examples and the lungs is that it's never too late to buy a new pair of jeans for your kid sister; and the lawn can be mowed when it's tall—it'll be harder, but it can be done. If the lungs are let go for too long, it may be impossible to get them back in shape again. You may be able to gain some control over infection and inflammation, but the parts that have been replaced by scar tissue can never be made into healthy lung tissue again. Just as important, when the cure is found for CF, it is very *unlikely* that the cure will work on scarred lungs. Since it is very likely that you will have excellent new medications and even a cure for CF in your lifetime, it is important that you keep your lungs as healthy as possible.

One big problem with the older (and still useful) ways of clearing mucus from the lungs, like CPT, was (and is) that for these to be done well, you had to have someone else do them to you. That "someone else" was almost always a parent. That's fine when you're a baby or young child, but gets harder when you and your folks may not see eye-to-eye on everything, including exactly *when* something is supposed to be done. You have your schedule of activities, friends, and so on, your parents have their own schedules, and the two might not coincide. This can be an area of conflict between teenagers and parents (ever notice how a *lot* of things can be an area of conflict between teenagers and parents?). If this has been a problem for you, there's very good news. There are some treatments that are as effective as (maybe even *more* effective than) the old CPT. You can read more about these in Chapter 3 and in Appendix C. Here's exactly what Chapter 3 says about one of these techniques, namely, the Flutter valve.

"This is a hand-held device, small enough to carry around in your pocket, which looks a little like a kazoo. It has a stainless steel ball in it that vibrates up and down (flutters, you might say) as you blow into the tube. The vibrations are transmitted backward down through the patient's mouth into the trachea and bronchi, where they shake mucus free from the bronchial walls. Many teenagers and adults who have undergone traditional CPT for years have become "Flutter converts," saying that the Flutter is more effective in helping them bring up mucus, letting them feel when there's excess mucus there, and to know when they've cleared their airways. The Flutter has the advantage of enabling patients to work on airway clearance without help."

Much the same kind of thing can also be said about a newer device, the vibrating vest—although it's much harder to move from one place to another than the Flutter or Acapella, and is very expensive (as much as $17,500!), it too can give very effective airway clearance for teenagers, without help or interference from parents.

Autogenic drainage, the PEP mask, and the active cycle of breathing are all airway-clearance techniques that also can be done independently. These last three techniques are used more in Europe than they are in the United States and Canada. They seem to work well, but you need to be taught how to do them by someone with a lot of experience in using them. The point is that there are several different options. If one is not working for you and your lifestyle, ask your CF doctor about others that may work (and work into your life) a little better.

Exercise

Exercise is another thing that also helps to clear mucus. Many of you have no doubt noticed that you cough and bring up mucus when you exercise hard. Right now, most CF doctors recommend that exercise be used *in addition to* one of the other airway-clearance techniques (and not instead of them), but it is clearly helpful.

Mucus-Thinning Drugs

CF mucus is hard to clear because it's so thick and sticky. Thinner mucus should be easier to move up out of the lungs. There are a couple of drugs available (and some others that might be available before too long) that make CF mucus thinner. These drugs work extremely well, in a test tube. It's hard to know ahead of time which actual patients these drugs will help, but for *some* people they *do* seem to be very good. The main drug in this family is DNase (aka Pulmozyme®, aka dornase alpha). DNase is breathed in once a day in an aerosol. One study with 900 patients showed an overall small improvement in lung function in patients with CF who took DNase once a day for 6 months, compared with no change in lung function in those who took a *placebo* (a drug that looked and tasted like DNase, but had no effect). Some patients definitely feel better when they take DNase, and some say they breathe easier. Almost no one is hurt by the drug (except financially, since it costs anywhere from $10,000 to $25,000 a year). A very few patients who have more severe lung problems and lots of thick mucus stuck in their lungs have trouble when the DNase has freed huge amounts of newly thinned mucus all at once. For these few patients, it's too much fluid in their airways for them to handle comfortably. One surprise about DNase is that it helps improve pulmonary function tests (PFTs) even in patients who do not seem to have a lot of thick sticky mucus in their airways. We're not sure why it helps those people, but it might have other effects in addition to thinning mucus.

Inhaled saline (salt water) can also help dislodge and thin mucus in people with CF. If you think about the reason why mucus is thick in the first place, it makes sense that saline would work. In the air tubes of the lungs (and for that matter, other tubes in the body), the channel that conducts chloride out of the cell is absent or doesn't work well. If chloride does not get out of the cell into the airway, then there is a lack of chloride in the airway. When chloride doesn't get out, neither does sodium. If sodium chloride (salt) is missing from the airways, water doesn't get into the mucus and thin it out. Inhaled hypertonic saline (super concentrated salt water) helps replace that missing chloride, sodium, and water in the air tubes, making mucus easier to cough out. Just ask your surfer friends. And if you don't believe them, check out the study that looked at the effect of inhaled hypertonic saline in people with CF. It found that those who were treated with hypertonic saline twice a day for 48 weeks had higher lung function values and less chance of getting sick than those who were treated with low-concentration saline.

Treating Bronchial Infection

Antibiotics are the main tools for fighting infections, including bronchial infections, that people with CF get. (We often call these times of bronchial infections *pulmonary exacerbations*, which just means times when the lungs are worse than usual.) Antibiotics kill bacteria. They don't kill viruses, but they are often prescribed when someone with CF has a viral infection (like a cold), too, because the viruses can throw off the lung defenses enough that bacteria can take hold there more easily. Antibiotics come in different preparations, including pills, liquids, aerosols, and intravenous (IV) infusions. Usually, with a new infection, oral antibiotics are used. Antibiotics are prescribed to go in your nebulizer if the oral antibiotics aren't working well enough, and if the nebulized and oral antibiotics aren't controlling the infection, then IVs may be needed. IV antibiotics are usually given in the hospital, for at least 2 weeks, and sometimes as long as 3 or 4 weeks, depending on how long it takes to get you back to normal (back to your "baseline" is what we often say, meaning back to where you were before this particular *exacerbation* started).

The steps here are pretty easy to understand. It's *not* always easy to know when to start treatment at any of the steps, when to move on to the next step, or even when you've gotten back to your baseline. The reasons for this are a bit like what we just said about bronchial obstruction: You can't always tell when you've got worsened infection in your lungs or when it's improved as much as it can. Doctors can't always tell that easily, either.

How to Tell If You Need More Treatment

The amount of cough you have is the main clue for most pulmonary exacerbations. Someone who usually has no cough may start with a morning cough, while someone who usually does have some cough may have more cough. Your parents, brother, sister, or roommate may tell you that they heard you coughing during the night (or the cough may actually awaken you during the night). Just like your dad/brother/roommate may not realize that he snores, you may not notice that you are coughing or coughing more. Your family and friends may be more "attuned" to an increase in your cough.

Your mucus is the next clue. Someone who doesn't usually feel like there's extra mucus inside the chest might start to feel some or start to bring it up. People who are used to bringing up mucus may have more, or it may be darker, thicker, or harder to bring up. Some people may have some trouble catching their breath (they are short of breath) when they go up stairs or run or even just sitting there. There are some signs that aren't obviously connected to your lungs that often go along with a pulmonary exacerbation, including being tired, losing weight, and having a crummy appetite. You might find that you're feeling irritable. All of these changes can signal worsened lung infection (and inflammation). But it may be hard for you to detect any small changes from your baseline, particularly if the changes have developed gradually.

That's where your doctor can help. He or she may be able to tell some things by examining you. Listening with a stethoscope can help. If your lungs are usually clear, but now have *crackles* when your doctor listens, or perhaps more crackles than usual, it suggests extra mucus and infection. (If you're wondering what crackles sound like to the physician, reach up to next to your ear, take a few strands of your hair, and roll them back and forth between your fingers. The sound the hairs make rolling over each other is what crackles sound like: Now you're a doctor! Well, maybe not, but now you know what we hear when we say we hear crackles.) But if you have no crackles, or only in the same places you always have them, the listening might not have told the whole story. Your weight will be important: If it's down, without another explanation, the most likely cause is your lungs (lung infections make you lose weight several ways; if you're breathing harder, your breathing muscles use up energy and calories, just as any other prolonged muscular exercise can do; your body also uses calories to fight infection; and finally, having a lung infection can often make you lose your appetite, so you won't feel like eating as much as usual).

Finally, PFTs (breathing tests) can be a big help. You've probably had these a bunch of times: You blow into a tube and a machine records numbers. These numbers mostly tell how quickly you've been able to blow air out of your lungs and that tells how much blockage there is: the more blockage, the slower the air comes out. If the larger bronchi are blocked, that will affect the first part of the breath, and if the small bronchi (the ones further out in your lungs) are blocked, that will have more of an effect on the last part of the breath. The PFTs are a much more sensitive tool than your doctor's stethoscope, or your ability to feel how hard it is to exhale, for telling just exactly how much obstruction you have in your lungs. Just as it's important to pay attention to how you feel, it can be very helpful if you know a little about your PFTs. Get to know your "personal best" numbers. It can help you and your doctor decide what needs to be done if you are not quite at your "personal best."

Since the doctor (with or without the PFTs) can often detect changes that you hadn't been aware of, it's usual for regular checkups to be scheduled somewhere around four to six times a year. If an unexpected problem shows up at one of the regularly scheduled clinic visits, it's usually possible to start effective treatment before irreversible lung damage has set in. If you waited a year between appointments, it is certainly possible to have some lung damage that's gone beyond the stage of recoverability, *even if you feel pretty good*. That's why it's important to keep those clinic appointments. A lot of people think of doctors' appointments as what you do when you're sick, but there is now good evidence that patients with CF who are seen more frequently—even when they're well—stay healthy longer than those seen less frequently.

Fighting Inflammation

The main way to fight inflammation is to fight infection. For most people, controlling infection with antibiotics will also control inflammation. But some people with CF (and lots of people with asthma) do better if they also get specific *anti-inflammatory* treatment. There are a couple of different kinds of anti-inflammatory medications. *Steroids* are the first kind, and *prednisone* is the most common form of steroids used for people with CF. These drugs are very powerful and control inflammation very well. There are many people whose breathing is a lot more comfortable when they take prednisone. Unfortunately, prednisone (and all other steroids, too) has some side effects that are unpleasant or even dangerous. The two side effects that probably bother teenagers the most are that they can cause acne and they can cause some puffiness, particularly of the face ("chipmunk cheeks").

Another anti-inflammatory medication that's being used is *ibuprofen*. You've probably used ibuprofen on occasion for headache or other minor ache or pain. A study has shown that ibuprofen taken in fairly high doses over a 4-year period seemed to slow the deterioration in lung function in patients with CF. It did not *improve* lung function, but it slowed how quickly lung function got worse. So, this is not a medicine that is going to make you feel better after you've been on it for a day or so. Even if it helps, you won't be able to tell. There are some other problems with the drug, too. Ibuprofen can cause kidney problems and can cause stomach ulcers. It's possible that your CF doctor will want you to take this drug, and it might be good for you, but be sure you understand the possible side effects, and also understand that—even if it's helping—you probably won't *feel* any better on it.

There are a couple of anti-inflammatory inhalers that are very effective for people with asthma, and might also help in CF. One family of these drugs is inhaled steroids, including budesonide (Pulmicort), fluticasone (Flovent), Advair [a combination of fluticasone and salmeterol (Serevent)—which is a long-acting bronchodilator, like albuterol, but longer lasting], and Symbicort [a combination of budesonide and formoterol—which is also a long-acting bronchodilator]. One of the differences between these steroids and prednisone is that these are not absorbed into the bloodstream (or absorbed in tiny amounts), so as a rule they don't cause side effects (no acne, no chipmunk cheeks). Another difference is that they are not as powerful and don't do very much to make you feel better *right away* (even in people with asthma for whom they work extremely well, they *prevent* problems, and don't cure problems once they've started).

Complications of Lung Disease

Problems that are the indirect result of CF include *pneumothorax* and *hemoptysis*, and both are discussed in Chapter 3, *The Respiratory System* and in Chapter 14, *Cystic Fibrosis and Adulthood*. Pneumothorax is a great name for a band, but it's already taken, so you'll have to come up with something else. In addition, *pneumothorax* is a collapsed lung, and can be serious, but is quite uncommon. Anyone who develops a very sudden sharp pain on one side of the chest, along with being short of breath, should call the CF center because this might be a pneumothorax and need quick treatment.

Another problem is *hemoptysis* or coughing up blood (also a great name for a band, but taken. Can you believe it?). It's not uncommon to have some blood streaks in the mucus, and a few people have pure blood. This is very scary but usually not nearly as dangerous as it might first appear. See Chapter 3 for more details.

Gastrointestinal System

There's not very much difference in the gastrointestinal (digestive) system for teenagers with CF. The main thing is the need for enzymes with all meals and most snacks (all the ones with fat or protein in them; see Chapter 6, *Nutrition* for details). About 90% of all patients with CF need to take enzymes for full digestion of their food. You're probably already familiar with what happens if you miss your enzymes or don't take enough: abdominal pain, loose, greasy, smelly stools, and maybe more gas. Surprisingly, some teenagers may need slightly fewer enzymes than they needed as children. Intestinal blockage, called DIOS (distal intestinal obstruction syndrome and also the name of a band—Who are these people?), is more common in teenagers than in children and can be extremely uncomfortable (abdominal pain, no stools). This kind of intestinal obstruction can often be treated by drinking a glass of water or juice with a powder called Miralax, but some people may need a special enema (in the radiology department of the hospital) or even surgery. If the problem is caught and treated early, it's easier to avoid the more invasive treatments. So, if you're having "stomachaches" and fewer bowel movements than normal, let someone know.

Diabetes

About 15% to 20% of teenagers with CF develop diabetes, a condition where the pancreas does not make enough insulin, and therefore the amount of glucose (sugar) in the bloodstream increases, and some glucose is lost in the urine. Losing sugar in the urine means several things: You lose calories, so you might lose weight and energy (before diabetes is diagnosed and treated, people often feel drained and dragged out without knowing why). In addition, sugar in the urine makes you lose a lot of urine, and you're likely to notice that you're getting up in the middle of the night to pee, and you're thirsty all the time. If you have these symptoms, you should be checked for diabetes. Diabetes is usually treated with a special diet (mostly cutting down on soda, candy, and other "concentrated sweets"). Most people with CF diabetes end up getting insulin shots one to three times a day. These shots are surprisingly easy to get used to and make an amazing difference in how good someone feels. Developing CF diabetes is often a case of "good news disguised as bad news." Hearing that you have *another* problem—and one that needs several shots a day!—certainly at first seems like bad news. But it's good news in a couple of ways: First, diabetes in people with CF is usually less severe than diabetes in young people without CF. Second, studies have shown that people with CF who start insulin shots often improve their nutritional status *and* their pulmonary function.

Liver

Some patients also have liver problems, and these are discussed more in Chapter 4, *The Gastrointestinal Tract.*

Other Systems

Sweat Glands

You probably know that people with CF have extra salty sweat. You may have even noticed that some people with CF get "salt rings" on their face and clothes after a hard workout (by the way, Salt Rings is not a name for a band, so go for it). Salty sweat is what makes the sweat test such a good test for CF (analyze sweat, and if there's a lot of salt in it, that means the person has CF). It also means that people with CF lose more salt than normal when they sweat and will have to take in more salt in their diet than others, especially during hot weather, and particularly if they're exercising a lot. This is something that your taste buds are pretty good at telling you: In most cases if you *need* more salt, you'll *want* more, and you'll find yourself heading for the chips or pretzels or pickles, or just using the salt shaker more at meals. It's not necessary or useful to take salt pills.

Reproductive System
General

Both boys and girls with CF may be delayed in going through puberty (growing and developing). This can be a big worry for young teenagers when their friends (or not-friends) are bigger and look more mature. Locker rooms make the differences and delays in development embarrassingly obvious. It's good to keep in mind that almost everybody with CF will catch up, even if it's a year or so later.

Males

Everything about the reproductive system in men with CF is normal, except one little tube. That tube, the *vas deferens*, is the tube that takes sperm from where they're made (the testicles) to the penis, and in 98% of men with CF it's blocked or even absent. That means that men with CF can and do have a completely normal sex life, but there are no sperm in the semen when they ejaculate. In almost every case this means that men with CF are *sterile*, that is, they cannot get a woman pregnant. You can have your semen analyzed to see if there are sperm present (as there will be in 2% of patients). There's more about this in Chapter 14, *Cystic Fibrosis and Adulthood*.

Females

Everything about the reproductive system in women with CF is normal, except for thick mucus in the cervix (the opening to the uterus). This makes it harder for women with CF to get pregnant. Yet, hundreds of women with CF have gotten pregnant. Some women with CF have irregular menstrual periods. These can be regulated with various birth control methods. Many young women have vaginal yeast infections (with itching and burning, especially during urination). Women with CF may be somewhat more likely to develop these infections than women without CF, probably because taking antibiotics makes it easier for the yeast to take hold. These infections can be treated, but only if your doctor knows and gives you a prescription. Some women also have the nuisance problem called "stress incontinence"—leaking a little urine with a cough, sneeze, or laughing. See Chapter 14 for more details.

YOUR MEDICAL CARE: WHO'S IN CHARGE?

Your medical care is like so many other aspects of your life where you're between childhood (where your parents take care of everything for you) and adulthood (where you take care of everything yourself). Ideally, during the teenage years (actually, *early* in the teen and pre-teen years), you should be starting to take charge. That means knowing your medications (names, doses, times, side effects you've had, and so on), being able to report your symptoms correctly (being honest with your doctor and—a necessary first step—yourself about new or worsened symptoms). That means making a call (yourself) to your doctor to report new symptoms, get a new prescription, or arrange for a new appointment. It's extremely common for a teenager to tell the doctor, "I'm fine," leaving it to the parents to point out that the teenager has been coughing a lot more in the past week or two and needing a nap in the afternoon. This inaccuracy on the part of the teenaged patient is almost never *lying*, but rather a kind of *optimism* that sometimes is called "*denial*" by physicians. The kind of optimism and positive outlook on life that so many people with CF have is very important and healthy, *if it doesn't blind them to symptoms that need attention.* We'll talk a little more about denial and optimism later in the chapter.

Your medical care team is going to include you, your parents, and your physician (as well as other folks at the CF center), and needs to be a cooperative venture. You may not always know when you need more care, more antibiotics, or a clinic visit. Your parents won't always know for sure, and, in fact, your doctor can't know either, without good information from you. It's very common for parents to have a hard time giving up their control over their child's medical care. And it's not uncommon for their teenagers to resent this refusal to turn over responsibility. If the resentment is great (as it often is), there are two different ways teenagers express it. One is just to tune out and *let their parents and doctors get away with doing all the talking and making all the decisions for them.* The other is to refuse to have anything to do with treatments, medications, and so forth. By refusing to do treatments, some patients feel that they are taking over control of a part of their lives ("They can't make me do this!"). But it's an unfortunate mistake that ends up almost being: "I'll show you, I'll get sick!" And this approach actually hands control over to *the disease*. A way a patient can really take control of this important part of his or her life is to learn about CF and say: "*I'll do the front-line monitoring of how I'm doing; I'll call when I'm doing worse; I'll make sure I get more treatments to keep myself healthy.*" You can't get rid of CF, but there's lots you can do with your life, including getting as good control as possible of your CF.

At some point, you will be ready to be out on your own and taking care of CF by yourself. When you become an adult, most adult CF doctors will expect that you have a good understanding of CF and your body. Hopefully, you will be prepared for this challenge. One way to know how you are doing is to think about the skills that adults with CF need to take care of themselves. A useful tool is the ADULT mnemonic (fancy word for a shortcut that helps you remember stuff). It helps address five main categories for preparation:

A—access to care. Is there an adult CF clinic that you can go to and do you have the means to go there (is it close to your home and do you have the health insurance that they will accept)?

D—decision-making capabilities. Who is making most of the decisions about your health and life? Is it you or your parents?

U—understanding of CF. How smart are you about CF and your body? If you're feeling a little shaky, check out the beginning of this chapter or other chapters in this book.

L—life skills. Do you have a plan for your life and how you are getting there? Are you going to school? Do you have a job? Do you have that winning lottery ticket?

T—timing. Is now a good time? Changing to a different doctor when you are sick may not be the best time. On the other hand, if you are married, have a job, and are contributing to a retirement plan, then it's probably time that you see a doctor who feels comfortable addressing adult issues.

Know that you are probably the least apprehensive about transitioning to the adult clinic. Real scientific studies have shown that parents and pediatricians are more anxious about their children/patients transitioning to the adult clinic than the children/patients themselves. Your parents/pediatricians will need your help getting through this transition period as you become an adult. So, go easy on them. Even after you have left the house/pediatric clinic, you may need their help someday. Remember, that after you become an "adult" with CF, you are not out there on your own. We all have times when we need a little help from families and friends.

PSYCHOLOGICAL AND FAMILY ISSUES

You and Your Parents and CF

Although most parents and teenagers get along reasonably well, some are constantly at each other's throats. Even the families that get on well together have times when they get on each other's nerves. The teenagers are embarrassed by and feel nagged and harassed by their parents, while the parents feel exasperated that the teenagers don't listen and don't have a sense of responsibility. These occasional or constant irritations and disagreements can affect CF care. Some teenagers feel that their parents restrict their activities because of CF and are always "on their case" about their diet or doing their treatments.

It's worth keeping in mind that parents who don't care about their children don't nag them about medications or treatments. So, most nagging parents nag because they care (not that that's the best way to show it, and not that nagging is easy to put up with, but it's worth checking back in with that fact now and then). One way a lot of teens with CF have found to get their parents off their case is to grab control of treatments and CF in general away from their parents: Show that you can be more attentive and reliable about your treatments than they ever were. Show that there is no need or point to nagging you, and you've won! They leave you alone, you've gotten control, and your health improves, all in one.

Your Parents, Prenatal Testing for CF, and Abortion

A very few teenagers will have the experience that their mother has gotten pregnant, had prenatal testing for CF, and decided to have an abortion because the test showed that the baby would have been born with CF. Others will have heard their parents discuss this question. Sometimes when this happens, the person who's already alive with CF gets the feeling, "Do they wish *I'd* never been born? Do they hate me *that* much?" Of course, this is seldom the case. Almost always when parents make the decision not to have another child with CF (either by not taking the chance and deciding not to have *any* more kids at all, or by using prenatal testing and having an abortion if the prenatal tests show positive for CF), it's not because they regret having had the child or children they already have, but because they want to spare future children the hardships (and there are some, as you know) that come along with having CF.

You and Your Siblings and CF

Sometimes CF can seem to cause tension between siblings. Every single person on earth occasionally gets into a "poor me" mood. People with CF are no exception, and you may on occasion think of the unfairness of CF: Why did you get it, and not someone else? If you have a healthy brother or sister, they are obvious examples of the "someone else" who could have gotten CF instead of you. Try to keep in mind that just as it wasn't *your* fault that you ended up with CF, it wasn't *their* fault that you did, either—or that they didn't. Many brothers and sisters of patients with CF also feel (particularly when they're in their own "poor me" moods) that they've been dealt an unfair hand too. It may seem to them that you get all your parents' love and attention, since your parents spend a lot of time giving you treatments, going to the doctor's with you, and perhaps visiting you in the hospital. If you've been in the hospital, you may have gotten gifts from friends and relatives, too, that siblings didn't get. All this might seem to confirm that you're luckier or more loved than they are. You can reduce these feelings by trying to include them in your life and making it clear to them that they are important to you. Of course, this isn't always easy, because younger siblings *can* be a royal pain sometimes.

You and Your Own Attitude Toward CF

There are almost as many different approaches to one's own CF as there are people who have CF. Most people have a very strong healthy positive outlook that serves them well. Psychologists who have studied groups of patients with CF are always impressed with what an emotionally healthy group of people they are. In practically all areas of life, a positive outlook brings positive results. You might have heard of "self-fulfilling prophecies." This means that if someone is convinced they'll succeed at something, it makes their success that much more likely. (Certainly, the reverse is true: If you go into something convinced you'll fail, you will.) So, someone with CF who approaches life with optimism and determination (as most people do) ends up doing better and being happier than those who have a more pessimistic approach.

If you find that you just can't seem to get that optimistic attitude and are sad or depressed a lot of the time, you should let someone know, because you can be helped by talking with someone (your doctor, a social worker, a psychologist, or a psychiatrist) or by some very effective medications. If you feel you are depressed, you are not alone. In fact, there may be more people with CF who are anxious or depressed than we realize. Sometimes CF can take its toll, and people with CF can feel overwhelmed by everything that comes with having CF. This is a normal reaction to a stressful situation. In addition, sometimes parents, doctors, and nurses are not too good at picking up on when someone may be overwhelmed, anxious, or depressed. Just like you, we like to maintain an optimistic outlook and this can be very annoying when you are feeling down in the dumps. Find someone who you can talk to honestly about your feelings. You will not be letting them down if you tell them that you are having a hard time keeping a positive attitude. They will be happy to help and likely will be relieved to find out that there is something that can be addressed to improve your health.

Most teenagers with CF are able to go on about their lives without paying undue attention to CF. In fact, when CF rears its ugly head, for example, with an article in the newspaper about CF being a "fatal disease," or with a friend dying, or even with a parent nagging you about taking your aerosols, most people are able to push aside the darker thoughts about dying and go on with their lives. By thinking, "this person who died isn't me," you are able to go on about your business. Some professionals call this "denial," meaning that somebody is denying that they have a disease, or refusing to face reality. Actually, though, this approach can be seen as *optimism* and a very healthy, positive way to live your life, with one qualification (see below). People who don't push away negative thoughts and who dwell only on the depressing parts of life (CF or other) get stuck in a quagmire and will not have a very rewarding life.

The only qualification about this approach is that you can't be so unrealistically optimistic about life that you ignore (or deny the importance of) signs that you might need more treatment to maintain or improve your health. Don't dwell on them, don't let them run your life, but face them, deal with them, and move on. If you've got more cough, don't pretend you don't, but increase your treatments, contact your doctor for an antibiotic, and get on top of the problem. If your parents nag you about treatments, don't react to the nagging by skipping health-maintaining treatment.

Your Body Image

Body image means how you feel about your body. This is a problem for some teenagers with CF, which shouldn't be terribly surprising because it's a problem for lots of teenagers without CF, too. Many people think they're too short or fat or whatever. Very few people think that they are *too* good looking (believe us, these are the people with *real* problems). In addition to the doubts about their bodies that most teenagers have, the teenager with CF may have some specifics to focus on: finger clubbing that might seem ugly to him or her (and likely not very much noticed by others); big chest because of overinflated lungs; and skinny, or perhaps puffy chipmunk cheeks from prednisone. For many of these things, nothing can be done other than to try your best to accept them as part of who you are and what you look like, remembering the dedication at the front of this book ("it's not just what you're given, but what you do with what you've got"). For some things, you may be in a position to do something [e.g., a number of teenagers with CF were upset enough about being short and skinny that they agreed to have a gastrostomy tube placed (see Chapter 6, *Nutrition*) for overnight feeds]. Many of these people have liked the results of their taking some control over their bodies.

Friends

Friends Who Do Not Have CF

Most of your friends don't have CF. You should be able to do everything with your friends that they do. There are just a few qualifications to that last statement: If your friends are smoking and drinking, you shouldn't. It's not a great idea for *anyone* to smoke at all or drink heavily, but these can be more trouble for people with CF than for people without CF. Cigarette smoke is clearly very harmful to the lungs of people with CF, whether they are holding and sucking on the cigarette themselves or whether they're breathing in the *sidestream* or *secondhand* smoke from someone else's cigarettes (sidestream smoke is the smoke that comes from the lighted end of a cigarette that's just sitting there; secondhand smoke is what's exhaled from a smoker's lungs). Too much alcohol can depress your breathing, and even a small amount of alcohol can react badly with certain antibiotics and make you feel very sick. If you're old enough to drink, and plan to have a glass of wine or a beer, ask your doctor if that will be a problem with any of your medications.

Late nights, meals out, even trips away, shouldn't be a problem *if you continue to take your enzymes, antibiotics, and other medications, and get in your airway-clearance treatments.*

Whom Should You Tell that You Have CF?

This is a hard question that everyone with CF has to decide for him- or herself. People worry that if others know they have CF, they'll be treated as "a case of CF," or a freak, and not be treated for who they really are. And there certainly are horror stories of kids asking, "why aren't you dead if you have CF?" or teachers announcing on a school-wide announcement system that someone has CF and asking the whole school to pray for them (these are true stories). Most CF physicians, social workers, and psychologists believe that if you are just open and matter-of-fact about your CF, you will do much better overall, including dealing with the occasional jerk who does or says something stupid. It's a lot easier just to go about living your life, not carrying around a deep dark secret. Keeping a secret is very difficult, anyway. If you tell *some* people, like your very best friends (and you *should*), it'll be hard for you to know who knows and who doesn't. Instead of going around scared that someone who knows might spill the beans around someone who's not supposed to know, if everyone knows (or at least if you don't care if they know), your life is a lot easier. This doesn't mean defining yourself as *a case of CF*, (you're *not*; you're a person who happens to have CF). And it doesn't mean going up to strangers on the street and saying, "Hi, I'm Arthur (or Anna); I have cystic fibrosis." It just means not hiding the fact and being comfortable with discussing it. For example, you might meet somebody who complains about needing to take an inhaler for asthma. You can say, "Yeah, I know what you mean. I have cystic fibrosis, and I have to take inhalers too."

Friends with CF

Often people with a lot in common can support each other. We tend to seek out people with similar interests and experiences. CF is no exception, and many people with CF get comfort from knowing others with CF—people who can understand what it's like to have a hard coughing spell in the middle of class, or what it's like to have to swallow capsules with a pizza, and so on. (Some people choose *not* to associate with a lot of people with CF, because they don't want to define themselves too much as "Someone With CF", and that's fine, too.) A recent change has occurred to make this a little more difficult for people with CF: Physicians and families worry that patients with CF can give each other possibly dangerous bacteria (the most notorious of which is *Burkholderia cepacia*, or just *cepacia;* see Chapter 3, *The Respiratory System*). Because of this concern, there is less opportunity to meet and mingle closely with other people with CF. This limited contact is a bother (and the reason for it can feel scary), but it has probably saved some people from getting sicker. Limiting contact does not mean eliminating it completely, so you still should be able to have friends, perhaps electronically, with CF.

Seeing Other Patients with CF Get Sicker

This can certainly be hard. Some of your friends with CF will undoubtedly be sicker than you, and you might see some get sicker who you know didn't need to because they didn't take care of themselves. Some others might do every single treatment and still get sicker. Your job is to be as supportive as you can and to keep in mind for yourself that CF affects different people very differently. Let your friends talk to you if they want, about anything, including their fears and wishes. Sometimes people who are worried about their health—perhaps even worried that they might die—have trouble finding people to talk to about their fears. It might be hard for their parents, who might tell them, "nonsense, you're fine, don't even think about it," and their friends can do them a big service by letting them talk and being supportive and understanding. It can be sad for you to see someone you care about get sicker and especially sad if he or she dies. You may find a lot of different feelings arising, including sympathy, guilt that you're healthier than your friend, fear that you might get sicker, and so forth. You yourself may need someone to talk to about the feelings their sickness brings up for you. Parents sometimes *are* good people to talk with about this. Other friends may be able to help by listening to you. Your physician or CF social worker has a lot of experience with people going through exactly what you're going through, and they may be able to help.

Seeing Yourself Get Sicker than Your Friends

This too can be hard and sad and can raise "it's not fair" feelings. It is almost never too late for increased attention to your health to make some difference; so if you've not been taking good care of yourself and you realize that you're sicker, start taking care of yourself *now*. You won't be able to heal scar tissue, but you can slow deterioration, and you will probably make yourself feel better. There is an excellent chance that you'll be able to feel better *about* yourself if you've adopted a positive "I'm going to take control now" attitude.

DATING, MARRIAGE, AND FAMILY

Some of these topics are also discussed in Chapter 14. CF should not keep you from having friends, including boyfriends or girlfriends. People with CF have the same wishes as everyone else, and dating and forming intimate relationships with others are important parts of life for many people. There is nothing about CF to prevent this, although there are a few little points to keep in mind.

If You're Dating, Should You Tell Him (Her) that You have CF?

As you have seen, most people think it's a whole lot easier if you are open about having CF. There certainly are cases where a possible boyfriend or girlfriend has hit the road as soon as he or she found out that the person they were dating had CF. Clearly, if that is the way someone will react to hearing about CF, it's better to find that out sooner rather than later in a relationship. If you are close to someone, they need to know. If they are close to you and care about you, they will *want* to know. Their knowing about CF will help avoid a lot of otherwise awkward times and explanations: Why you might have to excuse yourself more often to go to the bathroom; why you take those pills with your meals; what was that embarrassing explosive coughing spell just as you were getting ready for (or worse, in the middle of) a good-night kiss?

Sex

Most of the same things that are true about sex for all teenagers are true for teenagers with CF as well. In addition, there are a few special considerations. Some of the things that apply to *anybody* include being sure not to get pressured into having sex. Being physically close to someone else can be very special, and many teenagers feel, correctly, that that closeness (whether it's actual sexual intercourse or holding, hugging, and kissing) shouldn't be entered into lightly and certainly not done without a full understanding of the possible consequences. In addition to the tremendous emotional commitment that having sex with someone entails, there are definite medical consequences as well. The risk of pregnancy is the first that should be considered. You've already learned that *most* young men with CF cannot get someone pregnant, although they can have sex just the same as any other man, and that women with CF are less likely than other women to get pregnant. You absolutely must be clear that some men with CF *can and have* gotten women pregnant, and many women with CF have become pregnant. *Having CF is not adequate birth control.* For young women with CF, it also is essential to keep in mind that there are reasons not to get pregnant in addition to the huge responsibility that anyone would have if they got pregnant. Those additional reasons include the fact that pregnancy can, in some cases, be very harmful to a young woman's health. (Don't despair; if your lungs are in good shape, you may well be able to have a baby later, when your living situation is stable and you're able to take care of one; this is discussed in the next chapter.) Men can have a semen analysis done to see if they have sperm. If they do not have sperm, they might not need other birth control, *but* anyone having sex should be practicing safe sex. Using a condom can protect against STDs (sexually transmitted diseases), including acquired immunodeficiency syndrome (AIDS), as well as protecting against pregnancy.

EDUCATION

Many young people with CF decide to further their education after high school. Many have gone away to college, and lots have even earned graduate degrees. Your CF certainly doesn't interfere with your ability to think, and many patients with CF are outstanding academic successes. Plan your education so that it fits your lifestyle, and so that your health doesn't suffer.

Home or Away?

The decision to move away from home when in college is a big one, especially for someone with CF. For many people—with or without CF—it's not something they want to do, and it certainly is not something that *needs* to be done. But, if you want to attend college away from home, it can be a wonderful experience and an opportunity to establish your independence and, in certain ways, even to define anew who you are. If you decide to take the plunge, you must be certain that your CF care doesn't suffer. You will be in a place where your parents won't be reminding you to eat properly (and providing the food), to take your enzymes, to do your treatments, and to insist that you go to (or call) the doctor if you have new symptoms. They won't be there to do your airway clearance. All of these things must be done, though. One of the saddest things any CF doctor sees is his or her favorite patients going off to school full of enthusiasm and coming back with irreversible lung damage because they neglected their health while they were away. One of the *nicest* things is patients going off, full of enthusiasm, and coming back grown up *and healthy*, because they took care of their health as well as their education! It can be done. Ask your doctor who has done it before you and see if you can ask them what was their secret to success.

CAREER DIRECTION

CF does not need to dictate your career choice. People with CF have successfully held a broad range of jobs: doctors, lawyers, businessmen and businesswomen, secretaries, school teachers, coaches, construction workers, grave diggers, housewives, husbands, computer repair technicians, and so on. So if you really want a particular career, you can probably have it. It is worth keeping a few things in mind. It's not a great idea to have a job with heavy exposure to airborne pollution, smoke, dust, chemical fumes, and so forth. You should also keep in mind that very heavy physical labor might be difficult to sustain over a period of many years. There are people available who can help you make career decisions. Some of these people include CF social workers and people connected with your state's Office (or Bureau) of Vocational Rehabilitation. (There's a lot more about careers and employment in the next chapter.)

SUMMARY

The teenage years are full of challenge for people with CF, just as for people without CF. However, for those with CF, the stakes are higher—if they neglect their health during these important years, they might never regain it. If teenagers with CF take good care of themselves, these years can be wonderfully happy, healthy, productive, and fun.

Cystic Fibrosis and Adulthood

14

Joseph M. Piliewski, David M. Orenstein, Jonathan E. Spahr, and Daniel J. Weiner

THE BASICS

1. Most patients with cystic fibrosis (CF) live well into adulthood; death in childhood is uncommon with aggressive maintenance care.

2. Most adults with CF study, work, marry, and do most of the other things that adults do.

3. Adults may have more health problems than younger patients with CF.

4. Adults have to deal with some difficult questions, including what kind of work they can do, whether they can or should have children, and how long they will live.

Until fairly recently, adults didn't have cystic fibrosis (CF); children had it, and they died. Today, most patients with CF can plan to live well into adulthood, with the pleasures and responsibilities that come with adulthood. In fact, nearly 12,000 (nearly half) of all patients with CF today are 18 years or older, compared with only 624 (8%) in 1969. Patients now live to an average age of about 37 years, and some experts have predicted that survival will increase to over 40 years for someone born in the 1990s (even without any of the many new treatments that are on the verge of becoming available).

Adults with CF are living fulfilling lives. In 2008, 92% of patients with CF, 18 and older, graduated from high school; this compares with the national rate of 87%. Many (66%) of those CF high school graduates went on to college and some to graduate school. Only 7% of patients with CF over 18 years old listed themselves as unemployed or disabled, whereas 25% were students, 36% were working full-time, and 17% were working part-time; 40% of these adults were married.

Upon reaching adulthood, people with CF must contend with some special issues, in addition to those faced by all people as they approach adulthood and in addition to the CF issues facing younger patients and their families. Since the lung problems with CF are progressive (that is, they tend to get worse, slowly, as time goes by), many adults with CF have more symptoms and limitations than they had as children and teenagers. What is true of the lungs is also true to some degree for the other body systems affected by CF: More CF-related problems happen in adults than in children. For this reason, we will have a brief discussion in this chapter of the different organ systems and how they may be affected differently for adults than for younger patients with CF. We'll also discuss some other issues, including medical care, health insurance, employment, marriage and family, disability, and psychological issues.

Newspapers, television, and "the public" (whoever *they* are) often refer to CF as "a fatal disease," which forces even healthy adults to consider the issue of death and dying, which we will address with a brief discussion of death and the adult with CF. More complete discussions of each of these topics can also be found in other chapters. Patients' attitudes and outlook on life have a tremendous influence on what they are able to do, and indeed, on how long they live. Patients with CF typically have a strong, positive outlook, and therefore are able to accomplish many of the normal tasks and enjoy many of the normal pleasures of adulthood, despite having to contend with some difficulties.

DIFFERENT ORGAN SYSTEMS

Respiratory System

Upper Airway: Nose and Sinuses

There is little difference about the involvement of the nose and sinuses in adults with CF compared with CF children and adolescents. In all ages, the sinuses will look abnormal on radiographs (x-ray films), and patients may develop nasal polyps, which may or may not respond to nasal sprays and may need to be removed surgically. The sinus abnormality is more apt to bother an adult with CF than a child with CF, and some adults will have problems with chronic (long lasting) sinusitis. Headache, constantly stuffed nose, and even increased cough may signal infection of the sinuses, which will usually improve with antibiotic treatment. If sinus problems persist despite antibiotics, sinus surgery (to open up the sinuses and make it easier for them to drain) may be helpful in some cases.

Lower Airways: Lungs and Bronchial Tubes

The lungs, especially the bronchial tubes, are the main source of problems for anyone with CF, with buildup of secretions, infection, and inflammation that, if untreated, can lead to permanent damage of the lungs. The lung problems are more likely to occur, and be more difficult to manage, in adults. By the age of 15 years, about one half of all patients with CF cough up mucus each day, and 85% bring up mucus from their lungs occasionally. Adults have more episodes of infection for which they need to be treated with intravenous (IV) antibiotics, either in the hospital or at home. While pulmonary function tests (PFTs) do not tell the whole story, they can help give a general picture of this situation: You may recall from Chapter 3 (*The Respiratory System*) that the forced expiratory volume in 1 second (FEV_1) is the amount of air that can be blown out of the lungs in 1 second, and is a measure of how much bronchial blockage there is (the higher the FEV_1, the higher the airflow, and the less blockage there is). The average FEV_1 for 7-year-olds with CF is 95% of normal (meaning that the average 7-year-old with CF can blow out 95% as much air in 1 second as a healthy 7-year-old without CF), the average FEV_1 for 18-year-olds is 82% of normal, and for 30-year-olds it is 60% of normal. What this shows is that adult patients are more likely than younger patients to have considerable bronchial blockage and generally serious lung disease. Adults are more likely than children to have difficulty exercising; however, regular exercise continues to be a very important means of maintaining lung function for adults. Adults are more likely than children to need to use oxygen (although most will not). Adults are more likely than children to be referred to a lung transplant program for possible lung transplantation (see Chapter 8 , *Transplantation*). But, not everyone continues to get worse and worse after they reach adulthood. Some patients remain quite healthy, and even those who have gotten sicker as they have become adults may be relatively stable for a long time. Some adult patients tell us that they don't get sicker each year, but feel that they have to work harder to stay the same.

Of specific *complications* of lung disease (see Chapter 3), adults are more likely than youngsters to have hemoptysis (coughing up blood) and pneumothorax (collapsed lung caused by a hole in the lung). It is fairly common for an adult with CF to have blood streaking of the mucus that they cough up and spit out, but bringing up a large amount (enough to require hospitalization, for example) is much less common: about 2.5% of patients older than 21 do so (this compares with fewer than 0.4% of children under 15 years). Although pneumothorax is three times more common after the age of 15 years than before, only about 1% of older patients suffer this problem in a given year. So, even though both of these problems are more common in adults than in children, neither one is a major problem for most adults with CF.

Gastrointestinal System

The symptoms and signs from the gastrointestinal system vary in their effects on adults. Most patients, young and old alike, need to take pancreatic enzymes for the digestion of their food. For some strange reason, it seems that many adults have less abdominal discomfort from their pancreatic problem (and may need fewer enzymes with meals) than children with CF. We don't know why this is so: it may be simply that by the time they are adults, patients have learned how to take their enzymes better, or they've learned to avoid problem foods. It may also be that with age, there is a change in their diet or a change in the pancreas, stomach, or intestines that we haven't identified. There may be another explanation, too: It may be that some patients are just *used* to the discomfort, so they notice it less.

Distal Intestinal Obstruction Syndrome

Intestinal blockage (DIOS, standing for distal intestinal obstruction syndrome) occurs in as many as 20% of adults sometime during their adult lives. It's not known what causes DIOS, but one factor that has been blamed in many cases is not taking adequate enzymes. In addition, DIOS seems to occur more often when pain medications, in particular narcotics, are prescribed for pain that is initially unrelated to the intestine. Consequently, it is very important to be certain that bowel movements are regular while someone is on narcotic pain medications. DIOS can cause symptoms ranging from mild cramping to severe abdominal pain—that seems a lot like appendicitis—and lack of bowel movements. It can be very serious and occasionally may even require surgery. Because of the possible consequences, changes in bowel habits—especially having no bowel movements for a day—should make you call your CF physician right away. DIOS can usually be treated by drinking large amounts of special liquids (the best known is GoLYTELY) or, if that fails, by special enemas. Patients with CF should never undergo surgery for "appendicitis" without communicating with their CF physician, because DIOS can sometimes mimic appendicitis but usually can be treated without surgery. Only very rarely is surgery necessary. Fortunately, with better understanding of DIOS, pancreatic enzymes, and more liberal use of laxatives in patients who have had bowel problems in the past, DIOS appears to be less common than before. It is likely that people who would have had DIOS in the past are being identified and treated before a true obstruction occurs.

Antibiotic-Associated Diarrhea and Clostridium difficile Colitis

In recent years, diarrhea associated with taking antibiotics, particularly IV antibiotics, has become more of a problem for people with CF, particularly adults. Loose stools or diarrhea are common in adults on antibiotics, and this typically resolves when the antibiotic course is completed. CF physicians sometimes recommend live culture yogurt or other preparations of "healthy" bacteria to minimize diarrhea and maintain bowel health. Less commonly, diarrhea becomes more severe and difficult to control. When this occurs, it is very important to contact your CF physician or other professional, since an increasingly common complication of antibiotics is *Clostridium difficile* ("C. diff") colitis or inflammation of the large intestine (colon). C. diff results from overgrowth in the colon of a specific bacteria known as *Clostridium difficile* and requires a specific antibiotic to prevent further complications, which could even include the need for surgery to remove the colon.

Gallstones

Gallstones appear in about 10% to 15% of patients with CF at some time in their lives. This is more likely to happen in adulthood. Gallstones can be completely innocent or can cause pain or block drainage of liver secretions. If they do cause pain, they are usually removed by surgery (taking out the whole gallbladder).

Diabetes

As you saw in Chapter 5 (*Other Systems*), diabetes is more common in adults with CF than in children, with about 10% (or more) of patients with CF developing diabetes each decade after the age of 10 years: Almost no one with CF gets diabetes before age 10; as many as 26% of patients between 10 and 20 years old develop it; by age 30 years, as many as 35% of patients have developed it. Diabetes is well managed with diet and insulin injections (and in unusual cases, with diet alone). In some centers, oral medications are used to help control the blood sugar level. Usual complications from diabetes are of two major types: microvascular (small blood vessel) and macrovascular (large blood vessel). The microvascular complications affect blood vessels in the eyes (retinopathy), kidneys (nephropathy), and blood supply to nerves (neuropathy). Macrovascular complications can result in heart attacks and strokes. Fortunately, macrovascular complications (heart attack and stroke) do not appear to be common in people who have CF-related diabetes. However, the microvascular complications can occur, and so CF doctors will often recommend eye exams and kidney function tests (mostly just part of routine blood work) in people who have CF-related diabetes. More importantly, there is a correlation between CF-related diabetes, nutrition, and lung health. So, it is important to both identify and appropriately treat CF-related diabetes. Sometimes, making the diagnosis of diabetes can be that "Aha" moment that can explain why someone is having troubles with their weight or lung health, and starting insulin shots can improve both nutrition and lung health.

Liver Disease

Liver disease, including cirrhosis, used to be the second leading cause of death in patients with CF (after lung disease), accounting for about 2% of the deaths among people with CF. Experts predicted that as treatment for the lungs improved and patients lived longer, more patients with CF would develop liver disease; that is, as there were more adults, there would be more liver disease in patients with CF. This has turned out not to be the case. While most patients will not have liver disease that is life-threatening, a good proportion of patients with CF have enlarged livers or abnormal results of blood tests that check liver function. This is why CF doctors check liver health with blood tests at least annually. It seems that most patients who will develop severe liver disease (cirrhosis, or hardening of the liver) do so by their teens. Many adults with abnormal liver tests are managed with a medication, ursodiol, which helps to thin the secretions from the liver to improve liver functions tests and reduce the risk of progressive problems.

Bone Health

The density of bones of patients with CF tends to fall as patients age. The worse the patient's pulmonary and nutritional health, the lower the density of bone and the greater the risk of bone fracture. The problem is especially pronounced in patients treated with steroids and those who have undergone lung transplantation. Patients need to pay special attention to factors that help bone health, including overall nutrition (including taking pancreatic enzymes), vitamin D and calcium supplements, weight-bearing exercise, and adequate exposure to sunlight. Some patients may need special supplements of bone-building drugs, including alendronate sodium, pamidronate disodium, teriparatide, or calcitonin. This problem is discussed at greater length in Chapter 6, *Nutrition.*

Reproductive System

The reproductive system is more of a concern to teenagers and adults than to children.

Men

Some 98% of men with CF are sterile because of a blockage or incomplete formation of the *vas deferens*, the tube that takes sperm from the testicles to the penis. All other aspects of the sex life of men with CF are normal, but they cannot deliver sperm to their partners. This means that most men with CF are very similar to men who have had a vasectomy, where the *vas deferens* is cut and blocked for male birth control. Two percent of men with CF do not have this blockage, so you cannot assume that intercourse will not result in pregnancy. This possibility, although it is a very small possibility, of not having a blocked vas deferens may be good news for someone who wants to father children or bad news for someone who thinks that CF alone is adequate male birth control. A semen analysis can be done to see whether sperm are present. Men with CF have wondered whether there was a way to get around the blockage of the *vas deferens*, since the sperm are made normally in the testicles, but just can't get out. Recently, a new high-technology microsurgical technique has been developed for *in vitro* fertilization, which has enabled some men with CF to father children. This technique is called MESA, for microsurgical epididymal sperm aspiration. Here's how it works: Using a special surgical operating microscope and tiny needle (because the structures are so small), a urologist aspirates (uses suction to pull out) some sperm from the man's epididymis (a crescent-shaped structure attached to the testicle). These sperm are then injected into one of the woman's eggs, which had previously been removed from her ovary and placed in a test tube. The injection technique is different from the usual *in vitro* fertilization procedures (not that *any* way of fertilizing a human egg outside the body can really be called "usual"). When *in vitro* fertilization is performed, most often the egg and sperm are just put together, with the hope that they'll hit it off and the sperm will enter the egg to fertilize it. But the sperm collected via MESA are generally not mature enough to fertilize an egg on their own, since they are removed before they have had a chance to take their normal maturing trip all the way through the epididymis. Since these somewhat immature sperm would not have much success at fertilizing an egg on their own, they are helped by being injected directly into the egg. The pregnancy rate with this technique may be as high as 50% per attempt. If the procedure works and the egg is fertilized, the tiny several-cell embryo can be analyzed to see whether it carries abnormal *CF* genes before it is implanted into the mother's uterus to grow and develop (the chances of the baby's having CF are shown in Table 11.1). The procedure is expensive (somewhere around $10,000), is not widely available, and is not covered by most insurance policies. Whether a couple in which the husband has CF wants to attempt this will depend on a number of factors, including (a) who will pay for it, (b) what will the couple do if the embryo is found to have two abnormal *CF* genes (most couples contemplating this procedure will decide to have the mother-to-be screened for the most common *CF* gene mutations beforehand), and (c) is the father healthy enough to be able to help raise the child?

Women

The reproductive tract is fairly normal in most women with CF, although a fair proportion of women with CF may have irregular menstrual periods. Women with CF are able to get pregnant (240 women with CF in 2008), and several hundred have carried their pregnancies to term and had babies, most of whom have been healthy. It is probably a bit more difficult for a woman with CF to get pregnant than it is for one without CF, for a couple of reasons. The first factor that makes women with CF less fertile than normal is that the mucus in their cervix (the opening to the uterus) is—like most mucus in people with CF—extra thick and sticky, making it tough slogging for a sperm trying to swim from the vagina through that cervical mucus to get to the uterus (womb) to unite with an egg. In addition, if a woman's nutrition is poor, or if she is in poor health otherwise (as, for example, from severe lung disease), her periods may not be regular, and the periods may be anovulatory (meaning that no eggs are released).

As we will discuss a little later in this chapter, the decision to have or not to have children is extremely important for any woman, particularly so for a woman with CF. Pregnancy can have a detrimental effect on the mother's lung and nutritional health, particularly if her lungs and nutrition were not in good condition at the onset of the pregnancy. (For most women whose lungs are in good shape, pregnancy does not usually seem to make the lungs worse than they would have been otherwise.) The general rule of thumb is that women with good lung and nutritional health can have successful pregnancies, and there is little (if any) compromise to lung health by having a baby. Women with CF who are considering pregnancy should know that pregnancy can stimulate formation of antibodies that can persist in the mother after birth. This would not ordinarily be a problem, but in women with CF who would later need to have a lung transplantation, these antibodies could be harmful to the transplanted lung.

In addition, both men and women with CF are often faced with the difficult proposition that CF may end their lives early. Of course, anyone raising a child is faced with the possibility that they may not see their children grow up, but this may be more concerning for someone with CF.

Birth Control

For many excellent reasons (some discussed later in this chapter), women with CF often decide they do not wish to become pregnant. They certainly should not become pregnant unless and until their ability to take care of themselves (particularly their lungs) and their baby is solidly established. This means that birth control is essential for many women with CF. Not counting abstinence (not having sex at all), the most effective birth control method is surgical: tubal ligation. Practically the only disadvantage is that if you change your mind, it will be difficult or even impossible to undo a tubal ligation. The pill is another reliable method of birth control that many women with CF have chosen and have used safely and effectively. The pill has the further advantage of regulating menstrual periods—a relief to those many women with CF who had had irregular periods. It is theoretically possible that the pill may not work quite as well in women taking antibiotics. This possibility can be avoided by talking with your CF doctor or gynecologist and arranging a special schedule of only 3 or 4 days (instead of the usual 7) each month taking a "placebo" pill. "Barrier" methods (diaphragms and condoms) are somewhat less effective than the other methods, mostly because they must be thought of and used each time a couple has intercourse. Condoms have the important advantage of providing excellent protection from sexually transmitted diseases, including acquired immunodeficiency syndrome (AIDS). You should discuss the pros and cons of the various methods with your physician.

Vaginal Yeast Infections

Somewhere around 75% of all women will have a vaginal yeast infection at some time in their lives. Women with CF are no exception and probably have more of them than other women because of CF women's frequent use of antibiotics. Women with CF would be expected to have more than their share of vaginal yeast infections (often referred to in the medical literature as thrush or vulvovaginal candidiasis—*Candida* species being the most common yeast causing this infection). This is because being on antibiotics increases anyone's chances of getting this infection, because antibiotics kill bacteria, including "good" bacteria in the vagina (and not just the bad guys in the lungs), which allows the yeast to multiply. One study from Australia showed this problem to be much more common in women with CF than women without CF, and for episodes of thrush to correspond to times they were taking oral antibiotics. Furthermore, diabetes also may make a woman more likely to develop a yeast infection, and more women with CF have diabetes. These infections are not dangerous, but can be extremely uncomfortable, causing terrible itching and sometimes burning. These infections can usually be treated successfully with antiyeast cream placed in the vagina. Occasionally, an oral medication might also be needed. Women with CF who get these infections whenever they go on antibiotics can be helped tremendously by starting treatment with vaginal antiyeast medications as soon as they start their antibiotics.

Urinary Stress Incontinence

Urinary incontinence (leakage of urine) is common in healthy women and is even more common in women with CF. As many as half of all women with CF may have urinary incontinence, usually associated with hard coughing or laughing. Some women with CF say that this problem sometimes interferes with their social life and often interferes with effective airway clearance. The problem with airway clearance is minimized by a trip to the bathroom before airway clearance sessions. Pelvic floor muscle exercises (Kegel exercises) are sometimes helpful for women with urinary incontinence. You should discuss this problem with your physician.

OVERALL HEALTH

Many adults with CF find that they are able to do less and less as time goes on, mostly because of the worsening health of their lungs. This can be very difficult, particularly for people who used to be very active. Recurrent courses of IV antibiotics may be needed, and if they are carried out in the hospital, these courses can have a huge impact on a person's ability to continue to carry out a normal work and home life. Permanent IVs such as portacaths and mediports (discussed in Chapter 7) can enable many adults to get their IV antibiotics at home, thus helping them to continue a relatively normal life.

One of the hardest parts for many people is getting used to using oxygen, something that was necessary for about 2.5% of all patients with CF in 2008, most of them adults. People—especially children—may stare at you if have this greenish tubing wrapped around your ears and plugged into your nose. Different patients have handled this discomfort in different ways, from ignoring it to answering questions with a gentle explanation of what the oxygen tubing is for ("it's oxygen to help me breathe better because I have a lung problem"). Oxygen is discussed more in Appendix B.

You may have less energy, find you need to take more time to do things, and schedule more time for rest. Some people may be helped by getting a handicapped parking placard and license plates. If you belong to American Automobile Association (AAA), they can help get you the necessary forms; otherwise, contact your local driver's license bureau.

MEDICAL CARE

The training of physicians in the care of adult patients with CF is just now catching up with the tremendous improvement in longevity. Until very recently, CF was a disease of childhood, and physicians who were trained to care for adults were not taught about CF. Today, there are still too few internal medicine physicians (general medical specialists for adults) who have had training and experience in the problems and care of people with CF. Fortunately, however, there are more and more adult pulmonologists (lung specialists) who have taken it upon themselves to become knowledgeable in the care of adults with CF, and medical training programs are beginning to pay more attention to the treatment of this important population. There has been a large effort over the past 5 years for CF centers to develop adult programs, and the CF Foundation has mandated that centers who care for more than 40 adults have an accredited adult program. As a result, most CF centers have a program for their adult patients, including physicians who are interested and knowledgeable in the care of adults with CF.

Care at an approved CF center, with its team of experts, is very important. Studies in Europe, Australia, and North America have shown clearly that *patients who receive their care at CF centers live longer than those whose care is not in centers; it's that simple.* This is not to say that the general internist or family doctor isn't capable of participating in the care of adults with CF. Quite the contrary: The primary care physician can be a wonderful ally in maintenance of the health of people with CF, just as with people without CF. But the CF care should be coordinated between the primary care doctors and the CF center and not done to the exclusion of the CF center. It is quite important to insist that you have access to center care, particularly in this era when costs may be more important than patient health to some health care plans.

HEALTH AND DISABILITY INSURANCE

Health insurance is a very important issue, because medical care for any chronic illness, including CF, is so expensive. Once a person reaches adulthood, he or she is usually excluded from his or her parents' family insurance coverage. Some states have "over 21" laws, which extend health insurance and/or state programs to adults with certain chronic illness, including CF. Some employers have excellent employee health insurance, but some plans exclude anyone with a "preexisting condition," meaning that they don't pay any expenses related to a problem that you had before you joined the company, which of course would include CF. Some policies limit how much they pay for a particular illness; many have a lifetime limit to how much they will pay. These two problems ("pre-existing conditions" and lifetime caps) have theoretically been eliminated in the health care reform act of 2010. You should find out whether a hospitalization for CF at one time will count as the same "illness" as a previous hospitalization that was also due to CF. Some policies or certifiers are liberal in their interpretation and might consider one pulmonary exacerbation (see Chapter 3) a separate episode of "bronchitis," "lung infection," or "pneumonia" and therefore pay for each of them, whereas others will be very strict and consider every episode to be part of CF and be less willing to pay for multiple admissions.

Health Insurance When Changing or Leaving Jobs

If you want to change jobs, for any reason, you may be scared off by the new company's having a "preexisting condition" exclusion in its health insurance that won't pay for medical expenses associated with a preexisting condition for the first 12 months the person is working for the company and is covered by the new company's insurance. Don't let that stop you. There is a federal law, referred to as COBRA (standing for Comprehensive Omnibus Budget Reconciliation Act), which requires that employees be allowed keep their medical insurance for 18 months after they stop working for an employer (unless they were fired for gross misconduct). That means you can start your new job, with the new insurance coverage, but retain your old insurance for the first 12 months. That way, if you have CF-related medical expenses within those first 12 months, the old company's policy will pay for them; then, once you've put in your 12 months, the new policy no longer excludes the preexisting condition. (There are some preexisting condition clauses that have a different 12-month exclusion: They won't pick up coverage of a condition until you've gone 12 months without any medical expenses related to that condition; those are very difficult to get around.)

That's the good news about COBRA and preexisting conditions. The bad news is that to continue your old insurance policy for the 12-month waiting time until the new one kicks in, you have to make the insurance payments yourself. This can amount to several hundred dollars a month, depending on the policy, and may be more than many patients can afford.

It is very important to look very carefully at insurance plans and possible exclusions before making decisions about employment. As we mentioned above, it is crucial to insist on being able to have access to a CF center for your care. Be certain that you will not be prevented from this specialized care. Try to stay up-to-date on what measures Congress considers and passes. Many people in the CF community were encouraged by recent changes that were enacted, limiting exclusion of patients on the basis of pre-existing conditions and eliminating lifetime caps. Yet, some politicians want to undo even some of these modest changes. Stay tuned and check with your CF center. The center personnel are likely to be up-to-date on these regulations.

UNEMPLOYMENT

If you must stop working because of your health, there are some programs that can help with income and some help specifically for medical bills.

Health Insurance If You Are Unemployed

The COBRA mentioned above is in force whenever you leave a job, whether it's to take another job (as discussed above) or to stop working entirely. In fact, if you are forced by your health to stop working, COBRA requires that you cannot lose your health insurance for 36 months after you stop working. Unfortunately, again, you can lose your health insurance if you can't pay for the premiums. People who have lost their jobs for health reasons may qualify for Medicare, which will pay some medical bills (but not prescriptions), but only after 2 years of being unable to work(!). So, some patients are caught in a difficult bind: too sick to work, unable to afford medical insurance, and with 24 months to wait until they can get Medicare. Some states have "over 21" programs that will pay for CF-related medical bills for people over 21 years in this difficult 24-month waiting period. These programs are a big help, although they don't have unlimited resources and have some arbitrary rules about what is and isn't covered. In Pennsylvania, for example, CF medical bills are covered (doctor's bills, most medications, etc.), but if you have CF diabetes, the state won't pay for your insulin or other diabetes-related expenses, even though the CF caused the diabetes. Your CF center staff is likely to be very knowledgeable about all these rules and is there to help.

Social Security Disability Insurance

Everyone who is employed pays into the federal Social Security fund, designed to help people who become unable to work. If you become unable to work, you may be eligible to receive income from Social Security. The amount you receive depends on how long you've worked and the amount of money you've put into the fund. A downside of this program is that—while it gives some income—it does not give health insurance for the first 2 years someone is on the program. After 2 years, you may qualify for Medicare, which is a form of health insurance (see previous paragraph).

Some patients who have lost their jobs because of their health may qualify for public assistance (Welfare), even if they are getting monthly Social Security Disability checks. For some, however, their income may be too high to qualify for public assistance. Your CF center social worker should be able to help you through the maze of public and private organizations set up to help. Or, you can call your local Social Security office or Public Assistance office.

EDUCATION

Many adults with CF choose to continue their education beyond high school, and some attend trade schools; many graduate from college and even get advanced degrees.

One of the main ways in which CF affects an adult's education is in the decision of whether to leave home to attend college. Leaving home is an exciting and valuable experience for many young adults, with CF or without. It is a time to establish one's independence and even to help "invent" a new personality. It can mean leaving unwanted parts of the past behind and fitting in with a new set of friends. Unfortunately, for too many people with CF that has meant trying to leave CF behind: Not wanting to be different, so not wanting to tell anyone about CF can also mean not doing treatments, not taking medicines, not taking care with nutrition, and so on. In too many cases, it has been possible to ignore CF until it's been too late. There are far too many young adults who have let their health slide and have realized what their parents and physicians had been saying all along about taking care of themselves only after they have suffered irreversible lung damage. Far too many adults have come to us and said, "I wish I had listened, and taken care of myself, but I thought I knew everything, and I never believed I could get sick. Now I wish I had it to do over again . . ."

Leaving home most often means leaving behind the people who perform (or at least remind you to do) daily chest physical therapy (CPT) treatments, which, in turn, means that a replacement must be found (either a replacement person to help with the treatments or a replacement form of airway clearance, using a technique you can do on your own). Much of the CPT can be done oneself, especially if you use the vest, acapella® or Flutter® (see Chapter 3), but some young adults feel more secure with a treatment performed by someone else and may feel that their parents do the best CPT. They are probably right. After all, it is very likely that no one cares as much about your health as you and your parents do. However, there are ways to get adequate help with CPT. Many college health services will offer assistance in this realm. Some schools that have PT students or respiratory therapy students may be able to arrange for these students to help give treatments. College students often have close friends who learn how to administer treatments. Others have placed more emphasis on an aerobic exercise program or on "huff" techniques that are easier to perform on oneself than the traditional CPT.

The acapella®, Flutter®, and the vibrating vest (see Chapter 3) have freed many people from dependence on others for effective airways clearance treatments. Some CF physicians will accept 15 to 20 minutes each day of vigorous exercise as a substitute for CPT. Whatever one chooses, it is extremely important to find some way to keep up with treatments and to not give in to the temptation to skip them in the excitement of being away on one's own, perhaps for the first time. There are always reasons to skip a treatment (test tomorrow, party tonight, etc.), and while it's fine to skip an occasional treatment, this cannot become a habit. A problem with many treatments, including CPT and other airway clearance techniques, is that you may not feel much better after them; what's important is their cumulative effect over many days, weeks, and months. So you may well skip a treatment and not notice any dire consequences. If this happens, it's easy to let yourself slip into a habit of skipping lots of treatments. Unfortunately, many people have noticed their lungs being worse from skipping treatments only after irreparable harm has been done to them. Then it's too late. So, it's important to try to keep up with all your treatments. It's also important to keep up with good nutrition, which many young adults have let slide when their parents (usually especially their moms) are not there to nag them or to cook for them.

While we're on the topic of nonhealthful temptations, it's important to mention two others, namely, smoking and drinking. It should be obvious (but isn't always) that smoking (cigarettes particularly, but also probably marijuana) is bad for anyone's lungs and especially so if one has underlying lung disease, like CF. There is definite evidence that secondhand cigarette smoke (that is, someone else is doing the smoking, and you're breathing in the extra smoke that just happens to be in the air around) is harmful to patients with CF; it stands to reason that active smoking is that much worse. Smoking will absolutely disqualify you for a lung transplant if you should ever decide that you want one. Alcohol in moderation is probably not bad, but you should discuss it with your physician, because there are some medications, including some antibiotics, which interact badly with alcohol, and alcohol is likely to aggravate any underlying CF-related liver disease (as described above).

Many states have vocational rehabilitation offices or bureaus [Offices of Vocational Rehabilitation (OVRs) or Bureaus of Vocational Rehabilitation (BVRs)] that provide educational and occupational counseling and financial assistance for students after high school. These programs used to be extremely helpful, with some of them automatically paying college tuition for anyone with CF, but many are now suffering from slashed budgets and may not be able to provide as much assistance as in years gone by. They may still be able to give helpful guidance on career selection, though, and are worth checking out. Your CF center social worker should be able to tell you about these resources, or you can call your state Department of Labor and Industry Office of Vocational Rehabilitation.

Many colleges and universities have an Office of Disabled Students. Many people with CF do not think to contact this office since they do not feel that they have a disability. However, the Office of Disabled Students can be very helpful in providing accommodations for students with CF by helping students with everything from getting a private room to air conditioning to reducing minimal hours needed per semester and providing plans for keeping up with classwork and rescheduling exams during times of illness.

Young adults with CF should know about the services the Office of Disabled Students can provide when looking at colleges and establish contact with the office prior to starting classes. Federal laws prohibit colleges (and any federally funded entity) from discriminating on the basis of disability. Colleges are required to provide accommodations for students with disabilities. So, there is no harm in finding out what services are available at each college.

EMPLOYMENT

Men and women with CF have had—and succeeded at—many different kinds of jobs, including physician, CF research scientist, lawyer, race car driver (at least one woman!), professional wrestler, basketball coach, school teacher, computer repair technician, farmer, homemaker, and so forth. CF may well influence one's career choices. It is important to consider your current physical condition and what your physical condition will be in several years as you make occupational plans. In general, a relatively sedentary job is better over the long haul than one that is physically demanding. This does not mean that a sedentary *life* is preferable, but rather that one should exercise during leisure time. It also doesn't mean that physical labor is bad, but rather it makes sense to plan for a time when you might not be as strong as you are when you are starting employment. Then, if you should become ill or weakened, it would not jeopardize your job and would only affect your leisure time exercise regimen. Jobs involving constant exposure to dust, chemical fumes, or smoke should be avoided. If you're thinking about teaching school, especially younger children, you should keep in mind the possible danger of near constant exposure to an ever-changing array of respiratory viruses.

CAREERS IN HEALTH CARE

Many people with CF are interested in careers related to health care. This makes a lot of sense and patients have much to contribute, as they have much knowledge of and experience with various aspects of the health care system. Jobs in health care often have good benefits, too. Furthermore, many health care careers have the possibility of transition to administrative roles, which are less physically demanding than active roles in direct patient care can be. This may be desirable if the patient/employee's health and stamina decline. However, there can also be a down side (can't there always?). As we just suggested, some health care careers are very physically demanding, perhaps too much so for someone with limited endurance. Infection control is another major consideration, for both the patient with CF and the potential employer. Frequent exposure to multiple respiratory viruses, as happens in pediatrics, is not helpful to patients with CF. The other side of the coin is that patients with CF who cough may pose a risk to patients they care for, particularly if those patients have any problems with their immune system. Thus, the decision to pursue a career in health care requires a great deal of thought.

If someone is not able to continue to do full-time work, some employers may be able to offer part-time work. Some patients have been able to do some of their work at home, particularly with the help of a computer modem and/or fax machine.

The Americans with Disabilities Act (ADA) of 1990 is a very important law for people with CF to know about. This is a federal law that protects people with disabilities from being discriminated against, including in the workplace. What "disability" means for this law is different from what it may mean in other settings. There have been many people who have applied for Social Security Disability (see below) and have been denied those benefits because they weren't sick or "disabled" enough. Yet, these people may still be covered by the ADA. For this law, the definition of a person with a disability is someone who:

- "has an impairment that substantially limits one or more major life activities; or
- has a record of such an impairment; or
- is regarded as having such an impairment."

People with CF, even those who are not dreadfully ill, may qualify. Here's how: CF may be considered to give a "substantial limitation" to the "major life activities" of breathing, eating, or walking. This may be true even if with treatment, you breathe, eat, and walk well. The disability determination must be made without considering the effects of treatments. Even for someone who has absolutely no limitation from CF, the ADA may provide protection for you from the situation where an employer or union official thinks you're limited. Of course, if anyone (from CF or other cause) becomes too sick to work, then the employer can fire that person. But before an employer can fire you because you are unable to do your job, the ADA requires that "reasonable accommodation" be made to allow you to continue to work. This "reasonable accommodation" includes such things as job restructuring, changing work hours, and giving additional sick time (paid or unpaid). This might mean allowing you to start work later in the morning, to allow for morning airway clearance. Unless there is something crucial about your job that requires it to be done very early, and doing it later would mean a hardship for your employer, you may have the right to have your work hours changed. Another possible "reasonable accommodation" would be getting 2 weeks more sick leave for a hospital admission.

The Family and Medical Leave Act (FMLA) also provides some accommodations for workers if they become sick. The act states that employees are allowed up to 12 weeks of unpaid leave per year due to serious illness that interferes with work without fear of being fired. This can be applied to parents, children, and spouses who have to take time off to care for loved ones. The FMLA applies to workers who work for employers who have more than 50 employees and who have worked for more than 1 year and 1,250 hours in the previous year. Health insurance must continue to be provided by the employer during these times of absence.

Applying for a Job

Patients often wonder what they should do about mentioning their CF in a job interview. Most lawyers and disability rights experts think it's not a good idea to volunteer the information during an interview. If you do mention your CF and aren't offered the job, it will be hard to know (or prove) whether it was the employer's feelings about CF that caused you to lose the job. On the other hand, if you don't mention CF and are offered the job, but then the job offer is withdrawn after the employer finds out you have CF, it's easier to prove that the offer was withdrawn because of CF, and that's illegal. If you are asked point blank during an interview whether you have a disability, it gets tricky. Employers are allowed to ask whether you will be able to do what's required for a specific job, but are not allowed to ask whether you have a disability. If you tell an interviewer that it's illegal to ask whether you have a disability (which is true), you could lose the job because of an "attitude" problem, whereas if you lie and say you don't have any problem, then you put yourself in a compromised position if and when it ever comes out that you have CF. In actual fact, in most cases, the question won't come up.

MARRIAGE AND FAMILY

About half the patients with CF over 25 years of age marry, and most of these marriages succeed, with a lower divorce rate than in the general population. Decisions about raising a family are definitely difficult if one partner has a life-shortening disease that limits fertility. Women with CF have a more difficult time conceiving than women without CF, and 98% of men with CF are sterile. Careful consideration must be given to the potential parents' long-term health, and difficult issues must be faced such as the possible death of one parent, which would leave the other a single parent and the child or children with only one parent. If it is the woman who has CF, the possible effects of pregnancy on her health must be considered. Pregnancy has often caused dramatic deterioration in the health of women with CF if their lungs were not in excellent shape at the outset. Similarly, in women with severe lung disease, the chances of having a miscarriage, stillbirth, premature birth, or birth of an abnormally small baby are increased. In addition, both parents must keep in mind that raising a child is hard, tiring work: occasionally up all night with crying or minor illnesses, giving the child attention for much of the day, and being exposed to the many different viruses that all children bring home from day care or school. These can be difficult stresses and strains on the parent with CF, especially if he or she is the one doing most of the child care. Finally, with either parent having CF, the baby might have CF. The child will have gotten one abnormal *CF* gene from the parent with CF, and whether he or she ends up with CF depends on whether the other parent passes on an abnormal *CF* gene as well. The chances of this happening are presented in Table 11.1. Because of the dangers to the mother and baby, a number of women with CF lung disease have been advised not to get pregnant or to terminate a pregnancy. This can be hard advice to hear and has made some women sad and/or angry, particularly if they had their hearts set on having children. Many couples in which the husband has CF have decided to adopt children, and some have decided to have children through artificial insemination. New, expensive, high-technology methods have made it possible for a few men with CF to father children, as discussed earlier in this chapter. Both partners must be willing to discuss all the issues around the important decision of whether to have children or not. It certainly is okay to decide not to have children.

Infant Feeding: Breast Versus Bottle

Breastfeeding a child after birth can require 500 more calories per day from the mother. For the most part, women with CF who are healthy enough to deliver a child can tolerate this increased expenditure, and therefore intake of calories (and are probably used to eating gallons of ice cream at midnight). Breast milk from women with CF is perfectly normal and healthful for the infants. Breast-feeding may put a strain on the mother, however, and may put both a nutritional and energy drain on her. If a woman is having trouble maintaining her own nutrition, breast-feeding may add to her difficulty of keeping her weight up. Bottle-feeding infant formulas will also provide excellent nutrition for the baby and will spare the CF mother that extra calorie drain. It will also make it possible for both parents to share the joy (and work) of feeding, including middle-of-the-night feedings.

Sex

Most couples with one partner with CF are able to have fulfilling intimate relations, including an active healthy sex life. As you've already learned, most men with CF have blocked or incompletely formed *vas deferens*, making it as though they had had a vasectomy. They can have sexual intercourse normally, only no sperm come out. Similarly, although women with CF have more difficulty getting pregnant than women without CF, they too usually have normal sex lives. For both men and women, coughing spells can be disruptive during intimate times, and this may on occasion be a problem. Some patients with CF with more advanced disease have a harder time breathing when they are lying flat on their backs. If this is a problem that interferes with sex, different positions can be used. Just as oxygen can help people breathe more easily when they exert themselves in other ways, it can also be helpful for people who otherwise become short of breath during intercourse. Other small adjustments can make a big difference to the partner with CF if he or she has advanced lung disease that has interfered with a couple's sex life: Consider timing your sexual activities for when you feel good. Many people with CF lung disease are not at their best in the early morning before a good aerosol and airway clearance session, so sex as the first thing in the morning may not be such a good idea for such a person. Similarly, some people feel short of breath and tired after a big meal, so think about giving yourselves a while to digest before planning exertion of any kind, including in bed. Finally, an aerosol and airway clearance may help make sex less taxing for the patient with CF and therefore more enjoyable for both partners.

PSYCHOLOGICAL ISSUES

The overall psychological health of patients with CF is excellent. Professionals have been impressed at the low rate of depression and the excellent ability to cope among patients with CF who have a life-shortening disease that—for some—makes employment difficult, decreases fertility, and presents so many physical and financial obstacles. Most patients do extremely well psychologically and emotionally. They are models of a very realistic, healthy, positive outlook.

Nevertheless, some patients with CF will be sad, and some will be depressed. These feelings can interfere with people's ability to work, to sleep, and to function in many different ways. These feelings should not be ignored, because in most cases, they can be helped with counseling or medication. If you experience depression or other difficult emotions that make it hard for you to carry on, you should let your doctor or social worker know, because you are certainly not alone, and there is an excellent chance that you can get effective help.

DEATH

This book contains a whole chapter on the difficult subject of death (Chapter 15). We mention the subject briefly here because it is an area of particular concern to adults. More adults than children with CF die each year, and the death rate for adults is much higher than that for children (in 2008, 96% of patients with CF who died were 18 years or older). However, perhaps surprisingly, the chances of dying at any given age do not seem to keep increasing for every year you age: In one recent year, the mortality rate for 10-year-olds with CF was 0.012 (meaning that of every 1,000 10-year-olds with CF, about 12 died), while it was 0.054 for 20-year-olds, but only 0.047 for 30-year-olds, and 0.045 for 41-year-olds. Furthermore, if you look at PFT results to try to predict who will die, you find big differences between children and adults, in favor of the adults: For any given PFT number, a child with that number will be more likely to die than an adult with the same number. An example is the FEV_1: about 27% of children 6 to 17 years old who had an FEV_1 between 30% and 40% of normal died within 2 years, while only 18% of those aged 18 to 44 years died within 2 years. The same difference holds between children and adults for most PFT values. Experts speculate that a child who has a low PFT (bad bronchial blockage) may be sicker and have somehow more rapidly worsening lungs than an adult who has taken up to 30 more years to develop the same amount of blockage. So, adults with CF, even with fairly severe lung disease, have staying power. Nonetheless, some do die, and adults with CF have to face the issue.

Adults may have spouses, children, and jobs to consider and personal and financial affairs to get in order. Adults will also be forced to confront issues like life support when they are hospitalized, since federal and state laws now require any adult who is admitted to the hospital to be informed of his or her right to make "advanced directives." These are decisions about what medical treatments they will or will not accept, including "artificial ventilation, artificial feeding, and artificial hydration."

Adults may have to decide whether they want to consider lung transplantation. Many patients have found this decision to be the most difficult they've ever faced and thinking about it to be among the most stressful tasks they've ever undertaken. The stakes are so very high, with possible positive outcomes so positive, and possible negatives so very negative (these are discussed at some length in Chapter 8, *Transplantation*). Add to this the seeming irreversibility of the decision and the time pressure patients have felt to make the decision, and you have a recipe for a difficult and emotional time. It must be stressed that either decision—for or against transplantation—can be the right one for different people.

COMMUNICATING WITH OTHER ADULTS WITH CF

Many people with CF are interested in meeting others who might be going through similar trials and tribulations. Some communication with other CF adults happens through the CF center, just through the coincidence of being in the clinic waiting room at the same time or being hospitalized at the same time. CF center physicians, nurses, and social workers can give you names of other patients/families who have expressed a similar interest. (Of course, not everyone wants to get together with other patients.) Many local Cystic Fibrosis Foundation branches used to have get-togethers for families, but because of increased concern about sharing bacteria that may be dangerous along with sharing good times, there are many fewer of these social functions these days. Since it appears that physical contact, or extremely close proximity, can result in person-to-person transmission of bacteria, CF centers now encourage their adults to avoid physical contact with other patients with CF and, for example, to forego the usual handshake when they meet other patients with CF. There are several newsletters and Internet websites that are aimed particularly at (and run by) adults with CF. Newsletters come and go, and are often driven by one dedicated person, so your CF center or the Cystic Fibrosis Foundation may be able to give you up-to-date information on these newsletters and websites. The opinions expressed in the newsletters and on the websites do not always coincide with what CF physicians might believe, so we urge you to discuss treatment issues with your physician. We include here several websites and newsletters that have been helpful to some adults with CF:

1. Newsletter of Cystic Fibrosis Worldwide: write to the editor c/o 1, The Cottages, Southill Road, Cardington, Bedfordshire, MK44 3TF, England; e-mail her at: editor@cfww.org; the website for this organization is: www.cfww.org (Cystic Fibrosis Worldwide)
2. CF Roundtable (a publication of the United States Adult Cystic Fibrosis Association: http://www.cfroundtable.com/).

SUMMARY

Most patients with CF now live well into their adult lives. Adulthood with CF brings challenges of living independently, perhaps facing declining health and the possibility of dying but also the satisfactions that can come with approaching life with a positive attitude and succeeding at many different tasks in one's personal, family, educational, recreational, and career paths.

Death and Cystic Fibrosis

15

Elisabeth P. Dellon and David M. Orenstein

THE BASICS

1. Many people with cystic fibrosis (CF) think about dying.

2. Most people with CF will die from their disease, and not of old age.

3. People with CF do not choke to death on their mucus.

4. Death is seldom sudden or unexpected for people with CF, but the exact timing of death is often difficult to predict.

It has been stressed throughout this book how well people can live with cystic fibrosis (CF) and how much better and longer their lives are now than they were just a few decades ago. Advances in treatment and exciting research progress promise even better things to come. In the meantime, people do still die from CF. In fact, until a cure is found, it is probable that most people with CF will die from their disease, and not of old age. In order to dispel some common misunderstandings and fears about dying, this chapter will discuss what happens when someone dies from CF.

Most people who die from CF die because their lungs have become so damaged that they can no longer perform the work of bringing in oxygen and eliminating carbon dioxide. This means that oxygen levels in the blood will be too low and carbon dioxide levels too high. All body tissues need oxygen to stay alive, so when the oxygen level is too low, tissues and organs cannot function appropriately. In some people, low oxygen level is the factor that is most apparent near the end of life. "Air hunger" is a term that is used to describe how someone feels if the oxygen level is too low. Air hunger is very uncomfortable and can be quite distressing, both for the patient and for family and friends who find themselves unable to relieve the suffering. Fortunately, even when the lungs are so damaged that nothing can be done to prevent the person's death, most often oxygen and medications can help to relieve air hunger.

When the carbon dioxide level in the blood rises, it acts like a sedative, causing drowsiness and difficulty in communicating. People with high carbon dioxide levels are not usually uncomfortable, as they are relaxed and often asleep much of the time. If carbon dioxide levels become extremely high, the person may sleep so deeply that the breathing efforts become very weak. In this situation, the person may be difficult or impossible to awaken, may not respond to people in the room, and may die in his or her sleep. This is more difficult for people who are watching and waiting than for the person who is dying, since he or she is not uncomfortable.

WHAT CAN BE DONE?

If someone's oxygen level is low enough to be causing air hunger and distress, one relatively simple thing to do is to give more oxygen to breathe. Although this is an obvious thing to do, it is not always done because of physicians' concerns about its effects on how the brain controls breathing. You'll recall from Chapter 3 that when someone's lungs are badly damaged, and the carbon dioxide level has been high for some time, a low oxygen level may become the brain's main signal to keep breathing. Physicians may be concerned that if extra oxygen is given, it may raise the blood oxygen level enough that the brain will respond by inhibiting the signal to breathe hard. Breathing will then get progressively shallower, and the carbon dioxide level will build higher, putting the patient to sleep, perhaps so deeply that he or she will die.

There are some important fallacies in these concerns. When someone's carbon dioxide level has been high for some time, receiving extra oxygen rarely impairs breathing. Sometimes it even improves it, probably by giving needed oxygen to the breathing muscles. The primary concern should be for the patient's comfort, such that sedating him or her slightly by allowing the carbon dioxide to build up may actually be helpful. The extra oxygen may change the situation from one in which low oxygen dominates, making the patient suffer, to one in which high carbon dioxide dominates, making the patient sedated and comfortable.

Another treatment for people who are suffering from low oxygen levels is the careful use of medications that can relieve anxiety and discomfort. Morphine and other opioid medications are the best drugs for this purpose and can be extremely effective. The main danger of medications like morphine is that too much can cause excessive sedation to the point where the patient falls asleep so deeply that he or she does not wake up. Given carefully, these drugs are not likely to cause this problem and are very likely to relieve otherwise unbearable suffering. The effects are often like those just discussed of administering oxygen: Morphine (or other opioid medications) and/or oxygen can sedate someone whose oxygen levels are low, making that person much more comfortable. Almost always, if a person is dying, the primary concern should be the person's comfort.

MYTHS ABOUT DYING WITH CF

There are a number of well-known myths about dying with CF. Many of these are inaccurate and are important to discuss and to understand.

"People with CF May Choke on Thick Mucus and Die."

It is certainly true that thick mucus is a problem for people with CF and that some children and adults with CF have very severe coughing spells. During these spells, it can look (and feel) as though they won't be able to catch their breath. However, people with CF do not die by choking on their mucus. In fact, a sudden unexpected death in CF is extremely rare. People with CF do not go to bed well and die during the night.

"Doctors Know When a Person with CF Is Going to Die."

It is possible to know that someone is getting sicker and that his or her pulmonary function has been declining for several months. While statistics enable physicians to estimate that someone with certain numbers for pulmonary function tests has a 50% chance of dying within the next 2 years, these statistics apply to the entire population of people with CF and there is individual variation in the rate of progression of CF lung disease. In extreme conditions, experienced CF physicians may be able to say that someone is so sick that he or she is not likely to live many more hours or days. It is not possible to predict the exact timing of death. Physicians who treat patients with CF have seen patients who they thought could not possibly make it through the night recover sufficiently to live for months or even years. For this reason, some CF physicians believe that when someone is extremely ill and is unlikely to survive, it is still worth giving as much treatment as possible to enable the lungs to recover (usually antibiotics, aerosols, and airway clearance) if these treatments do not interfere with the patient's comfort. Invasive and uncomfortable procedures and treatments that are not likely to sustain life, such as using a breathing tube in the trachea and a mechanical ventilator, may not be justifiable if the chances of recovery are extremely small. On the other hand, relatively simple treatments, such as intravenous (IV) medications, which might give a patient the slight chance of recovery and which would not interfere with comfort, should be offered.

"Dying from CF Is Very Painful."

If someone is dying with a very low oxygen level, the sensation of air hunger can be extremely uncomfortable. However, that sensation can most often be lessened considerably by giving oxygen and sometimes medications such as morphine.

While physical pain, particularly chest pain, back pain, and headaches, may occur, these are usually well treated with pain medications and become less bothersome during the dying process.

"It's Better to Die at Home than in the Hospital."

Don't all of us want to die among loved ones, in a familiar setting, without strangers being present and without suffering intrusive treatments? While many people feel this can only be achieved at home, it is important to recognize that dying in the hospital can also be peaceful. When the patient, family, and medical providers have had discussions about dying and patient and family preferences are understood, the procedures and medications necessary to keep the patient comfortable can be readily handled in the hospital. For many patients with CF and their families, the support of the hospital staff can be very comforting. For patients who would prefer to die at home, hospice agencies may be able to provide the necessary services, medications, and support with ongoing involvement of the CF care team.

"It's Important to Keep Fighting."

When someone with CF is dying, that person has lived for many years with the disease, has done much to stay well (exercise, airway-clearance treatments, medications, etc.), and has been recognized by others as fighting against the odds. Family, friends, medical providers, and the patients themselves think of them as "fighters," in the very positive sense of that word. Too often, however, in a family's grief over losing a very special person, they may convey to that person the idea that they must keep fighting and not "give up." The message may come across that if the patient dies, he or she has let down the family. Patients may need permission from their loved ones to let go, and to rest. They need to know that they don't have the burden of supporting their surviving family.

LUNG TRANSPLANTATION AND DYING

While the advent of lung transplantation for patients with CF has brought hope to many and has extended the lives of some, it has greatly complicated the dying process for many others. If someone is dying and is awaiting a transplant, there can be conflicting goals: For the dying patient, the traditional approach has been to stress comfort, even if that meant fewer days of life. For the patient awaiting a lung transplant, the goal sometimes changes to extending life day by day as long as possible until donor lungs become available. For some patients, this life extension has included measures as drastic as tracheostomy and mechanical ventilation, often in a lung transplant center hundreds of miles from home. Patients and families can be in a very difficult bind: Do they forego the chance of extended life that transplant represents in favor of a peaceful and relatively comfortable death, or do they forego that peace and comfort for the possibility of a longer and possibly healthier life? The time spent on the waiting list for donor lungs, which may be months or even years, during which CF lung disease progresses and health continues to decline, makes this decision all the more difficult.

PATIENTS' CONCERNS ABOUT DYING

Adolescents and adults with CF (and even younger children with CF) may worry about death and dying. It is important for them to be able to talk about these concerns. The death of a friend or an acquaintance with CF may cause great concern, and it may be reassuring for patients to hear of ways in which they are different from the person who died and that they are not in danger of dying soon. On the other hand, it may be that their concerns are very realistic and that they are in fact close to the end of their lives. In either case, it is extremely important for them to be able to confide in someone, express their fears, and have their questions answered.

It is tempting for people who care a lot about patients with CF to reassure them and to try turn their thoughts away from death and dying. It's fine to be hopeful and optimistic, but refusing to acknowledge and talk about a person's worries does them a great disservice. It may be that just listening and being supportive can relieve someone's worries tremendously. Many people have thoughts and worries about their own death, and it is helpful for those thoughts to be discussed openly. It is not helpful, however, to force a discussion of death on someone who is not ready for it. Family members, close friends, and medical providers may be the people chosen to share in this kind of discussion. The questions that children have about death may range from whether they will be in pain to whether they will be remembered and missed to whether they will see their dead relatives after they die. A family's religious beliefs may influence how they answer these questions.

REACTIONS TO THE DEATH OF SOMEONE WITH CF

When a person with CF dies, family and friends have many different kinds of feelings. Sadness and grief for the lost loved one, and for the suffering that he or she might have gone through, are often accompanied by feeling sorry for oneself for having to go on without the person who has died. There is also commonly a feeling of relief, especially if the death comes after a prolonged difficult period. This relief may cause guilt, but it is a perfectly normal and healthy feeling. Parents who have lost a child with CF may have some renewed sense of guilt for having "caused" the CF, or for not having done more for their child. Again, these feelings are normal, but must be balanced by the realization that no one causes a genetic disease and that, in most cases, families have done everything possible in caring for their children.

Parents with other children with CF may be especially sad to think that what one child has just gone through will be repeated for the surviving sibling(s). This may be true. It is also true that treatment for CF continues to improve, and surviving children may be able to be spared some of what their sibling has just gone through.

Surviving brothers and sisters have complex reactions, which may be confusing to them. They will be sad, of course. They may have a frightening feeling that they were somehow to blame for their brother's or sister's death because of having had "bad thoughts." It is important for them to know that all children at some times wish that their siblings were dead, or out of the way, so that they can have their parents' undivided attention and love. They might be feeling especially guilty for wishing these things and for believing their parents favored the sick child.

They need to know that these thoughts are normal, that they are not bad for thinking them, and that they did not cause their sibling's death. It can be helpful to point out ways in which the surviving child was special to the sibling who has died. If the surviving sibling has CF, he or she may be especially frightened about his or her own fate. In this case, it is helpful to assure him or her that everything will be done to keep him or her well for as long as possible. It is important to give the child the chance to express worries and to seek support from others with experience in helping grieving children.

POSTMORTEM EXAMINATIONS

After a person with CF dies, a physician may request permission from family members for a postmortem examination, also called an autopsy. This is very difficult for many people to think about. In cases where it is not clear exactly why the patient died, important information may be discovered from a postmortem examination which may make it somewhat easier for surviving family members and friends to cope with the loss of their loved one. It is also possible that something will be discovered that could benefit other people with CF.

ORGAN DONATION

When patients with CF are dying, it may comfort them and their families to know that they may be able to help someone who is alive but suffering. Organ donations for transplantation may offer this solace. Patients with CF have been able to donate their eyes to enable others to see and their hearts to enable others with terminal heart disease to live.

RESEARCH

As everyone who is reading this book now knows, the basic defect in CF is still not completely understood, and there is no cure for CF, but many scientists around the world are working toward these ends. In some cases, research that furthers the understanding of CF can only be carried out with tissues from someone with CF. This means that it may be possible for organs from someone who dies from CF to be donated to a research laboratory in order to help future generations of people with CF. The fact that many, many patients and their families have asked that their organs or tissues be donated for CF research has been part of the reason we've learned so much about CF, and have developed more effective treatments for CF, to the point where we can think about a cure.

Research and Future Treatments

16

Christopher Penland, David M. Orenstein, and
Daniel J. Weiner

THE BASICS

1. Cystic fibrosis (CF) research has increased our understanding of CF and has led to the development of new treatments.

2. Basic researchers (scientists in the laboratory) are now examining the different CF gene mutations, how to cure CF cells with gene therapy, how CF interferes with salt and water transfer, how CF cells might be made to act like they do not have CF through drug therapy, why germs can live within the CF lung, and why CF lung inflammation is more active than non-CF inflammation.

3. Clinical researchers (researchers working with patients) are evaluating new ways of delivering normal CF genes into patients' cells, bypassing or correcting the defective CF protein, making CF mucus easier to cough up, fighting infection, and decreasing airway inflammation.

4. Soon new treatments will likely be available for making mucus easier to clear, fighting infection, reducing inflammation, and digesting food and absorbing its nutritional components, continuing to improve the outcome for patients.

5. New, powerful approaches to treat CF are in development that may be able to prevent CF symptoms by correcting the function of the defective CF protein or using alternative chloride channels in cells to get the job done.

6. As new medicines become available, clinical researchers will need to identify the optimal treatment strategies for CF patients to minimize the burden of care for patients.

7. Both researchers and patients have important responsibilities for CF research.

Since the *CFTR* gene was discovered in 1989, there have been major advances in our understanding of the basic defects in cystic fibrosis (CF) cells and how the disease progresses. During these same years there have been tremendous improvements in the quality and length of life of patients with CF. The improvement in the quality and quantity of life enjoyed by CF patients today is due to prior research. To continue seeing such improvements, new and improved therapies must be identified and tested. This chapter reviews the main areas of current CF research and progress, the direction for future research, and the potential future treatments that are being explored.

Medical research is divided into two general categories—basic and clinical. Basic research, sometimes called "bench" research because it usually takes place in a laboratory, concerns itself with tissues, cells, and even molecules. Clinical research deals directly with people, examining the effects of diseases or treatments on individual patients or groups of patients. Scores of clinical research projects related to CF are continually being conducted. They may deal with any one of the problems seen with CF or its treatment. Some of the projects involve very few patients; others involve national or even international cooperative efforts involving many researchers and hundreds of patients.

Both basic research and clinical research are essential for a complete understanding and satisfactory treatment of any disease. In the current era of CF research, there is great cooperation and overlap between basic and clinical research; for example, basic scientists work in the laboratory on ways to alter cells or deliver genes to cells, and, if successful, these techniques are carefully evaluated by clinical researchers to see if the new therapeutic approach is effective and safe in people with CF. You can read about the Cystic Fibrosis Foundation-supported network of research centers set up to facilitate this translation of basic research discoveries into new treatments, the Therapeutics Development Network (TDN), in Chapter 17.

In the following sections, we discuss basic and clinical research approaches that are being carried out in different CF-related areas. You can think of these areas as the steps of the disease, beginning with the defective gene and ending with associated symptoms. Sometimes treatments in one area may affect another area. For example, a drug that helps clear CF mucus may also lead to improved control of airway infection and inflammation. Likewise a drug that corrects the basic defect [i.e., the gene or the cystic fibrosis transmembrane conductance regulator (CFTR) protein] may prevent the other symptoms from even developing. Much of the background for this chapter can be found in Chapters 1, 3, and 11. More information about the new medicines being developed for CF can be found on the Cystic Fibrosis Foundation website (www.cff.org).

DEVELOPING NEW DRUGS FOR TREATMENT

For any new drug treatment that's being studied, there are several steps, or "phases," of study that are required before the drug can be approved for general use, with possible pitfalls at each phase:

After basic laboratory studies, and usually (but not always) studies in lab animals, a drug goes into Phase I clinical trials, mostly to test for safety in relatively small numbers of volunteers. Those compounds that make it through safety trials then go to Phase II clinical trials in patients with CF, to fine tune the dosage and search for evidence that the drug works as expected. For those drugs that successfully complete Phase 2 trials (that is, drugs which appear to be safe and effective), the last crucial steps are to confirm in larger numbers of patients, during Phase 3 trials, the promising early results and gain approval from governmental regulators. Unfortunately drug development through clinical trials is a battle of attrition, and many of the drugs that enter clinical development never make it to the commercial market.

Now we'll examine different fields of research that might lead to new treatments.

THE CF GENE

Basic Research

Because CF is an inherited disease, finding the gene that causes it in 1989 was an extremely important step toward unraveling the mysteries of the disease and coming closer to solving them. As you'll recall from Chapter 11, the *CFTR* gene directs the production of the CFTR protein. You might say that the gene carries the blueprint for the CFTR protein. The normal blueprint is actually a series of DNA letters. When the letters are joined together, they form words and sentences. If letters are scrambled, then the sentence no longer makes sense. In the cell, if the DNA letters are changed, the resulting protein will no longer "make sense" or work properly.

Scientists have identified more than 1,800 different separate changes (mutations) in the *CFTR* gene's DNA that can be abnormal and produce CF. (A vast majority of these mutations are quite rare—only 27 mutations account for more than 90% of mutations seen in patients.) As more patients are identified and mutations in their *CFTR* genes examined, a greater understanding of how different mutations affect function of the CFTR protein is developing. This work is important and will be discussed later in this chapter.

But (as you'll recall from "Different Mutations: Different Diseases?" in Chapter 11, *Genetics*) the types of *CFTR* gene mutations probably do not tell the whole story behind the characteristics of an individual patient's disease. Researchers across the world are also working to identify other genes and environmental influences (such as secondhand smoke exposure) that may modify the course and the severity of CF. These modifying influences may help explain why two patients with exactly the same *CFTR* gene mutations may develop different symptoms or levels of disease progression. Identification of key modifier genes may lead to the development of exciting new ways to treat CF or perhaps in the case of environmental influences suggest relatively simple measures that patients and their caregivers can adopt to slow the rate of disease progression.

Shortly after the *CFTR* gene was identified, basic researchers showed that they could place normal, healthy *CFTR* genes into CF cells and restore chloride transport (a hallmark of CFTR protein function). This early success in the laboratory led to clinical trials that attempted to place normal *CFTR* genes into CF patients. Although it was found that a normal *CFTR* gene could be placed into patients' cells, the effects were very short-lived. While frustrating, this setback has not prevented basic researchers from continuing to work to make gene therapy a reality for people with CF. In the laboratory, researchers are developing various methods to transfer healthy genes into airway cells. They are also working to overcome the barriers to the success of this complicated process, maximizing safety for the patient, and extending the length of time the healthy gene will continue to work once it has gotten into the CF cell.

Scientists have come up with several creative methods of getting healthy *CFTR* genes into CF cells. First, scientists have to find something that can carry a healthy gene into the affected cells. This "something" that carries a gene into target cells is called a "vector." Most gene transfer research has been performed using viruses as vectors. These viral vectors are attracted to cells lining the airways (epithelial cells). By attaching the healthy *CFTR* gene to modified versions of these viruses and aerosolizing this virus–gene combination into the lung, scientists hope that the healthy gene can be delivered directly and safely to airway cells. The viruses need to be modified so that they do not cause infection, which is what viruses are used to doing, do not multiply out of control, and do not cause inflammation.

Gene therapy for CF has turned out to be more complex than expected, but researchers are working to surmount every obstacle that arises. For example, some viral vectors, although modified, were found to trigger an immune response in patients' airways, causing inflammation, and limiting adequate transfer of the healthy gene. Therefore, scientists are working on ways to modify viruses to make them less likely to be recognized by the body as a "foreign invader," to tone down the body's immune response, or to use a nonviral vector to carry the gene into CF cells.

Progress is being made using specialized fat particles called "liposomes" instead of viruses as the vectors to which a healthy gene could be attached and which could carry that gene into affected cells. Another approach is to use specially compacted DNA which makes the genetic material so small that a vector is not needed to get healthy *CFTR* genes into the target cells.

Clinical Research and Future Treatments

Several clinical trials have been conducted in North America and Europe using various vectors to deliver healthy *CFTR* genes to the airways of patients with CF. Although these studies had the eventual goal of paving the way to *CFTR* gene therapy, it would be inaccurate to say that these trials were actually gene "therapy" trials, because these trials were not really therapy (treatment); no one who went into the trials expected to be made more healthy. Rather, these were experiments primarily to see if it was possible to get the healthy gene into cells in living patients with CF and to make the cells act as though they no longer had CF. Importantly these experiments also examined whether transfer of healthy *CFTR* genes into the cells of CF patients might cause harmful reactions. Therefore, we refer to these types of experiments as gene "transfer" trials and try to avoid calling them gene "therapy," so that we do not give the mistaken impression of being a lot closer to a treatment than we really are.

In many of these studies, the nose was the first site targeted, followed by the lung. The nose is used initially because the cells lining the nose are very similar to those lining the inside of the lungs and are relatively easy to study.

At the time of this writing, one method of *CF* gene transfer is being examined in a clinical trial of CF patients in the United Kingdom. This trial is designed to test whether a liposome can safely carry the *CFTR* gene into cells lining CF patients' lungs and result in a clinically meaningful response. The trial began in early 2009 and is divided into three parts. The first part is examining whether a single dose of the gene–liposome combination is safe when placed on cells within the nose of CF patients. After establishing that the single dose is safe and following a multiple-dose safety examination, the final part of the trial will test whether the gene–liposome combination is effective when administered to the lungs of CF patients. No data are available yet from this trial to know whether the approach will be successful in altering the function of cells in the CF lungs or whether there are measurable changes in the way CF patients feel.

CFTR GENE AND PROTEIN FUNCTION

Basic Research—CFTR Protein

As we've already discussed, one of the main problems in CF cells is that the CFTR protein does not permit chloride to move properly out of those cells. At the same time, sodium is moved into CF cells at a greater-than-normal rate. Because water follows the movement of salt (sodium chloride), not enough fluid is moved into spaces that are lined by CF cells, and fluid that is already there is removed too quickly. Exciting research is being conducted in laboratories worldwide to figure out exactly how the malfunctioning CFTR protein blocks chloride movement through CF epithelial cells and why sodium seems to be overabsorbed. Scientists are learning why these defects lead to the problems that occur in the organs and glands affected by CF and, finally, what might be done to reverse these salt and fluid movement abnormalities. Some scientists are also investigating whether the transport of other ions (tiny particles that carry an electric charge) besides chloride and sodium are affected by the abnormal CFTR protein.

You may recall from Chapter 1 that the CFTR protein is produced within the cell, then must fold into a particular shape so that it can be transported to the cell membrane, where it does its job of allowing chloride to exit the cell. You may recall further that some of the *CFTR* gene mutations create a situation where the CFTR protein does not get to the cell membrane, but if it is artificially placed there by researchers, it is able to work, to a certain degree. Various chemicals and conditions (e.g., cool temperature) have been identified that help get the altered CFTR protein from where it is made to where it belongs. Research is being conducted to identify and assess chemicals that patients might be able to take as medications that could get the CFTR protein to the cell membrane in millions of airway cells, when otherwise those proteins would be stuck in the interior of the cell where they are ineffective.

Besides those *CFTR* gene mutations that adversely affect how the CFTR protein folds and moves to the cell membrane, other *CFTR* gene mutations allow the CFTR protein to reach the cell membrane, but affect how it opens to allow chloride movement, while still others seem to prevent the production of any protein at all. Other mutations may not even truly cause CF disease! Of the 1,800-plus mutations that have been described so far in the *CFTR* gene, many are very rare, occurring in only one patient or one family, so little is known about them. To get a better understanding of what the different mutations mean, researchers are looking at databases worldwide to accumulate genetic (CFTR mutations) and clinical (pulmonary function, pancreatic function, etc.) data within a single resource that will be accessible on the Internet. By gathering this information and describing what a population of patients with rare mutations looks like, researchers will be better able to understand which CFTR mutations are truly associated with CF disease, and the ways in which the different mutations affect CFTR function. That information can then be used to help inform which potential future treatments might restore CFTR function and directly help patients.

In fact, researchers are examining approaches to understand how to restore function to defective CFTR proteins. One approach that basic researchers are using to find new ways to "fix" defective CFTR proteins is called *proteomics*. Proteomics is the science of the complete analysis of proteins to uncover their locations, control, and functions. It is believed that many other proteins interact with the CFTR protein to determine how it folds, moves through the cell to the cell membrane, and once there how its function is regulated. By identifying and studying the function of these other proteins in CF cells, researchers hope to identify which ones play a role in maintaining a healthy CFTR protein's normal functioning and which ones contribute to an abnormal CFTR protein.

A complementary approach to cataloguing proteins via proteomics is currently restricted to work in the laboratory, but might one day have clinical significance, and that is to regulate the amount of individual proteins in cells to understand their role. Scientists can specifically reduce or eliminate a non-CFTR protein and then determine whether that protein improves the function of mutated CFTR. Those proteins that affect CFTR function can then become targets for potential new drugs, with the goal of making the mutated CFTR protein behave normally, regulating a healthy balance of salt and water at CF cell membranes.

Another strategy to fix the faulty CFTR protein is called *structure-based drug design*. Through this process, chemical compounds are designed to change how a protein works by attaching to it. But, in order to design a chemical that can attach to CFTR, scientists have to know its exact three-dimensional shape. So far scientists have been successful at making lots of CFTR protein, but isolating it to determine its three-dimensional shape has proven extremely difficult. Therefore, another approach being tried uses advanced computer programs to predict the structure of the CFTR protein based upon what is known about the structure of other similar proteins and then to design chemicals that will fit into areas of the CFTR protein the computer program predicts.

Clinical Research and Future Treatments

Scientists in universities and industry have developed special "screens" to identify chemicals that could make mutated CFTR proteins behave normally or to find other means to improve the salt and water transfer by CF cells, potentially preventing CF symptoms from developing. Just in the last few years only, three drugs aimed at restoring function to mutated CFTR proteins have moved forward into clinical testing.

The first drug is called VX-770 (Vertex Pharmaceuticals, Cambridge, MA). This drug was found to activate CFTR proteins that have the *G551D* mutation. This mutation results in a CFTR protein that makes it to the cell membrane but does not open properly. Therefore, chloride does not move out of CF cells. When patients with the *G551D* mutation took one VX-770 pill twice a day, there was strong evidence that their CFTR proteins began to function much more normally: remember the "nasal PD" from Chapter 1? That's a way of measuring the electrical charge inside the nose, which is a very good measurement of the movement of chloride in and out of the cells lining the nose (which are just like the cells lining the trachea and bronchi). Well, in patients with the *G551D* mutation, their nasal PD was nearly normal after they'd been taking the VX-770 pills for just a few weeks. Not only that, their sweat tests had changed to very close to the normal range! Additionally, most CF patients who had changes in their nasal PD and their sweat chloride also had significant improvements in pulmonary function. This last measure is important, as it is one clinical measure of wellness that the United States Food and Drug Administration (FDA) requires before it can approve a new drug. Patients involved in the early trials of VX-770 also had very few side effects, which suggests that the drug is safe; this is also required for FDA approval and, of course, for clinical use. At the time of this writing, VX-770 has started the first of three final trials that are required by the FDA before it can be considered for approval. Approximately 7% of CF patients in the United States carry the *G551D* mutation. Scientists assume that CF patients who have other mutations that enable CFTR to reach the cell membrane (but not allow it to work normally) will also respond to this drug. About 90% of the U.S. CF population carry at least one copy of the Δ*F508* CFTR mutation. With this mutation, as you'll recall from Chapter 1, the CFTR protein does not make it to the cell membrane. And, even if it's artificially moved to the cell membrane, the protein does not open properly to allow chloride to pass through. Another drug from the Vertex company, VX-809, seems to help the mutated form of the CFTR protein to move to the cell membrane, at least in cell cultures in the laboratory. VX-809 has entered Phase 2 clinical trials, to test if it also works in real live patients. At the time of this writing, no data are available to determine how well this compound works in CF patients. It seems likely that VX-809 by itself might not be enough to restore normal chloride and water movement across cell membranes, since getting CFTR protein to the cell membrane isn't enough, if the protein doesn't open properly once it's there. Therefore, VX-809 might need to be tested along with a compound that restores opening of the ΔF508 CFTR protein, perhaps VX-770.

Some CF patients (approximately 10% of the U.S. CF patient population) carry a mutation that causes the CFTR protein's manufacture within CF cells to be stopped prematurely. Many of these mutations' names end with an "X" (*W1282X* is one of the most common) and they are known as nonsense mutations or "stop" mutations. For these patients an oral compound known as Ataluren (PTC Therapeutics, South Plainfield, NJ) has entered Phase 3 trials. In earlier trials Ataluren improved the nasal PD in CF patients carrying nonsense mutations and decreased the number of coughs of these CF patients. These results suggest that CFTR production was able to proceed, and not be stopped prematurely.

AIRWAY FLUID/MUCUS COMPOSITION

Basic Research

Although you cannot see the abnormal *CF* gene and protein with the naked eye, you can certainly see the results of the disordered salt and water balance in the CF airway. Abnormally thick and sticky airway mucus characterizes CF and encourages chronic infections. Scientists are closely examining the composition of the fluids in CF airway, including the proteins found in the mucus, to understand the disease process in CF, and to find new ways to treat it.

The movement of salt and water into the airway is extremely important to keep mucus that is present in the airways sufficiently hydrated so that it can be moved up and out of the lungs. The job of mucus in the lungs is to trap germs (technically bacteria, viruses, fungi, and protozoa), dust, and other small particles we breathe in every day, and the movement of mucus up and out of the lungs is an essential part of the body's defense system. When the CFTR protein does not function properly, the mucus becomes sticky, making it difficult to move. The stationary mucus still traps the germs that are breathed in, and eventually infection develops. It has been known for a long time that CF patients develop infections in their lungs, but it took a number of years after the *CFTR* gene was identified to put many of the puzzle pieces together to understand how the lung is supposed to keep itself infection-free and why this process does not work in CF.

Mucus that is made in the lungs comes from specialized cells and glands found throughout most of the lung. The main component of mucus is a long stringy protein called "mucin" that is decorated with sugars. You might imagine it looking like a pipe cleaner. When the mucin protein with its sugars is inside the cells it is folded up tightly into a very compact structure. However, when the mucin protein is released from the cell it expands rapidly and weaves itself in with other mucin proteins, forming a protective net above the cells lining the airways.

In CF, because the CFTR protein does not function properly, there is not enough fluid within the airway, and some scientists believe that the fluid that is there is missing some vital components that are needed to allow mucins that have just been released to unfold and join properly with other mucins. Scientists from the United States and Europe have banded together to understand how mucins are supposed to unfold and analyze the small amount of fluid on top of CF airway cells for missing components. Through these studies scientists will learn how mucins are supposed to unfold and what is needed to make this happen correctly. This information will provide a more complete understanding of how lung disease begins and open up new avenues for treatment that promotes the movement of mucus up and out of the lungs.

Defective CFTR results in too little chloride secretion *into* the airways from the cells and too much sodium absorption *from* the airway into the cell. The net result is dehydration (drying) of airway secretions, making airway mucus harder to clear, and setting the stage for airway infection and inflammation. Therefore, correcting these abnormalities should improve the ability of CF airways to be cleared.

Clinical Research and Future Treatments

Besides the CFTR protein there are other proteins in cells of the lung that can move chloride into the airway space. These channels can be thought of as a backup system. An inhaled compound called denufosol created by researchers at Inspire Pharmaceuticals (Durham, NC) activates these backup chloride channels. Denufosol was evaluated in several early CF clinical trials where it was found to be safe and improved lung function. Unfortunately larger and longer Phase 3 trials of denufosol did not demonstrate the same benefit and the company has stopped development of the drug. Another inhaled compound that moves chloride into CF airways is Moli 1901 (Lantibio, Inc., Chapel Hill, NC). This compound has completed some early-stage CF clinical trials in the United States and Europe.

Besides playing an important role in moving chloride out of cells in the lung, the CFTR protein also controls the activity of another protein called the "epithelial sodium channel" (ENaC) that serves as a pathway for sodium to be absorbed. Exactly how CFTR controls the activity of ENaC is unclear. Nevertheless, shortly before scientists found that the *CFTR* gene was the cause of CF, they recognized that CF cells absorb sodium much more rapidly than non-CF cells. Building upon this understanding of robust sodium absorption, some very early CF clinical trials examined whether amiloride, a drug known to block sodium absorption, could improve lung function in CF patients. Unfortunately, inhaled amiloride's effect did not last long enough to see any improvement in lung function. Parion Sciences (Durham, NC) took this information and partnered with Gilead Sciences (Foster City, CA) to create a new inhaled compound called GS9411. This compound has entered early-stage CF clinical trials. It is not yet known how well any of these compounds will work, and ultimately a combination of therapies, such as a backup chloride channel activator and sodium absorption blocker, may be used to improve salt and water transport into the CF lung.

There is another way to move fluid into the CF lung without using backup chloride channels, and this is by placing an *osmotic* agent into the airways. An osmotic agent draws water to itself. A simple way to think about this is remembering what happens to a salt shaker outside on a humid day. The salt crystals are osmotic agents and they draw water from the air into the salt shaker that then clogs up the holes in the top of the salt shaker. In CF this simple principle is being explored with two separate approaches.

The first approach was examined when teenagers and adults with CF inhaled a salty water (hypertonic saline) solution. When the salt arrived in the airways, it drew water into the airway spaces and improved the movement of mucus out of the CF lung. Patients participating in these studies also had fewer pulmonary exacerbations. Many teenagers and adults with CF now inhale hypertonic saline as part of their normal treatment. A follow-up study called the Infant Study of Inhaled Saline (ISIS) trial is examining whether infants who inhale a salty solution also see benefits. This trial has only recently begun in the United States, so no data are available yet as of this writing.

Another similar approach is examining whether inhaling the sugar mannitol (Bronchitol; Pharmaxis Ltd., New South Wales, Australia) improves pulmonary health. Bronchitol has been examined in clinical trials in Europe and Australia, where it was found to improve pulmonary function. Bronchitol has begun a Phase 3 clinical trial in the United States, but no data are currently available.

All these agents provide potential opportunities to improve the movement of mucus out of the lungs and improve pulmonary health. Because they are inhaled, delivery of these agents into areas of the lung blocked by mucus plugs could be difficult.

CHRONIC CF LUNG INFECTIONS

Basic Research

Basic scientists are increasing our understanding of why the CF airways are prone to chronic infections, especially with the bacteria *Pseudomonas aeruginosa*. Using traditional microbiology tools along with new tools such as gene chips, researchers are probing why the *P. aeruginosa* bacteria are so capable of colonizing and infecting the CF lung. All of *P. aeruginosa's* genes were recently mapped on a tiny computer chip. Using this gene chip, researchers are determining the functions of each of the nearly 6,000 genes that make up this organism. It may be possible to use those genes that are found to be essential for survival of *P. aeruginosa* as targets for new antibiotics to kill *P. aeruginosa*.

A special set of *P. aeruginosa* genes that are receiving a lot of attention among CF researchers are referred to as quorum-sensing genes. Quorum sensing is the process whereby bacteria send out chemical signals that other bacteria nearby sense, and these organisms then understand how many of their kind are in the vicinity. When *P. aeruginosa* bacteria sense that a certain density of their own kind are nearby [a certain number in a particular location (i.e., a quorum)], the bacteria can respond by creating a protective coating, called a *biofilm*, which shields the bacteria from antibiotics and the body's own defenses. Researchers are looking for ways to target the protein products of these genes or the signaling systems that are stimulated by quorum sensing in a way that would allow antibiotics to work more effectively. For example, a new antibiotic might be able to fool the bacteria into thinking there was not a "quorum"—there were not enough similar bacteria around—to start making the protective biofilm. In this case, without the protective biofilm, even old antibiotics might be able to penetrate into the bacteria and kill them.

Other basic scientists are examining how *P. aeruginosa* adapts to live within the CF lung. Normally *P. aeruginosa* lives in places that are dark, humid, and oxygen-rich such as sink drains. In the CF lung, *P. aeruginosa* lives within the mucus, surrounded by human immune cells trying to kill it. Studies have also found that CF mucus is very low in oxygen. To thrive in such a harsh environment *P. aeruginosa* not only creates protective biofilms but also must alter the way that it processes nutrients (metabolism) due to the low oxygen. By understanding how *P. aeruginosa* adapts its metabolism, approaches could be designed to literally starve the organism.

Like humans, bacteria need iron, but cannot produce it. Humans obtain iron from their diet and nutritional supplements, but researchers have found that *P. aeruginosa* must scavenge iron from its environment. Iron is used by bacteria for multiple processes involved in growth and is an important cofactor for multiple enzymes used by bacteria to protect them from harm or to repair damage. Research has also found that iron promotes biofilm development. Interesting new work has found that gallium can be used as a "Trojan Horse" to kill *P. aeruginosa*. Gallium is a transitional metal that *P. aeruginosa* believes is iron and the bacteria rapidly takes it up. Unlike iron though, gallium cannot be used as a cofactor for *P. aeruginosa* enzymes; therefore, the bacteria become poisoned. Gallium has successfully been used in animal models of *P. aeruginosa* infection, suggesting that this may be a possible new avenue for treating CF *P. aeruginosa* infections.

There are other bacteria, fungi, and protozoa that infect the airways of CF patients, and basic researchers are using all the tools available to them to understand these, too.

Clinical Research and Future Treatments

Although new antibacterial therapies that are produced from basic research are probably still years away from being used in the clinic, other new anti-infective approaches against *P. aeruginosa* and other bacteria and respiratory viruses are being evaluated in clinical trials today. These approaches include novel anti-infectives such as gallium (Genta Inc., Berkeley Heights, NJ), vaccines (KB001; Kalobios Pharmaceuticals Inc., South San Francisco, CA), and new ways of delivering existing antibiotics already used in CF such as ciprofloxacin (Bayer Schering Pharma, Berlin, Germany), levofloxacin (Mpex Pharmaceuticals, San Diego, CA) and amikacin (Transave Inc., Monmouth Junction, NJ), and tobramycin (Novartis Pharmaceuticals, Basel, Switzerland).

Many CF clinical researchers are working to evaluate antibiotics that are already on the market for other diseases and conditions to see if they have value in treating CF. For example, the widely prescribed oral antibiotic azithromycin was successfully added to the CF physician's medical arsenal because a large study showed it could improve lung function and body weight and decrease hospitalizations in patients with CF. Likewise the antibiotic aztreonam has been revised by Gilead Sciences so that it is appropriate for inhalation and has been approved by the FDA for use in CF.

Another avenue being pursued is combining two existing antibiotics into a single medicine. The antibiotics—fosfomycin and tobramycin—are being combined into a single inhalation mixture by Gilead Sciences. The many efforts to create inhaled versions of existing antibiotics follows the lead of TOBI®, which was found to be effective at delivering very high concentrations of the antibiotic tobramycin at the site of infection. Significant improvements in pulmonary function of CF patients taking TOBI® resulted in this being the first inhaled antibiotic specifically approved by the FDA for use in CF.

INFLAMMATION

Basic Research

In the airways, inflammation naturally results from the body's defense against bacteria and other invaders. The body produces an immune response, usually a beneficial and necessary reaction, to fight infection or other perceived threats. This immune response includes inflammation, with white blood cells being sent to the site of invading bacteria. These white blood cells release chemicals that can help kill bacteria. However, in CF, the immune response, including the release of chemicals from white blood cells, is more intense and prolonged than in people without CF, and injures lung tissue as well as killing bacteria.

The overactive and prolonged immune response of CF is an area of very active investigation. Presently, researchers are trying to understand why the immune response in the CF lung does not slow down and stop, as it should. In addition, scientists are examining which chemical signals from the lung are important in starting the CF immune response. Blocking these signals would decrease the destructive overactive inflammation process.

Clinical Research and Future Treatments

Inflammation is a part of many other diseases besides CF. In the same way described in the lung infection section, anti-inflammatory therapies that are already on the market for other conditions are also being tested for their use in CF. In particular, researchers are looking at drugs being used for conditions such as rheumatoid arthritis, Crohn's disease, high cholesterol, and malaria, because the biological pathways these drugs influence probably play a role in CF airway inflammation.

One new treatment approach being pursued in CF is designed to decrease the activity of neutrophils, which are bacteria-fighting cells that move out of the bloodstream and into the airways in response to lung infection. A compound called GSK SB 656933 (GlaxoSmithKline, Research Triangle Park, NC) blocks a signal that activates neutrophils, and has begun early-stage CF clinical trials.

OTHER CLINICAL RESEARCH

So far this chapter has focused upon research and potential new treatments important to improving the functioning of CF lungs. This is because a great majority of illnesses and deaths that accompany CF is due to lung disease, and altering the course of lung disease will add years to the life of most CF patients. However, as you know, CF affects other organs in addition to the lungs. Research continues to advance our understanding and treatment of these many other important aspects of CF, including nutrition, CF-related diabetes, CF liver disease, CF-related bone health, and reproduction. Furthermore, improvements are being made in the areas of medical treatment after lung transplantation and methods of airway clearance which are important, but not unique to CF. Lastly, strides are being made in better ways to measure patients' health status and the psychosocial aspects of coping with a chronic illness. Following are just a few examples.

Gastrointestinal System and Nutrition

Most people with CF must take numerous capsules containing pancreatic enzymes with every meal and snack to help them digest their food. Recently the FDA required all companies making pancreatic enzymes to adopt new standards that will increase the stability of enzymes, allow more precise dosing, and improve their safety. A new type of pancreatic enzyme is now in clinical trials for CF patients, and has the advantage that it is not made from the pancreas of pigs but is instead created from a controlled fermentation process. Liprotamase (Eli Lily, Indianapolis, IN) may allow CF patients to take fewer pills with every meal and may be available in a liquid formulation for infants.

Exercise Tolerance

Exercise tolerance has its own category (and its own chapter: Chapter 10) because it seems to affect—and be affected by—many other factors. Research into exercise has shown that exercise testing can be helpful in assessing a patient's progress before and after treatments of various kinds (hospitalizations, exercise training programs, etc.). Exercise testing can also identify patients whose oxygen level may drop while they are active.

Research in exercise tolerance has led to the understanding that most patients with CF can exercise safely and receive the same benefits that their classmates and friends receive from a regular exercise program. Important research with regard to salt loss during exercise in the heat has led to the recognition that people with CF can replace that salt perfectly well on their own without salt tablets or other forced salt replacement. Research also found that a patient's fitness level as measured in an exercise test correlated more closely than any other measure with the patient's likelihood of surviving for the next 8 years. Researchers continue to work to determine the type of exercise that is most helpful for patients with CF and whether exercise can improve lung function or delay its deterioration.

Psychology and Education

Research in several CF centers is examining the psychological adjustment of patients with CF and their families. Several studies have shown that individuals with CF and their families are remarkably well adjusted, and other studies are directed at understanding these strengths so that people with other chronic illnesses might benefit. Additional research is focusing on the best ways to educate children with CF about their illness.

FUTURE CHALLENGES

It is possible that in the next 5 years many new CF therapies will be approved by the FDA. While this is wonderful, in that they have the potential to add many years to the lives of CF patients, it also creates a problem. The medical regimen of CF patients is already time-consuming and expensive. The addition of new therapies will require CF researchers to determine which medical regimen is the most effective while allowing patients time to enjoy an improved quality of life.

RESEARCH ETHICS

Investigators' Responsibilities

Many medical researchers feel a responsibility to do what they can to answer questions that will ultimately lead to better health and less suffering for people. They also have the responsibility of conducting their research so that its drawbacks are clearly outweighed by the potential benefits. For clinical research, the drawbacks are expense, patients' inconvenience, discomfort, and possibility of toxic side effects. All federally funded research is evaluated for the balance of risks and benefits by Institutional Review Boards (sometimes called Human Rights Committees) of the hospital or university where the research is taking place.

Patients who are asked to participate in research must be given complete and understandable explanations of the research, including its possible risks and benefits. In most cases, patients or legal guardians must sign a consent form, saying that they do understand and that they are participating voluntarily.

To enhance patient safety in the clinical trials it supports, the Cystic Fibrosis Foundation formed the Data Safety Monitoring Board. This is an unbiased, independent group of CF physicians, an ethicist, pharmacists, and biostatisticians that serves in a "watchdog" capacity to protect patients and ensure the highest standards in clinical research. Among their duties, these clinical trial overseers review all research studies performed under the TDN (see above and Chapter 17) for reports of side effects, and can call for a clinical trial to be placed on hold or stopped if they have concerns.

Patients' Responsibilities

Patients and their families have responsibility, first of all, to themselves. People have an absolute right to refuse to participate in research, for whatever reason they might have. It is worth mentioning, though, that for a disease like CF, where there is no animal that has the exact disease, and where there are relatively few patients with the disease (approximately 30,000 in the entire United States), it is essential that some people with the disease volunteer to help with research. If no one volunteers, the encouraging progress that is being made will come to a halt.

Individuals who do participate in studies, and their families, often feel that they reap large benefits from being an essential part of the research team that will eventually control CF. Yet, it is unfair for the burden of all the research studies to fall on a small group of people who participate time after time, while others never help. Patients associated with a large CF care center are likely to have many research projects from which to choose, so they may easily participate in some, while skipping others. In 2008–2009, roughly 1,700 patients newly enrolled in interventional studies (those that are trying out new treatments), and 2,800 in observational studies (not taking any experimental treatments). This represents about 15% of all patients followed in accredited CF centers in the United States. Because of the recent discovery of promising new CF therapies ready for clinical evaluation, the TDN has expanded to 77 CF care centers across the United States to offer CF patients in nearly all geographic locations the opportunity to participate in an ever-expanding variety of clinical trials.

TISSUE NEEDED FOR CONTINUING RESEARCH

In laboratories around the world, investigators are working with tissues from the body to answer many of CF's critical questions. Progress has been phenomenal, yet it could be even faster if there were enough tissue to work with. Even now that there are genetically engineered animals with abnormal *CFTR* genes, and very good experimental CF cell lines, they are not the same as humans with CF. That means, for much of the research, tissue must still come from people with CF. Nasal polyps that are removed because they were blocking up the nose can be used, and lungs and livers that are removed from patients with CF who are getting transplants provide a rich source of tissue for research. Still more is needed. Organs can be used from patients who die, but few patients and families are aware of this possibility, and often CF physicians hesitate to bring up this potentially painful topic with a grieving family around the time of the death of a patient. Therefore, patients and their families are encouraged to speak with their CF physicians about donating tissues for research.

SUMMARY

The participation and collaboration of an ever-increasing number of superb scientists and patients with CF has meant that basic and clinical research has answered many questions about CF and its treatment. The research to date is paying off with improved treatment that will continue to enhance the length and quality of patients' lives. The continued enthusiasm of researchers and patients will ensure that we will eventually understand CF completely and this understanding will lead to optimum treatments. In many ways, the critical factor continues to be the willingness of the CF patient community to participate in ongoing clinical trials. Working together, patients, physicians, and researchers will turn CF into a disease that is lived with and not one that you die from.

The Cystic Fibrosis Foundation

17

Robert J. Beall

THE BASICS

1. The Cystic Fibrosis Foundation (CF Foundation) is a national organization that raises money to support cystic fibrosis (CF) research and specialized patient care throughout the United States.

2. CF Foundation-funded research has been very helpful in increasing our understanding of CF, and has led to the development of most of the new approved CF therapies.

3. The CF Foundation's approach to drug discovery has yielded a pipeline with more than 30 potential CF therapies in development, including those that combat the symptoms of CF and several that address the root causes of the disease.

4. The CF Foundation sponsors fellowships and other awards for physicians and scientists early in their careers.

5. The CF Foundation supports and accredits a nationwide network of approximately 115 CF care centers.

6. The CF Foundation provides patient education through its website (www.cff.org), YouTube channel (www.youtube.com/CysticFibrosisUSA) and presence on Facebook (www.facebook.com/cysticfibrosisfoundation) and Twitter (http://twitter.com/CF_Foundation); printed materials, e-mail communications and videos; and a general information hotline (800–344-4823 or info@cff.org) and CF Legal Information Hotline (800–622-0385 or CFLegal@cff.org).

7. The CF Foundation advocates for patients' rights in government legislation.

8. The CF Foundation has a mail-order pharmacy subsidiary to facilitate access to CF medications and equipments. This subsidiary also works with medical insurance companies to promote adequate insurance coverage for individuals with CF.

MISSION & BACKGROUND

The mission of the Cystic Fibrosis Foundation (CF Foundation) is to assure the development of the means to cure and control cystic fibrosis (CF) and to improve the quality of life for those with the disease.

History

When the CF Foundation was established in 1955, children born with CF were not expected to live long enough to attend elementary school. Little was known about the fatal genetic disease, and no effective treatments were available. In an effort to save their children and help all those with CF, a concerned group of parents established the CF Foundation. Their goals were to advance understanding of CF, create new treatments, and find a cure or control for this disease.

Since then and through the outstanding commitment of a wide community of volunteers and donors, the CF Foundation has achieved tremendous progress. Thanks in part to investments made by the CF Foundation in research and comprehensive care, the median predicted age of survival for people with CF is now in the mid-30s, and more than 46% of all people with the disease are aged 18 or older.

CF Foundation Milestones

- 1955—The CF Foundation becomes incorporated as the National CF Research Foundation.
- 1961—The CF Foundation launches a nationwide network of care centers, which it supports and accredits.
- 1962—The median predicted age of survival for people with CF is 10 years.
- 1966—The CF Foundation launches a patient data registry that collects health information on patients seen at Foundation-accredited care centers.
- 1980—The CF Foundation creates the Research Development Program (RDP), a network of research centers at leading universities and medical schools nationwide.
- 1988—The CF Foundation launches the Cystic Fibrosis Services Pharmacy, a specialty pharmacy designed to provide availability and access to CF medications, as well as assistance with insurance issues.
- 1989—A team of CF Foundation-supported scientists discovers the defective *CF* gene and its protein product [**c**ystic **f**ibrosis **t**ransmembrane conductance **r**egulator (CFTR)], opening the door to understanding the disease at its most basic level.
- 1994—The United States Food and Drug Administration (FDA) approves Pulmozyme®, which is proven to thin the tenacious, sticky mucus in the lungs and is the first drug developed specifically for CF.

- 1997—To bridge the gap between what researchers learn in the laboratory and the evolution of new therapies, the CF Foundation establishes the Therapeutics Development Program (TDP).
- 1997—The FDA approves TOBI®, the first aerosolized antibiotic designed for CF, which is proven to reduce hospital stays and improve lung function.
- 2000—Cystic Fibrosis Foundation Therapeutics, Inc. (CFFT), a nonprofit research affiliate of the CF Foundation, is established to facilitate drug discovery and development efforts.
- 2000—CF Foundation-supported scientists map the entire genetic structure of the most common cause of CF lung infections—the *Pseudomonas aeruginosa* bacterium.
- 2002—The CF Foundation launches its Quality Improvement Initiative to standardize and improve care at its nationwide network of care centers.
- 2004—CF Foundation-supported studies in Australia and at the University of North Carolina show that nebulized hypertonic saline helps clear CF mucus. It is proven to improve lung function and reduce hospital stays and becomes a therapeutic option.
- 2006—The predicted median age of survival for people with CF increases to the mid-30s.
- 2006—The first drug designed to target the faulty CF protein, developed by Vertex Pharmaceuticals with CF Foundation support, enters clinical trials.
- 2008—The CF Foundation and Vertex Pharmaceuticals achieve a "proof of concept," showing that it is possible to treat the underlying molecular cause of CF.
- 2008—The CF Foundation launches the Program of Adult Care Excellence (PACE) to enhance care for the growing number of adults with CF.
- 2008—The CF Foundation establishes the Cystic Fibrosis Patient Assistance Foundation (CFPAF), a nonprofit subsidiary dedicated to help CF patients get coverage for certain high-cost CF medications.
- 2009—Following the advocacy efforts of the CF Foundation, all 50 states and the District of Columbia screen newborns for CF.
- 2010—The FDA approves Cayston®, a new inhaled antibiotic developed with CF Foundation support by Gilead Sciences, Inc.
- 2010—The CF Foundation's therapeutic pipeline contains more than 30 potential drugs in various stages of development for the treatment of CF.

RESEARCH & DRUG DEVELOPMENT

To advance CF research that can expand knowledge of the disease and spur the development of new treatments, the CF Foundation offers a range of support, including grants to fund multidisciplinary research centers, individual grants for basic and clinical research studies, graduate and postgraduate research training programs, matching grants to biotechnology and pharmaceutical companies to pursue CF drug development, and support of small- and large-scale clinical trials to evaluate new CF treatments.

Over the course of five decades, the CF Foundation's medical research program has built a strong record of success, expanding understanding of the disease and translating advances in the laboratory to new treatments for patients. Since the 1980s, the CF Foundation has played an integral role in the development of CF drugs, such as Pulmozyme®, TOBI®, azithromycin, hypertonic saline, and, most recently, Cayston®.

The Research Development Program

To bring together top-notch scientists from varying disciplines to address the challenges of CF, in 1980, the CF Foundation established the Research Development Program (RDP), a network of CF research centers located in leading universities and medical schools throughout the country. By pooling their talents, RDP scientists have advanced our understanding of CF and the inner workings of the CF cell. In addition to bringing together intellectual resources, RDP centers also share research tools with CF scientists around the world.

Unlike many researchers in other fields, CF researchers work together to advance the science, readily sharing unpublished results at CF Foundation-sponsored forums, including the annual North American CF Conference. In addition, scientists at RDP centers have the opportunity to communicate directly with medical teams at nearby CF Foundation-accredited care centers. Through these collaborations, scientists are able to better understand the complexity of the disease process and gain an understanding of the larger context of their work.

An Innovative Business Model

It takes an estimated 10 to 15 years and costs more than $1 billion to move a drug from the discovery phase to market. Major pharmaceutical companies that develop drugs are primarily interested in diseases that affect large numbers of people because of the sizeable return on investment that may be possible from developing new drugs to treat them. Because fewer than 200,000 people have CF, it is considered a rare or "orphan" disease, and a less appealing target for investment.

To speed the development of new treatments, in 1997 the CF Foundation developed an innovative business model. This approach to drug development is based on offering drug companies incentives for taking on major CF drug development projects. To move promising drug compounds from laboratories to clinics, the CF Foundation created a cutting-edge research infrastructure.

Cystic Fibrosis Foundation Therapeutics, Inc.

Cystic Fibrosis Foundation Therapeutics, Inc. (CFFT), a nonprofit drug discovery and development affiliate of the CF Foundation, funds promising scientific research in academia and in the biotechnology and pharmaceutical industry. The CFFT

Therapeutics Development Program (TDP) supports a full spectrum of CF drug development—from the discovery of a promising drug to its evaluation in patients within the CF clinical trials network.

The TDP entices biopharmaceutical companies to apply their unique resources to CF drug discovery by providing CFFT funding and access to scientific and clinical expertise through CF Foundation-supported researchers and its accredited Care Center Network. When a drug is ready for clinical trials, the Therapeutics Development Network (TDN), a select group of care centers that are uniquely equipped with trained personnel and state-of-the-art technology for clinical trials, is ready to further a drug's development. CFFT is currently working with many companies and academic groups to develop and test new CF therapies at TDN centers.

Harnessing these innovative strategies and networks, the CF Foundation has built a dynamic pipeline of potential new CF therapies. There are currently more than 30 therapies in development—any one or a combination of which show promise for adding many years of life for those with CF.

CF CARE

The CF Foundation has revolutionized the standard of care for people with CF. To ensure the highest quality of care across the country, the CF Foundation accredits and funds a nationwide network of approximately 115 CF care centers and more than 55 affiliate programs, including 96 programs for treating adults with CF, located in major teaching and community hospitals. These centers provide diagnosis and comprehensive, age-appropriate care for more than 25,000 patients throughout the nation.

Specialized care for people with CF is critical because CF is a complex, multisystem disease, requiring lifelong treatment. To address all aspects of the disease, the CF Foundation brings together all relevant medical care specialties into one cohesive, total-care approach.

Multidisciplinary medical care teams at CF Foundation-accredited care centers have the knowledge and resources to keep patients with CF in the best possible health. Dedicated CF experts—such as pulmonologists, gastroenterologists, nurses, respiratory therapists, dietitians, psychologists, and social workers—work in unison to provide CF care tailored to meet each patient's unique needs. Care center teams also work together, gathering at annual CF Foundation-sponsored Learning and Leadership Collaborative meetings to work on finding ways to further improve CF care.

Early, aggressive medical intervention provided at CF Foundation-accredited care centers helps to slow the progression of CF lung disease. The array of inpatient and outpatient services includes laboratory tests, airway clearance technique instruction, nutritional assessment, therapies to fight lung infections and more. The centers offer additional services to patients and their families—from financial guidance through a social worker to family counseling referrals—that address other factors involved in living with CF or caring for someone throughout all stages of the disease.

Patient and family education is also a critical part of caring for those with CF, as informed patients are often better poised to manage their health and adhere to complicated but vital treatment regimens. To help inform patients and families and support parents of newly diagnosed children, the CF Foundation's care centers offer a range of resources, including hands-on training, family education days, and free informational printed materials and videos.

To ensure that high standards of care are maintained throughout the care center network, each center undergoes an evaluation by the CF Foundation's Care Center Committee before it receives accreditation and funding, and all accredited care centers are reassessed annually by the Committee according to requirements set forth in the CF Foundation's Clinical Practice Guidelines.

Patient Registry

For more than 40 years, the CF Foundation has maintained a comprehensive Patient Registry to track data on the health of CF patients in the United States. The CF Foundation analyzes health data from 25,000 patients at its 115 care centers and shares the registry report with the public, physicians, care providers, patients, and families. The data help identify best practices and areas for improvement, providing caregivers the firepower they need to make changes and improve care.

In 2007, the CF Foundation became the first and only rare disease organization to publicly publish comparative health outcomes of care for its nationwide network of accredited CF care centers. Accessible on the CF Foundation's website (www. cff.org), the data show how well patients as a whole are doing at each center, and how the outcomes compare both to national averages and to national goals set by medical experts. This ongoing data transparency enables the CF community to identify and adopt best treatment practices and improve overall patient care.

Widely recognized as an effective tool in the fight to control and cure CF, the CF Foundation's Patient Registry has become a model for many other chronic disease organizations.

Quality Improvement Initiative

To ensure that all care centers provide the highest quality care, the CF Foundation launched the Quality Improvement Initiative in 2002. The initiative works to identify best practices for CF treatment at high-performing centers and then provides training and tools to implement improvements at other centers, building stronger partnerships between people with CF, their families, and care center clinicians. The initiative has significantly improved the length and quality of life of those with CF by making optimal use of the tools available now for treatment of CF.

For its commitment to improving the quality of health care, the CF Foundation was honored with the Health Quality Award in 2009 by the National Committee for Quality Assurance.

Pharmaceutical Services

Cystic Fibrosis Services, Inc., a full-service pharmacy and wholly owned subsidiary of the CF Foundation, serves people with CF across the country by providing disease-specific drugs and an array of other medications. In addition, CF Services provides patient advocacy, patient education, and reimbursement support to the CF community.

Patient Assistance

To address growing problems of access to care and underinsurance, the CF Foundation has established the Cystic Fibrosis Patient Assistance Foundation (CFPAF), a nonprofit subsidiary that provides financial assistance for select FDA-approved medications and medical devices for the treatment of CF lung disease.

Legal Hotline

The CF Legal Information Hotline (800–622-0385 or CFLegal@cff.org) provides free information about the laws that protect the rights of individuals with CF, including insurance coverage and employment issues. Sponsored through a grant from a pharmaceutical corporation and administered by an attorney with CF, the hotline serves as a resource for CF care centers, individuals with CF, and their families.

Advocacy

One of the largest caucuses in Congress, with more than 150 members, the Congressional Cystic Fibrosis Caucus gives those with CF a voice in Congress. Volunteers from the CF community regularly visit their federal and state representatives and Caucus members, apprising them of important legislative issues, such as the Genetic Non-Discrimination Act, the Newborn Screening Saves Lives Act and legislation to improve clinical trials, and the need to increase federal funding of biomedical research at the National Institutes of Health, provide for a more streamlined drug approval process for treatments for rare diseases at the FDA, reauthorize the Small Business Innovation Research program, and expand access to quality health care.

A COMMUNITY OF SUPPORT

Hundreds of thousands of dedicated people—those living with CF, their families, caregivers, researchers, medical professionals, corporations, and other volunteers—devote their time and talents to cure CF. They are the engine that powers the CF Foundation, and their ongoing support makes progress in research and care possible.

The CF Foundation's more than 75 nationwide chapters and branch offices provide opportunities for the CF community to volunteer or participate in fund-raising events. These activities not only help in the fight against CF, but they also allow people with CF and their friends and families to meet others in their community and take part in informal support networks. The CF Foundation's Volunteer Leadership Initiative is aimed at identifying, recruiting, and engaging new volunteers and fundraisers.

Each year, more than 600 communities in nearly every state host the CF Foundation's GREAT STRIDES walks, raising millions of dollars for CF research and care programs. The CF Foundation's chapters and branch offices also host thousands of other special fundraising events year-round from signature galas and golf tournaments to bike rides and dinner dances.

In addition, generous support from corporations and business leaders helps the CF Foundation to continue funding groundbreaking research and provide the highest standards of care for all people with CF.

LOOKING TO THE FUTURE

Although people with CF are living longer and experiencing a better quality of life, there is still critical work to be done. The CF Foundation commits to working tirelessly until a cure and control for the disease are found, by functioning as:

- Scientific pioneers, blazing new trails in CF research
- Investors, funding drug discovery and development
- Caregivers, linking patients and families to specialized CF care
- Fundraisers, securing the money needed to support our efforts
- Advocates, keeping CF a top priority in government, industry, and research
- Family, offering support, information, and resources

HELPFUL RESOURCES

- For general information about the CF Foundation and to find a chapter near you, visit www.cff.org.
- To learn about the many ways you can support the search for a cure, visit www.cff.org/GetInvolved.
- To view the CF Foundation's most current drug development pipeline, visit www.cff.org/research/DrugDevelopmentPipeline.
- To find a CF Foundation-accredited care center, visit www.cff.org/LivingWithCF/CareCenterNetwork.
- To learn more about CF Services Pharmacy, visit www.cfservicespharmacy.com.
- To learn more about CF patient assistance programs, visit www.cff.org/LivingWithCF/AssistancePrograms.

Glossary of Terms

aerosol   A mist for inhalation, usually containing medicine. Aerosol mists may be made by an air compressor that blows air through a nebulizer, which contains liquid medicine, or may come from a handheld spray can.

airways   The tubes that carry air in and out of the lungs. These tubes begin with the nose and mouth and include the trachea (windpipe), bronchi, and bronchioles.

alveoli   The air sacs of the lung where gas exchange takes place.

anastomosis   A surgically created junction between two structures. An example of an anastomosis is the junction formed between the donor and recipient airways during a lung transplant.

anorexia   Lack of appetite.

anticoagulant   A drug that prevents blood clots.

atelectasis   Incomplete expansion of a portion of the lung, usually caused by mucus plugging.

BAL   An abbreviation for bronchoalveolar lavage.

baseline   One's normal state of health. The baseline or usual level of functioning includes a number of considerations, such as the amount of cough, exercise tolerance, and breathing effort. One's baseline health is often referred to for comparison. For example, after a pulmonary exacerbation, the goal of treatment is to return someone to his or her baseline state of health.

bicarbonate   An acid-neutralizing juice that is normally produced by the pancreas.

b.i.d.   An abbreviation meaning "twice a day."

biopsy   A small tissue sample of an organ. For example, after liver transplantation, the physician may wish to examine a piece of the transplanted liver; the piece obtained is known as a biopsy sample. "Biopsy" can also be used as a verb: Taking a small piece of an organ is called biopsy.

blood gas   The level of oxygen and carbon dioxide in the bloodstream, especially in the arteries. The term "blood gas" is also used to refer to the test and to the actual measurement of oxygen and carbon dioxide.

bronchi   The tubes through which air travels between the trachea and the bronchioles.

bronchioles   The smallest airways, connecting the bronchi to the alveoli. These airways differ from the bronchi in that they are smaller and have no cartilage to support them.

bronchoalveolar lavage   Washing a fluid (usually sterile salt water) into a small airway through a bronchoscope and then sucking the fluid back into a container. The fluid mixes with cells and other materials in the airway and allows them to be examined in the laboratory.

bronchoscope   An instrument that allows someone to look into the trachea and airways. There are two major types of bronchoscopes. The "rigid" bronchoscope is a steel tube that is placed through the mouth and into the trachea and airways. The "flexible" bronchoscope is a softer, flexible rubber and plastic bronchoscope that can be placed into the trachea and airways through the mouth, nose, or endotracheal tube.

bronchoscopy   Looking into the airways using a bronchoscope.

bronchus   Singular of bronchi.

cardiopulmonary bypass   A heart–lung machine used temporarily during cardiac or lung surgery to take the place of the heart and lungs.

cardiovascular system   The heart and blood vessels.

central line   A kind of intravenous catheter that extends into a very large vein, or even into the heart.

chromosome   Threadlike structures carrying all of the body's 5,000 genes.

cilia   The tiny hairs in the nose, trachea, and bronchi, which, through their coordinated movement, help keep the airways clean.

clubbing   An abnormal shape of the tips of the fingers and toes that is associated with different conditions, including cystic fibrosis.

corrector   A class of medication that helps move defective CFTR protein through the cell to the cell membrane, where it needs to be to function as a chloride channel (see also potentiator).

cyst   A fluid-filled sac.

dehiscence   The breakage of an anastomosis or any sutured surgical site.

diaphragm   The main breathing muscle. The diaphragm is located at the bottom of the lungs and separates the chest from the abdomen.

digestion   The process of breaking down foods into particles that are small enough to be absorbed through the intestinal wall into the bloodstream.

DNA   "Deoxyribonucleic acid"—the basic blueprint of the body's structure and function.

donor   A person donating tissue for transplantation; the person from whom a transplanted organ comes.

ectasia   Abnormal distention or enlargement. Bronchiectasis is abnormal widening of the bronchi.

-emia   A suffix meaning "in the blood." Thus, hypoxemia means lower than normal oxygen level in the blood.

enzymes   Chemicals that help perform biologic processes in the body; "enzymes" frequently refers to digestive enzymes, which are the chemicals formed in the pancreas that break down food into absorbable particles.

esophagus   The tube that connects the mouth to the stomach.

fellow   A physician in training for a subspecialty. A fellow has completed medical school, internship, and a specialty residency.

fibrosis   Scarring.

flaring   Nasal flaring.

gas exchange   The process of bringing oxygen into the bloodstream and removing carbon dioxide.

gastroenterology   The study of the structure, function, and diseases of the digestive system, including the esophagus, stomach (that's what the "gastro-" part refers to), and intestines (that's the "entero-" part). A gastroenterologist is a physician specializing in this area.

gastrostomy   A surgical opening through the abdominal wall into the stomach. A tube is placed through this opening, which allows feedings to be given through the tube.

gene   A unit of DNA that directs the production of a protein. Genes are responsible for directing everything all the cells in the body do.

genomics   The science of understanding how genes influence biologic activity.

GE reflux   Gastroesophageal reflux. A process in which fluid moves backward from the stomach into the esophagus.

graft   Tissue from one place placed into a second place. These places can be in one person's body, as when a vein is taken from someone's leg and used to replace a blocked heart blood vessel after–or to prevent–a heart attack. Or the places can be from different people, as with a lung graft, in which a lung from one person (donor) is placed into a second person (recipient).

heart failure   A condition in which the heart is not able to pump its full load of blood, resulting in the backup of fluid. Heart failure is *not* heart *stoppage*.

hemoptysis   Coughing up blood.

hep lock   (see "Glossary of Drugs" in Appendix B). An intravenous needle whose end can be plugged while it is not being used for medication administration.

hyper   A prefix meaning "more than normal." Thus, a hyperactive child is more active than normal.

hyperalimentation   This term literally means "overfeeding," but actually refers to the method of giving extra nutrition through an intravenous.

hypo-   A prefix meaning "less than normal." Thus, hypoxia means less oxygen than normal.

IM   Intramuscular. A way of administering medicine by injection into the muscle.

immunosuppression   Decreasing the immune response, usually using medications known as "immunosuppressives".

intern   A physician who has graduated from medical school and is in his/her first year of training in a medical specialty such as pediatrics, internal medicine, family medicine, or surgery.

internal medicine   The branch of medicine dealing with the general health of adults.

internist   A medical specialist in internal medicine (not to be confused with an intern).

***in vitro* fertilization**   A procedure for uniting a sperm and an egg outside the body, then implanting the fertilized egg in a woman's uterus.

-itis   A suffix meaning "inflammation." Thus, bronchitis means inflammation of the bronchi.

IV   Intravenous. This can mean the way a drug is given (IV) or the actual tubing used to give the drug ("the IV").

jejunostomy   A surgical opening made through the abdominal wall into the jejunum. This opening is used to hold a tube for feedings, as is a gastrostomy.

jejunum   The second part of the small intestine.

larynx   The part of the upper airway that contains the vocal cords—the "voice box."

LAS   Lung allocation score. A numerical score given to patients awaiting lung transplantation. The LAS is determined largely by the severity of lung disease. In general, the more severe the disease, the higher the score, and the more likely that person will be next in line for a lung transplantation, should suitable lungs become available.

lobe   The largest division of the lung. The right lung has three lobes and the left has two.

low-hanging fruit   The research strategy that targets possible solutions likely to give fast results, for example, exploring drugs that are already approved by the Food and Drug Administration for other diseases and may have potential for cystic fibrosis.

lumen   The inside of a tube. The lumen of the bronchial tubes is where the air flows.

lymphocyte   A type of white blood cell. Lymphocytes are important in immune function and are involved in rejection of grafts.

MESA   Microsurgical epididymal sperm aspiration. The procedure by which sperm can be removed from a man's testicle and used for *in vitro* fertilization.

motility   Movement. When used in reference to the intestines, this means the contractions of the muscles that help propel intestinal contents on their journey from esophagus to anus.

mucociliary escalator   A mechanism for keeping the lungs clear. Particles get trapped in the mucus, and the cilia move the mucus out of the lungs.

Mucoid   mucus-like. This term is often applied to bacteria (such as *Pseudomonas*) that form a protective slime layer over itself when growing in colonies. Often, mucoid forms of bacteria are harder to kill than non-mucoid.

mucous   Having properties like mucus. ("Mucus" is a noun; "mucous" is an adjective.)

mucus   The slimy fluid secreted in many glands of the body and whose function appears to be to protect and to lubricate.

mutation   A change or alteration. Most often used to refer to a change in a gene that makes it abnormal.

nasal flaring   Widening of the nostrils with each breath (often abbreviated as "flaring"). This is a sign that someone is working harder than normal to breathe.

nebulizer   A device used with an air compressor which directs the compressed air past liquid medication, lifting the medication into a mist ("aerosol") for inhalation.

NG tube   Nasogastric tube. A tube that passes through the nose into the stomach. This tube is used for feeding someone who can't eat, for continuous feeding during sleep, or for the administration of other substances such as medicines.

panresistant   Resistant to all tested antibiotics.

peak   The highest concentration that a drug reaches in the bloodstream.

PFT   Pulmonary function test.

PICC   Periperally inserted central catheter. A long intravenous (IV) catheter inserted in the arm, with its tip ending in the large vessels that go to the heart. Often redundantly called as "PICC line."

"pipeline"   A term used by the Cystic Fibrosis Foundation to describe the flow of new medications for cystic fibrosis from early experimentation to widespread use by patients.

pneumothorax   Collapsed lung caused by a hole in the lung. Air escapes from the lung through this hole, collects within the chest, and presses in on the lung.

potentiator   A class of medication that increases the effectiveness of a slightly defective CFTR protein that is already correctly positioned in the cell membrane (see also corrector).

proteomics   Proteomics is the science of the complete analysis of proteins to uncover their locations, control, and functions.

pulmonary exacerbation   An episode of worsening of lung disease, usually caused by worsened bronchial infection.

pulmonologist   A physician specializing in the care of patients with lung problems.

pulmonology   The branch of medicine dealing with lung and breathing problems.

recipient   A person receiving tissue for transplantation.

reflux   The backward movement of fluid; this term is often used to refer to gastroesophageal reflux.

rejection   The body's attempt to destroy transplanted tissue. Rejection is carried out by lymphocytes, which are immune cells capable of causing damage to foreign cells.

resident   A physician who has completed medical school and is undertaking further training in a medical specialty.

resistant   This term means "not killed by" when used to describe bacteria's relation to an antibiotic. For example, the statement, "*Pseudomonas* bacteria are resistant to penicillin," means that, in the laboratory, penicillin does not readily kill *Pseudomonas* organisms.

respiratory failure   The condition in which blood oxygen levels are too low and blood carbon dioxide levels are too high.

retracting   The pulling-in of skin between the ribs with each breath, indicating hard breathing.

saline   Salt water (see Appendix B).

sedation   A state of reduced excitement, anxiety, and (often) a state of mildly reduced consciousness. Many drugs are used to produce sedation and are commonly used to decrease anxiety during medical procedures.

segment   The second largest division of the lung. Each lobe is divided into several segments.

sensitive   This term means "killed by" when used to describe bacteria's relation to an antibiotic. For example, the statement, "*Streptococcus* bacteria are sensitive to penicillin," means that, in the laboratory, penicillin kills *Streptococcus* organisms.

specialty (or medical specialty)   One of the main branches of medical practice in which physicians can become trained and qualified. The specialties are pediatrics, internal (adult) medicine, obstetrics/gynecology, surgery, psychiatry, and family medicine. Physicians may focus their skills and training in more specialized areas, called subspecialties, such as pediatric pulmonology, cardiology, and neurosurgery. (A pediatric pulmonary specialist must first become a pediatrician; a neurosurgeon must first become a surgeon.)

sputum   Mucus from the lungs that is coughed up and spit out.

stenosis   Narrowing. In transplantation, stenosis can occur at an anastomosis, for example, where a donor bronchus is attached to the recipient bronchus.

stoma   A hole, usually one created purposely by a surgical procedure. This word is often used as a suffix: tracheostomy is a hole made in the trachea; gastrostomy is a hole through the abdominal wall into the stomach.

TDC   One of the centers in the TDN (Therapeutics Development Center).

TDN   Therapeutics Development Network of the Cystic Fibrosis Foundation of the United States. A system of clinical research centers established to perform collaborative studies, especially on new drug treatments for cystic fibrosis.

toxicity   Harmful effect(s). This term is often used to refer to the undesirable effects of a medication.

TPN   Total parenteral nutrition. This term refers to nutrition given through an intravenous catheter (same meaning as hyperalimentation).

trachea   The tube that carries air from the mouth and throat into the chest, where it connects with the bronchi from each lung.

tracheostomy   A hole placed in the trachea.

trough   The lowest concentration that a drug reaches in the bloodstream (this level is found immediately preceding a dose of the drug).

urologist   A physician specializing in problems of the urinary and genital tracts.

ventricle   One of the two main portions of the heart. The right ventricle pumps blood through the lungs, and the left ventricle then pumps the blood to the rest of the body.

Medications

Your physician knows the most about your treatment needs and will prescribe the best medications for you. *You should not take any medications without the advice of your physician.* Contact your physician if you have questions about the medications described.

The very exciting thing about cystic fibrosis (CF) in the 21st century is that the development of very good medications to treat CF is taking place more rapidly now than at any other time in history. That is great for people with CF and not so great for this section of the book. In the time it takes to write this section, publish the book for you to read it, there may be many medications for CF that are new. The most reliable and up-to-date listing of medications for CF can be found on the CFF.org website. Check out the "Drug Development Pipeline" to find out what medications are available and what exciting therapies are on their way.

This appendix is organized according to the systems of the body; for example, the antibiotics used to combat lung infection are discussed under *Respiratory System Medications: Lungs*, and digestive enzymes are discussed under *Gastrointestinal and Digestive System Medications*. There is a separate category for medications used specifically by people who have received an organ transplant. For each medicine discussed, there is information on how the drug is taken as well as possible side effects or dangers.

The most common method of taking the drugs described in this Appendix is by mouth. Some medicines can be given by injecting them into a vein (IV, for *intra*venous) or into a muscle (IM, for *intra*muscular). Others can be taken as aerosols, and breathed into the lungs or sniffed into the nostril, while still others may be applied directly to the skin. There are times when physicians will even prescribe medications to be used in a way that was not intended by the manufacturer. This is called off-label usage. This most commonly occurs in the care of patients with CF when IV preparations of antibiotics are given by nebulization.

A word about side effects: Every medicine has potentially serious side effects. There is no drug that has only good effects and absolutely no dangers. However, all the drugs discussed here have passed numerous tests, which, to most doctors and scientists, will mean that the drug's benefits outweigh their risks. Most people are able to take most of the medicines in this book without experiencing any serious problems. The "undesirable effects" noted for each drug are not meant to frighten you but to help you be as well informed as possible about your medications.

Drug names (generic names and the trade names given by the drug companies) are listed in the *Glossary of Drugs* at the end of Appendix B.

RESPIRATORY SYSTEM MEDICATIONS

Lungs

In order to prevent disease in the lungs, therapies target three main problems that occur in CF: (a)—retention of thick/sticky mucus, (b)—infection, and (c)-inflammation. What happens is that mucus can get trapped in the lungs. Bacteria love to live in warm places with a lot of food (in this case, mucus) and so infection can occur if mucus is present in the lungs. Then, in order to fight infection, the body sends cells to the site of infection, causing inflammation. Sometimes this inflammation can get out of hand leading to more mucus and more infection and more inflammation leading to more mucus and, well, we think you see the point. Eventually, damage to the lung can occur. By using medications that help thin out and remove mucus, treating infections before they become problems, and appropriately calming down inflammation, treatments for the lungs can prevent lung damage.

Mucus Clearance Agents—Mucolytics

Lysis means destruction or decomposition of a substance, so *muco*lytics are drugs that destroy or break down mucus. Since much of the lung trouble in CF has to do with extra thick mucus, a completely safe and completely effective mucolytic for the lung would be wonderful. There isn't such a drug now. However, one comes closer than anything previously available.

Dornase-Alpha/DNase/Pulmozyme®

When DNase (Pulmozyme®) is put in a glass test tube with CF lung mucus, it breaks down the mucus, making it much more watery, and easier to move. When cells from the body go to the lungs to fight infection, they eventually die and release DNA. DNA is very sticky. DNase (-ase means to break down) breaks down DNA in mucus and makes it easier to cough out. It seems to help some patients and even has improved lung function in several hundred patients over a period lasting 6 months. Other patients have not had measurable improvements in pulmonary function but have felt better. Very few patients are harmed by it. Not everyone with CF is helped by it, and it is impossible to predict who will benefit. This difficulty in predicting response goes both ways. That is, you might expect it to help only those patients who are clearly bothered by a lot of thick mucus. And, it does help many patients like that. But, it also helps improve pulmonary function in some patients whose lungs are in quite good shape, without lots of extra thick mucus. It is expensive (anywhere from $10,000 to $25,000 per year).

How it is taken: This drug is always given by inhalation.

Undesirable effects: Some patients may experience a sore throat, but this goes away with time in most instances. A very few patients with very severe lung disease and a large amount of thick mucus may have trouble handling that mucus if it is suddenly all liquefied at once. This is uncommon.

Hypertonic Saline/Hypersal®

If we understand the basic problem with CF correctly as there being a lack of chloride and water in the airways, then adding chloride and water to the airways should fix the problem. That is what hypertonic saline aims to do. It adds sodium and chloride to the airways that should help in hydrating the mucus and making it easier to cough out. When given to patients with CF over a long period of time, hypertonic (7%) saline appears to improve lung function and prevent patients from exacerbations (getting sick).

How it is taken: This drug is always given by inhalation.

Undesirable effects: The usual saline content in our bodies is about 0.9%, and hypertonic saline is over seven times that amount. Because of this, our bodies are not used to this much salt, especially in the lungs. Therefore, most people cough when inhaling hypertonic saline. This is a good thing because coughing will help get the mucus out, but sometimes coughing can get out of hand and bronchospasm (coughing and wheezing) may occur. Because of this, most people take albuterol (see below) prior to hypertonic saline to open up the airways and prevent problems. Sore throat can also occur with hypertonic saline. Usually this goes away with time.

Acetylcysteine (Mucomyst®)

This is another mucolytic, one that's been in use for decades. Like DNase, it is highly effective in breaking down CF mucus in the test tube. Unlike DNase, it seems to have adverse effects in a number of patients. In many people, this drug causes bronchial irritation with production of more mucus. In others, it causes bronchospasm. Some physicians prescribe an aerosolized bronchodilator along with Mucomyst to try to prevent bronchospasm. Mucomyst smells like rotten eggs and is expensive.

Bronchodilators ("Asthma Medicines")

We can talk about bronchodilators in this section since opening up the airways helps to get the mucus out. Also, some people with CF also have asthma, or a condition like asthma, where the bronchi can become partly blocked for a time when the bronchial lining becomes inflamed and swollen, and the muscles surrounding the bronchi squeeze down. Bronchodilators are medicines that open (dilate) the bronchi by relaxing the muscles around them. The medicines are effective in treating bronchospasm once it starts and help to prevent it from occurring. Some of these drugs can be taken by inhalation, some by injection (either IM, IV, or under the skin), some by mouth, and some by several different methods. Bronchodilators seem to help some people with CF, while not being effective in others.

Beta-Agonists/Albuterol

This is the name applied to a class of very helpful bronchodilators, including albuterol (that's what it's called in the United States; it's called salbutamol in the rest of the world) and others. Levalbuterol (Xopenex) is newer preparation of albuterol, very heavily marketed, which is not needed for most patients.

How they are taken: These drugs are best taken by inhalation (either from a handheld canister-type nebulizer—usually called *a metered-dose inhaler* or just MDI—or from the air-compressor type of aerosol machine). They can also be taken by injection or by mouth (pills or liquids), although the beneficial effects tend to be less and the side effects more than if they are used by inhalation.

Undesirable effects: The three main undesirable effects of this class of drugs are (a) shakiness, which often goes away with continued use of the drugs; (b) overactiveness (getting "hyper"), a fairly uncommon side effect; and (c) stimulation of the heart, causing it to speed up, which can be somewhat annoying. It may also cause an irregular heartbeat, which can be dangerous. Dangerous effects are uncommon if the drugs are taken by inhalation. In the 1960s, a number of deaths were reported in patients with asthma who used their handheld nebulizers of beta-agonists too much. It's not clear what caused these deaths, but there are two likely reasons: It may have been the chemical used to make the aerosol, and not the bronchodilator itself, or, it may have been that patients got such good relief from the inhalations that they didn't see their doctor for a very serious asthma attack, but instead kept puffing on their aerosols, even when the effect lasted a shorter and shorter time. When they finally did try to go for help, they were too sick. Today, the vehicle for delivering the aerosol is safer. However, there is still a danger if a patient with asthma or CF tries home-prescribed antibiotics, bronchodilators, and so forth. While they may seem to work at first, they can lead to serious consequences. Talk to your doctors about medicine changes in order to avoid dangerous combinations or dosages and to avoid overlooking a serious problem for which you should be examined.

Antibiotics

Antibiotics are drugs used to fight infections caused by bacteria. They do not kill other kinds of germs, such as viruses and fungi. There are many different families of antibiotics, several methods of taking antibiotics, and certain unwelcome effects with which you should be familiar. These areas are all discussed below.

Perhaps two introductory words should be said about antibiotics and undesirable effects: The first is that antibiotics kill or control bacteria, which is their job, and they are usually very good at it. However, antibiotics can't tell good bacteria from bad. Everyone does have some good bacteria in the body, especially in the mouth and intestines. Among other things, these good bacteria keep people from becoming overrun with fungi and yeasts. Sometimes while a person takes antibiotics, the good bacteria are killed along with the bad. When this happens, a yeast infection can take hold, with a cheesy-looking material in the mouth or vagina. The condition is referred to as *thrush* when it occurs in the mouth. Generally, these yeast infections are easily dealt with, but your doctor needs to know about them in order to prescribe the right medicine (usually nystatin). The same problem of killing the good bacteria can also cause trouble in the intestines, and some patients develop diarrhea from antibiotics. Many people choose to eat yogurt while they are taking antibiotics in order to replenish the good bacteria in their intestines.

The last point to mention is that with the availability of so many new medicines, it is possible that new side effects can appear that have not been seen or recorded. If you develop any disturbing symptoms or problems shortly after you've started taking a new antibiotic, it may be from the new drug, and you should let your doctor know about it.

Penicillins

This family was first used in the early 1940s and was one of the earliest groups of drugs to be used to fight infection in people. The number of drugs included in this family has grown tremendously over the past 30 years. New members of the penicillin family keep appearing, so it is impossible to list them all. Although the members of the penicillin family have distinct, individual personalities, there are a number of shared characteristics. The most important of these is that if you are allergic to any one penicillin, there is a strong chance that you will be allergic to all of them.

1. *Penicillin.* The first in its family (as you might have guessed from the name), this drug kills many germs, especially *Streptococcus* (*Strep*) and *pneumococcus* (the "pneumonia germ"). These bacteria are not the major problem bacteria for patients with CF. The most common causes of bronchial infections in patients with CF are *Haemophilus*, *Staphylococcus* (*Staph*), or *Pseudomonas* organisms, and penicillin is usually not effective in treating these infections.
    How it is taken: Penicillin can be given by mouth, intravenously or intramuscularly.
    Undesirable effects: Allergic reactions to penicillin can be mild but can also be very serious. Any of the drugs in this family can cause a reaction in someone who is allergic to penicillin. Penicillin injections are painful. Other than

these two problems, penicillin is remarkably gentle to the human body while being brutally hard on the unwelcome bacteria.

2. *Ampicillin.* Ampicillin kills most *Haemophilus* (also called *H. flu*) in addition to the bacteria that penicillin kills. It does not usually kill *Staph* or *Pseudomonas* organisms.

    How it is taken: Ampicillin is most commonly taken by mouth. It can also be given by IV or IM injection.

    Undesirable effects: Loose stools are fairly common in people taking oral ampicillin. A skin rash may appear in some people, too, even if they are not actually allergic to the penicillins.

3. *Amoxicillin.* This is a slightly different version of ampicillin; it kills the same bacteria, but is less likely to cause diarrhea.

    How it is taken: Only by mouth.

4. *Augmentin®.* This combines amoxicillin with another chemical, clavulanic acid, and makes it effective against *Staph* in addition to the usual bacteria that are killed by amoxicillin.

    Undesirable effects: Augmentin® can cause loose stools even more than amoxicillin on its own. Usually this is tolerable.

5. *Methicillin, oxacillin,* and *nafcillin.* These three drugs have been modified so that they kill *Staph* very well. They do not usually kill *Haemophilus* or *Pseudomonas* organisms.

    How they are taken: These drugs are used mostly by IV but can also be given by IM injections. Oxacillin and nafcillin have some effect if taken orally (but not as much as cloxacillin or dicloxacillin, discussed next).

    Undesirable effects: These drugs are irritating to the tissues where they are injected. They can cause discomfort as they go into a vein.

6. *Cloxacillin* and *dicloxacillin.* These are also good anti-*Staph* drugs, used only by mouth. Otherwise they are similar to the other anti-*Staph* penicillins.

7. *Carbenicillin, ticarcillin, piperacillin, mezlocillin,* and *azlocillin.* These are anti-*Pseudomonas* drugs. They generally do not kill *Staph*, but they do kill *Haemophilus.*

    How they are taken: Almost always given intravenously; they can be given intramuscularly, but most people feel this is not a practical way to administer the drugs over the relatively long period of time (1 to 3 weeks or longer) for which they are usually used. Carbenicillin can also be given by mouth for treating bladder infections, but none of the drug gets to the lungs if it's taken by mouth. Therefore, orally, it is not effective in treating CF *Pseudomonas* bronchial infections. Occasionally, these drugs are given by inhalation.

    Undesirable effects: In addition to the possibility of allergic reactions in people who are allergic to penicillin, and the irritation these drugs can cause when they are injected, there are some other problems that occasionally arise. These medicines can make liver tests appear abnormal; fortunately, however, the problem is only with the laboratory result and not with the liver itself.

The liver continues to function normally, and if the medicine is continued to be given, the test results will return to normal. These antibiotics can also interfere with the function of platelets (blood cells that are responsible for proper clotting of blood).

8. *Timentin®*. This combines clavulanic acid with ticarcillin, the way Augmentin® combines it with amoxicillin, to make the ticarcillin effective against *Staph* in addition to *Pseudomonas* and *Haemophilus* organisms. Timentin is administered by IV like ticarcillin and has similar side-effects.

9. *Zosyn®*. This is similar to Timentin®, in that it takes an anti-*Pseudomonas* penicillin—piperacillin, in this case—and combines it with a chemical (tazobactam in this case, instead of clavulanic acid) that enables the drug to kill *Staph* in addition to *Pseudomonas* organisms. Zosyn is administered by IV like piperacillin and has similar side-effects.

Cephalosporins

This family of antibiotics is growing even faster than the penicillins. Most members of this family are helpful in combating infections with *Strep*, *Staph*, and *Haemophilus*. Some of the newest members of this family have some activity against *Pseudomonas*. To preserve space, only a few of the more commonly used cephalosporins are listed here (but a more complete listing is in the glossary).

How they are taken: Cephalexin, cefdinir, cefprozil, and cefaclor are taken by mouth only. Cephalothin, cephaloridine, ceftazidime, cefepime, and cefotaxime are given only by injection (IM or IV). Cefuroxime can be given by mouth or by injection.

Undesirable effects: About one third of people who are allergic to penicillins will also be allergic to cephalosporins. Other problems are fortunately not common but include diarrhea or other stomach/intestinal upset.

Sulfa Drugs

These were the first antibiotics ever used to fight infections in people, and they still have many uses.

1. *Sulfisoxazole.* This drug can help in some infections with *Haemophilus*, but it is of little use in fighting *Pseudomonas* organisms.
   How they are taken: By mouth.
   Undesirable effects: Problems with this drug are not common. Some people have allergic skin reactions.

2. *Trimethoprim–sulfamethoxazole (TMP-SMX).* This is a combination of two drugs. Trimethoprim is not a sulfa drug, but the combination is quite effective in treating several kinds of bacteria, usually including *Haemophilus*. It is not usually effective for infections caused by *Staph* or *Pseudomonas*.
   How they are taken: By mouth (rarely by IV).
   Undesirable effects: Problems with this drug are not common.

3. *Erythromycin/sulfisoxazole.* This is another combination product including a sulfa drug (sulfisoxazole) and a non-sulfa (erythromycin) that is quite effective in treating several kinds of bacteria, usually including *Haemophilus, Strep,* and *Staph.* It is not usually effective for infections caused by *Pseudomonas.*

> *How they are taken*: By mouth.
> *Undesirable effects*: Problems with this drug are not common although the erythromycin component may cause some upset stomach.

Aminoglycosides

This family includes gentamicin, tobramycin, neomycin, kanamycin, amikacin, and netilmicin. Many kinds of *Pseudomonas* infections can be treated effectively with these drugs, especially with gentamicin, tobramycin, and amikacin. These drugs seem to be particularly helpful in killing *Pseudomonas* if they are given with an anti-*Pseudomonas* penicillin.

How they are taken: Almost always given by aerosol or IV or IM injection since these antibiotics are not absorbed well into the bloodstream if they are taken by mouth. Shots into the muscle with these drugs are not as painful as those with the penicillins.

Undesirable effects: The two main problems with these drugs are their effects on the kidney and the ears. These problems are usually (but not always) avoidable if the blood levels of the drug are checked and dosages adjusted to keep the blood levels in what is considered the safe range. (Levels do not need to be checked if gentamicin or tobramycin is used by inhalation, since almost none of the drug gets absorbed into the bloodstream from the bronchi.) The kidney problems are usually not uncomfortable for the patient. The ear problem is worsened hearing. The harmful kidney effects usually disappear if the drug is stopped (or the dosage reduced). If the drugs are continued after the hearing or kidney damage has begun, there can sometimes be serious and permanent damage.

Macrolides

These drugs include erythromycin, clarithromycin, and azithromycin. They are commonly substituted for penicillin in people who are allergic to penicillin. They kill *Strep,* many *Staph* and *Haemophilus* organisms, and several other bacteria that aren't big problems in CF. They may or may not kill *Pseudomonas* and may decrease the inflammation caused by *Pseudomonas.* It is possible that one or more of the macrolides will kill *Pseudomonas* in the airways even though they don't kill it in the bacteriology laboratory.

How they are taken: Macrolides are most often taken by mouth, but IV forms are also available.

Undesirable effects: Abdominal cramping is sometimes an effect of these drugs, and some years ago, there was a scare about liver damage with some macrolide preparations. It now seems that liver damage is not very likely with this medicine.

Tetracyclines

The tetracyclines (tetracycline, doxycycline, minocycline, and tigecycline) were among the first drugs available that had any effect against *Pseudomonas* organisms. They are no longer as helpful as they once were because many bacteria have become resistant to their effects. There are still some *Pseudomonas, Staph, Haemophilus,* and *Strep* bacteria that are sensitive to tetracyclines. Also, with less common infections such as *Burkholderia* cepacia, Alcaligenes (also called *Achromobacter*), and some forms of mycobacteria, the tetracyclines may have some use.

How they are taken: The tetracyclines are usually taken by mouth but can be given by IV or IM injection. Tigecycline is available only in IV form.

Undesirable effects: The main undesirable effect of tetracyclines, one that's known to those CF patients in their 40s and older, is that if it's given to people between the ages of approximately 4 months and 8 years, it can permanently stain their teeth a grayish/brownish/yellow color. Thirty years ago, physicians knew about the tooth problem, but often didn't have any other antibiotics to give, so they had to use a tetracycline. Fortunately, today there usually is another antibiotic available, and tetracycline should almost never be used in young children. Other side effects include allergic reactions, intestinal upset, and a rash that is made worse by being exposed to the sun.

Quinolones

This family of antibiotics has some activity against *Pseudomonas* organisms in the lung, even when the drugs (especially ciprofloxacin) are taken by mouth.

How it is taken: Several of these medications can be taken by mouth and intravenously.

Undesirable effects: Remarkably few side effects have been recognized with these antibiotics. To date, intestinal upset has been seen occasionally. Another problem seems to be that bacteria become resistant to the quinolones very soon after the patient starts to take them (within a week or two). Young animals given these drugs have developed some problems with the cartilage in their joints, so most physicians are reluctant to prescribe the drugs for young children. These drugs may also cause a skin rash with sun exposure.

Vancomycin

Vancomycin is an effective antibiotic against strains of *Staph* that are resistant to penicillin antibiotics, specifically methicillin-resistant *Staphylococcus aureus* (MRSA).

How it is taken: Vancomycin is effective for CF lung infection only by injection. It can be given by mouth but has no uptake from the gut, and so it is given by mouth only to treat infection in the gut.

Undesirable effects: Vancomycin can have effects on the kidneys and needs to be monitored with blood levels in order to make sure that levels are not too high.

Linezolid

Linezolid is an effective antibiotic for MRSA and can also be used for some strains of mycobacteria.

How it is taken: Linezolid can be given by mouth or injection.
Undesirable effects: If given for more than 2 weeks, linezolid can affect the production of blood cells. Therefore, a blood count may be needed during long-term use of linezolid.

Imipenem and Meropenem

These drugs have activity against *Pseudomonas, Staph,* and *Haemophilus* organisms and seem relatively safe and effective.

How they are taken: These drugs are given intravenously.
Undesirable effects: *Imipenem* can make the vein tender and may cause nausea, particularly while it is running in; meropenem seems less likely to do either.

Aztreonam

This drug is one with some anti-*Pseudomonas* activity; it seems to be safe and effective.

How it is taken: Aztreonam is taken by IV injection and is now available in an inhaled preparation.
Undesirable effects: The side effects of this drug have been few and not very serious. They have included diarrhea, nausea, allergic reactions, and tenderness at the site of injection.

Colistimethate/Colistin®

This drug has activity against *Pseudomonas, Staph,* and other bacteria that can live in the lungs of people with CF.

How it is taken: Colistimethate can be given by injection (IV or IM), but the undesirable effects prevent many doctors from prescribing it this way. Although not approved by FDA (Food and Drug Administration) to be given by aerosol, there are many patients with CF who safely use this medication by aerosol.
Undesirable effects: When given by injection, colistimethate can have serious effects on the kidneys and the nervous system (headache, numbness, tingling in the extremities). Therefore, close monitoring is needed when colistimethate is given by injection. When aerosolized, colistimethate has very few side effects.

Antiviral Medications

Although antibiotics do not kill viruses, a few drugs do.

Oseltamivir, Amantadine, and Rimantadine

These drugs are used to treat or prevent influenza, especially in a person who has not received the flu vaccine (especially those who can't receive the flu vaccine because of severe egg allergy).

How they are taken: These are taken by mouth, starting (for treatment) immediately after influenza has been diagnosed, or (for prevention) throughout the flu season. There is an influenza medication (zanamivir) that is available by inhalation. Because this inhaled medication can cause bronchospasm, it is not recommended for patients with CF.

Undesirable effects: These medicines are generally well tolerated.

Drugs for Respiratory Syncytial Virus

Respiratory syncytial virus (RSV) is a common respiratory virus that can cause severe disease, especially in infants with underlying lung problems. Three main drugs have been used: two for prevention, one for treatment; and none has been overwhelmingly successful.

1. *Palivizumab (Synagis®)*. Palivizumab (Synagis®) has been used to prevent RSV in sick tiny infants. It has been used in CF, but its benefit has not been proven.
   How it is taken: This drug is given by IM injection once a month for the whole RSV season (usually October to April).
   Undesirable effects: Although the drug is usually well tolerated, there can be local reactions at the site of injection, "cold" symptoms, rash, diarrhea, or vomiting.

2. *Ribavirin*. Ribavirin has been used to treat RSV pneumonia.
   How it is taken: This drug is given by aerosol. The treatments last 12 to 18 hours each day.
   Undesirable effects: Wheezing and shortness of breath can occur, and it is difficult to administer the aerosols for as long as they need to be given each day. The tubing used to deliver the medicine often clogs.

Antifungal Medicine

There is usually not much call for antifungal medicines in patients with CF, but in the case of ABPA (allergic bronchopulmonary aspergillosis), killing some of the *Aspergillus* organisms can help decrease the allergic reaction to these fungi. Two medicines that are available for this task are voriconazole (Vfend®) and *itraconazole (Sporanox®)*.

How they are taken: Both voriconazole and itraconazole are usually taken by mouth. In some cases, they can be given intravenously.

Undesirable effects: These drugs are usually well tolerated, but there is a long list of possible side effects, including fatigue, fever, itchiness, abdominal pain, and liver damage.

Anti-Inflammatory Medications

Steroids

Steroids, also called "corticosteroids," are cortisone-like drugs whose name strikes fear in the hearts of many people because of the serious side effects caused by improper use or even proper use where these medicines are needed at high doses for a long period of time. Actually, steroids can be extremely useful and very safe if used properly. In fact, everyone's body makes these drugs themselves, and they are extremely important in maintaining health. They are very potent agents for decreasing inflammation and swelling within the bronchi (and elsewhere). In asthma, they also seem to increase the sensitivity of the body to the effects of the beta-agonist drugs. The inhaled, non-absorbed steroids have become the "front-line" treatment around the world for people with asthma. It's not yet clear whether they will also be helpful for people with CF.

How they are taken: Steroids can be taken by mouth (pills or liquid), by IV injection, or by inhalation. The inhaled steroids, budesonide, fluticasone, beclomethasone, triamcinolone, and others, affect the bronchi by *preventing* inflammation and bronchoconstriction, much more than by reversing inflammation and broncho-constriction once they've started. Almost none of the inhaled steroid is absorbed into the bloodstream, so it has very little toxic effect on the rest of the body. There are preparations of inhaled steroids that are combined with long-acting bron-chodilators. Advair® and Symbicort® are two such medications. Advair® has fluticasone (steroid) and salmeterol (bronchodilator), and Symbicort® has budesonide (steroid) and formoterol (bronchodilator) in each inhalation.

There are many different schedules for taking oral steroids. They can be given several times a day, once a day, or once every other day. They can be given for a brief period—a 3- to 5-day "burst"—or for months. The schedule depends on the drug being used, what it is being used for, and the characteristics and needs of the person taking it.

Undesirable effects: The side effects of the inhaled steroids are relatively few. Some patients may get thrush (a yeast infection in the mouth). This can be avoided by brushing the teeth or rinsing out the mouth after inhaling the steroid. Some studies have shown a slowing of height growth in children taking inhaled steroids over a long time, but even in those studies, the children's eventual height is *not* affected.

The oral steroid preparations come with more side effects including greatly increased appetite and swelling ("chipmunk cheeks"), acne, slowed growth in height, increased possibility of developing diabetes, eye cataracts, bone brittleness, and difficulty in fighting infection. In general, the lower the dose and the shorter the length of time steroids are given, the less likely one is to develop side effects. When these drugs are used by mouth or injection for longer than a week or two, the body begins to detect them and seem to say, "Well, we don't need to make any more of our own." If the drug is then stopped abruptly, the body is left without the protection of its own steroids. For this reason, if steroids are required for more than a week or two, you can't suddenly just stop the drug; instead, you need to reduce (taper) the amount you take over several days or even weeks (depending on how long you've been on them and how used your body has become to receiving them from an outside source) so that your body gradually gets used to the idea of having to make steroids on its own again. If the drugs are used for less than a week (or even 2), they can be stopped abruptly with an extremely small likelihood of side effects. Another way to get around most of the side effects is to take the drugs every other day. This gives the body a day to recover between doses. In some cases, when steroids are really needed, a patient may not be able to tolerate being off them for that in-between day.

Ibuprofen

Ibuprofen is a non-steroidal anti-inflammatory drugs (NSAID). If given in high doses over a long time, ibuprofen can have anti-inflammatory effects in patients with CF.

How it is taken: Ibuprofen is taken by mouth.

Undesirable effects: In normal doses, ibuprofen can cause problems with bleeding, stomach upset, ulcers, and kidney problems in patients with kidneys that are not quite healthy. For CF, ibuprofen is needed in high doses, so these concerns are heightened. The high dosing and need for blood monitoring are two likely reasons why ibuprofen is not widely used for patients with CF.

Leukotriene Inhibitors

Leukotrienes are chemicals that are important in the cascade of reactions that cause inflammation. A whole class of drugs has been developed, which interfere with the actions of various leukotrienes, including montelukast and zafirlukast.

How they are taken: These drugs are taken by mouth.

Undesirable effects: Relatively few occur with leukotriene inhibitors. Headache can occur in patients taking these drugs.

Other Therapies/Medications for the Respiratory System
Oxygen

Most people with CF don't need any more oxygen than the amount that is in the regular air around us. Air is 21% oxygen, and at sea level, this generally provides plenty of oxygen for most people. If the lungs are severely affected by disease, or when someone is at high altitude—including in a commercial airliner, whose cabins are pressurized to be like an altitude of 5,000 to 8,000 ft—or when someone with moderate lung disease is exercising, it may be difficult for enough oxygen to enter the bloodstream. In these cases, people can breathe extra oxygen—air with 25%, 30%, 40%, or more oxygen. When someone's blood oxygen level is very low, it is remarkable how much better a little extra oxygen can make him or her feel.

How it is taken: This drug is always taken by inhalation (but you knew that). It can be delivered by nasal cannula (tubing that goes into each nostril) or by a mask placed in front of the mouth and nose. Oxygen can be kept in metal

TABLE 1

Oxygen Cylinders and their Specifications

Cylinder	Time (at 5 L/Min)	Size (Inches)	Weight, lb (Full)
B	44 min	3½ × 16	6
D	70 min	4¼ × 20	10
E	2 h	4¼ × 30	14
M	11 h	7⅛ × 46	82
G	17 h	9 × 51	127
K	23 h	9 × 55	150

cylinders of different sizes. Small "B-cylinders" are about 3½ inches across and 16 inches high and weigh about 6 lb when full. If someone is using 5 liters (L) per minute (see below), these cylinders last 44 minutes. Other cylinders are shown in Table 1.

Oxygen can also be stored in liquid form. Liquid oxygen tanks hold much more oxygen in the same space than oxygen gas. Different-sized tanks of liquid oxygen are also available (Table 2).

One other way of giving extra oxygen in the home is with an oxygen extractor or concentrator, which takes in regular room air and gets rid of the parts of air that are not oxygen (mostly nitrogen), resulting in almost pure oxygen. This method is expensive, and the machines are bulky and somewhat noisy, but for someone who needs oxygen much of the time, it may be cheaper and more convenient than using many small tanks.

Just how much extra oxygen you breathe depends on how the oxygen gets from the tank to your lungs. The main methods are mask and nasal cannula. The mask takes the pure oxygen from the tank and mixes it with varying amounts of room air to deliver 25%, 30%, 35%, 50%, or even 100% oxygen. Nasal cannulas, which consist of a flexible plastic tube with two short plastic prongs at the end that stick a short way into the nostrils, can deliver different amounts depending on how high you set the flow of oxygen from the tanks: for every liter per minute of oxygen flow, you add about 3% to 4% oxygen above room air. That means that if the flow

TABLE 2

Liquid Oxygen Containers and their Specifications

Cylinder	Time (at 5 L/Min)	Size (Inches)	Weight, lb (Full)
Stroller	3½ h	3½ oval	9.5
L-30	86 h	12 × 35	120

is set at 4 L/min, you get $4 \times 3 = 12\%$ or so above room air (room air has 21% oxygen) or $12 + 21 = 33\%$ oxygen. There are some newer methods that some adults are finding more convenient and less noticeable to other people than the old methods. These include nasal cannulas that come through eyeglasses (and therefore have just a little bit of tubing sticking out the end of the eyeglass nosepiece) and oxygen through a tiny tracheostomy (a small hole placed surgically in the neck; this way, the tubing can go under the clothes, and the tracheostomy itself can be hidden under a turtleneck or scarf). Other methods include oxygen tents, which surround the whole upper body; oxygen hoods, which surround the whole head; and single nasal tubes (with one thin tube going into the nostril). Most of these last methods are useful mainly for babies, and therefore are not used very much in CF, since babies with CF usually don't need extra oxygen.

Amount needed: Your doctor may want to do a "blood gas" or check a "pulseox" to see how much oxygen you have in your blood before he or she decides whether you need extra oxygen. The blood gas test involves taking blood from a finger stick, a vein, or an artery (usually the radial artery, at the wrist) and is therefore somewhat more painful than most blood tests, which are usually taken from a vein (closer to the skin surface than arteries). However, if some lidocaine or other local anesthetic—like EMLA cream—is used, this is not a painful test, and it can be very important. The pulseox is a less painful (and slightly less informative) test you've probably had done when you've done pulmonary function tests (PFTs). This shines light through the finger and the computer calculates your blood oxygen level. To understand how much extra oxygen is needed, you have to understand how the brain directs breathing. This is discussed in Chapter 3.

Undesirable effects: The main danger of oxygen is giving so much that it turns off the signal to breathe. As we have discussed Chapter 15, this is very unlikely. Oxygen is also very dry, even when it's been humidified (as it should always be before it's breathed), and can make the mouth and nose uncomfortably dry. Too much oxygen can be toxic to lung tissue (this is not a problem with less than 40% oxygen). The problem you might have heard of concerning eye damage from oxygen is true only in premature babies.

Addiction: Some people worry that once they start on oxygen they'll become addicted in the way that someone gets addicted to morphine or heroin. This does not happen. People whose lungs are bad enough that they need extra oxygen feel much better when they take that oxygen, and they won't want to stop taking it while their lungs are still in that condition. But if the lung disease improves, and extra oxygen is not needed any more, people don't continue to desire the extra oxygen because the body is now supplying it. If the lungs cannot improve, the person will continue to want to use the oxygen, but this is not an addiction.

Other worries about oxygen: Some people worry that needing oxygen is a bad sign— "the beginning of the end," or some such outlook. It certainly does indicate that someone's lungs are in worse shape, but many people need oxygen for a few days or weeks, and then are able to get back to doing well without extra oxygen.

Cough Medicines

There are two main kinds of medicines that usually are referred to as "cough medicines." One of these is the *expectorants*. Expectorants are intended to make it easier to bring up mucus from the lungs. This is a good idea; but unfortunately, these drugs don't work. The other kind of cough medicine is the *cough suppressant*; that is, a drug that controls the cough center in the brain and says, "don't cough, no matter what is in the lungs that needs to come up." This is usually a terrible idea, especially for someone with CF. Some drug preparations are available that combine these two types of cough medicine, which have opposite goals! In most cases, including most patients with CF, cough is an important defense mechanism that keeps the lungs clear of substances that shouldn't be there. Cough is a sign that something is wrong, but efforts should be directed at what is wrong. If a person is coughing because of bronchospasm, a bronchodilator will relieve the bronchospasm and thus stop the cough; in a sense, it is a good kind of cough medicine. Similarly, if someone with CF is coughing because infection in the bronchi has gotten out of control, antibiotics are probably needed; they may control the infection and thus stop the cough. Other kinds of cough medicines are rarely useful.

Upper Airway

Polyp Medicines

Many people with CF have nasal polyps, which are growths of extra tissue (not cancer) in the nose. Usually these cause no problems except mild stuffiness, but they can get large enough to be seen at the end of the nose or block one side of the nose so you can't breathe through it. A few medicines have been used to shrink polyps, and some people believe that they work. These medicines include antihistamines, decongestants (like Neo-Synephrine®), and steroid sprays (like Flonase®, Rhinocort®, Nasacort®, and Nasonex®). A person with nasal allergy symptoms may also be helped by some of these same nasal sprays.

Sinus Medicines

On radiologic (x-ray) examination, most patients with CF appear to have abnormal sinuses. Usually this bothers the radiologist more than it bothers the patient. Sometimes the patient may have symptoms from inflammation in the sinuses, in which case the nasal steroids mentioned above under *Polyp Medicines* can help. Occasionally, there can be actual sinus infection (sinusitis), which may be a nuisance to the patient. In these cases, doctors may prescribe antibiotics and/or a decongestant.

Allergy Medicines

Allergies can cause problems with the upper respiratory system (stuffy, sneezy nose) or lungs (congestion, wheezing) or both. Patients with CF are somewhat more likely to have allergies than are people without CF. It is often very difficult to tell if an upper or lower airway problem is caused by infection or by allergy. Complicating the matter is that either one can probably make the other worse, so that constriction of the bronchi from a pollen allergy will make it harder to clear mucus from the bronchi and make it easier for infection to get out of control.

Antihistamines

Histamine is a chemical that is released from white blood cells in response to different problems including irritation and allergy. Its release can cause many of the problems we associate with allergies: runny nose, itchy nose, constricted bronchi, hives. Antihistamines (such as loratidine, cetirizine, and diphenhydramine) do not stop the release of histamine from the blood cells, but they do help to block its action in the nose, skin, and so forth.

How they are taken: These are most commonly taken by mouth but can be given by injection.

Undesirable effects: The most common and often the most troublesome side effect from these drugs is drowsiness. They can also cause a dry mouth. At least one antihistamine, cyproheptadine (Periactin®), can cause an increased appetite. This can be good in some people with CF.

Decongestants

These drugs are supposed to make the nose less stuffy. Although they are used by millions of people, there is not very much scientific evidence that they work. Some decongestant nasal sprays can temporarily open blocked nostrils. If they are used for more than a few days, they can cause "rebound" inflammation and blockage of the nose that is just as bad as the inflammation the cold caused.

Allergy Shots

This is a very controversial topic. Most pulmonary specialists believe that allergy shots may be helpful for nasal allergies but not for bronchial allergies (asthma), while many allergists believe that they sometimes can be helpful for asthma too. There is nothing about CF that makes a person more or less likely to respond well to allergy shots than anyone else.

THE HEART

The heart is not directly affected by CF, and most people with CF have very good hearts. Therefore, there usually is no need for heart medications. However, if someone's lungs become badly diseased (from CF or any other cause), the heart may not be able to pump all the necessary fluid through the diseased lungs. When this happens, two types of medicines are sometimes used: diuretics and digitalis.

Diuretics

These drugs help the kidneys get rid of extra fluid that may have built up in the body because of the heart's inability to pump all of the fluid. Most doctors agree that when someone has heart failure because of severe lung disease, it is very important to cut down on the amount of fluid that the heart is asked to pump. This is accomplished through restricting the amount of salt and fluid consumed and through careful use of diuretic medicines.

Furosemide

How it is taken: Furosemide (Lasix®) can be taken by mouth (tablet, liquid) or by injection (either IM or IV).

Undesirable effects: Furosemide causes the body to lose potassium in addition to other salts, and this can upset the body's salt balance if used in high doses every day for too long. This effect can be lessened by an every-other-day schedule in people who tolerate this schedule. The drug can also do too much of a good thing—in eliminating too much excess fluid, it may actually dehydrate the patient. Furosemide has been associated with some cases of hearing problems, which are usually reversible. Occasionally, someone who is allergic to sulfa drugs may be allergic to furosemide also.

Spironolactone (Aldactone®)

This drug is less powerful than furosemide but keeps the body from losing potassium.

How it is taken: Oral tablets.

Undesirable effects: Any diuretic may cause excess loss of water (dehydration) and salt balance problems. Spironolactone may also give some gastrointestinal (GI) upset. A rash is sometimes seen. It may cause breast enlargement and/or impotence in men. These effects are nearly always temporary and disappear when the drug is stopped.

Thiazides

How they are taken: These diuretics are usually taken by mouth (tablet; although a liquid preparation is also available). Rarely, they may be given by IV but not by IM injection.

Undesirable effects: These are quite safe and usually there are no problems. Textbooks do list many possible reactions, including GI upset, dizziness, fatigue, headache, anemia, weakness, muscle spasms, and gout.

Digitalis

This drug has been known for centuries and is very effective in making the heart contractions stronger. It is not clear whether it is helpful in people whose heart problems are mainly caused by lung problems.

How it is taken: Digitalis preparations can be taken by mouth (tablets or liquids) or by IV injection.

Undesirable effects: Too much digitalis can be very dangerous and can cause heart beat irregularities, confusion, visual problems, vomiting, diarrhea, headache, and weakness.

Sildenafil

Sometimes when the lungs are really sick, it is harder for the heart to pump blood through the lungs (pulmonary hypertension). In this case, sildenafil (known more popularly as Viagra®) can be used to relax the muscles that surround the blood vessels in the lungs and take some pressure off the heart. It can also help improve oxygen levels.

How it is taken: Sildenafil is taken by mouth.

Undesirable side effects: Fast heart rate, low blood pressure, flushing, and the erection thing (remember why Viagra® was first developed).

GASTROINTESTINAL AND DIGESTIVE SYSTEM MEDICATIONS

The main problem in the GI and digestive system is the thick mucus that blocks the ducts of the pancreas and prevents the digestive chemicals (enzymes) from reaching the intestines where they mix with the food that has been eaten. If these digestive enzymes are not available, the food cannot be digested, that is, broken down into particles small enough to be soaked up into the bloodstream through the wall of the intestine. As a result, a lot of the food (especially the fat) will not be available to the body and will pass out into the stools. Most (but not all) patients with CF have this problem. Another GI problem is that the intestines' own mucus is very thick, which can sometimes lead to blockage of the intestines.

Digestive Enzymes

These enzymes come from the pancreas of animals. They have changed what used to be a serious, even fatal, problem into a nuisance problem. With enzyme type and dosage properly adjusted, most patients with CF are able to absorb most of what they eat (even the fat). Thus, they are able to get the nutritional value from the food that would be lost without the enzymes. Enzymes are discussed fully in Chapter 6.

Antacid Drugs

Excess stomach acid can cause several different types of problems in anyone and at least one additional problem if someone has CF. Too much acid interferes with the activity of digestive enzyme medicines. The way this happens is that stomach acid may spill over into the small intestine, preventing the coating around each enzyme bead from dissolving where and when it's supposed to, in the duodenum (small intestine).

Too much acid can also cause ulcers. Occasionally, the stomach acid can reflux (go backward) up into the esophagus, causing heartburn (the burning discomfort felt when the esophagus becomes irritated from acid). Drugs that prevent the stomach from making too much acid, or drugs that neutralize the acid once it is made, may be helpful for any of these problems. There are two main kinds of drugs that prevent the stomach from making too much acid: histamine-2 (H_2) *blockers* and *proton pump inhibitors* (PPIs).

Histamine-2 Blockers

In addition to playing an important (and nasty) role in allergic reactions, histamine also plays a role (sometimes nasty) in the production of stomach acid. One class of medications, the H_2 *blockers*, can help prevent this part of what histamine does.

Cimetidine

Cimetidine (Tagamet®) is very effective in decreasing the production of stomach acid.

How it is taken: Cimetidine is almost always taken by mouth, in a tablet or liquid form, usually before meals and before bed.
Undesirable effects: This is a very safe drug. Mild diarrhea, headache, or swelling of breasts have been seen in people taking cimetidine, but none of these problems is common.

Ranitidine

Ranitidine (Zantac®) is a close relative of cimetidine and is widely used for its antiacid properties. It can be taken at a lower dosage, less frequently, with comparable effects to cimetidine.

Nizatidine

Nizatidine (Axid®) is very similar to ranitidine in dosing and side-effect profile. Perhaps the advantage that nizatidine has over ranitidine is that the liquid form of nizatidine tastes better to most people than the liquid form of ranitidine.

Famotidine

Famotidine (Pepcid®) is yet another H_2 blocker antacid.

How it is taken: Famotidine is also taken by mouth.
Undesirable effects: This is also a safe drug, with side effects similar to the others
in its class.

Proton Pump Inhibitors

An important step in acid production depends on a pump in the cell membrane
of acid-secreting cells. Drugs that slow down or stop this pump are called PPIs
and are among the most potent acid blockers known. PPIs include *omeprazole*
(Prilosec®), *lansoprazole* (Prevacid®), pantoprazole (Protonix®), and *esomeprazole*
(Nexium®).

How they are taken: These drugs are taken by mouth.
Undesirable effects: These are safe drugs: mild diarrhea and headache occur in some
people taking them.

Various Antacids

These medicines, taken by mouth as chewable tablets or as the more effective liquid
form, do not influence how much acid is produced by the stomach, but they can
neutralize the acid once it's formed. They include Maalox®, Mylanta®, and
Tums®.

Antireflux Drugs

Several drugs may be helpful for patients with gastroesophageal reflux. Antacid
treatment is usually used, and even if it doesn't decrease the amount of fluid that
refluxes from the stomach into the esophagus, the fluid that does reach the
esophagus will be less acidic, and therefore probably less damaging. A few drugs
may actually decrease the amount of fluid that refluxes.

Metoclopramide (Reglan®)

This drug may help reduce gastroesophageal reflux by two of its effects: It strengthens the grip of the muscle at the bottom of the esophagus, and it increases the
speed with which the esophagus and stomach empty, leaving less matter there to
back up into the esophagus.

How it is taken: Metoclopramide is taken by mouth
Undesirable effects: This drug can cause diarrhea. Its most worrisome side effect is
that it can cause abnormal movement of the face and tongue. If the medicine
is not stopped when this symptom appears, the abnormal movements can
become permanent.

Erythromycin

Erythromycin, one of the macrolide antibiotics, increases the motility of the stomach, helping it to empty more quickly. An empty stomach has less fluid available to reflux.

How it is taken: Erythromycin is taken by mouth.
Undesirable effects: Too much erythromycin can cause abdominal cramping.

Anticonstipation Medicines

Constipation is seldom a problem in patients with CF, but it does occur occasionally. Failure to pass any stool can be an important sign of a dangerous intestinal obstruction called meconium ileus in a newborn infant and DIOS (distal intestinal obstruction syndrome) in a person older.

Enzymes

Before more drastic measures are undertaken, it usually helps to make sure the digestive enzyme dosage is appropriate, since very bulky, poorly digested stools may make blockage more likely.

Dietary Fiber

Someone who has difficulty passing bowel movements may benefit from increasing the amount of fiber in the diet. Foods high in fiber include fruits and some vegetables: bran is an especially good source of fiber. Breakfast cereals with bran should have at least 4 grams (g) of dietary fiber per serving to be effective (this information is included on the side panel of the cereal box; if the information isn't there, it's likely that there is very little fiber in the cereal).

Miscellaneous

1. Miralax® (polyethylene glycol): A powder that can be mixed with any liquid and then drunk. It works very well to "flush out" the intestines.
2. Lactulose (Cefulac®, Chronulac®): Medicines taken by mouth that pull fluid into the intestines to help make the bowel contents more watery and easier to move.
3. GoLYTELY®: A salty liquid that can be drunk in large quantities to "flush out" the intestines.
4. Colace: A stool softener.

Mineral Oil

On some occasions, a physician may prescribe oral mineral oil to help pass stools.

Bowel Stimulants

If someone is not completely blocked up, some medications that stimulate intestinal contractions may help the bowels to empty. Senna (Senekot) is one such laxative.

Enemas

With more blockage, enemas may be needed to help wash out the lower intestines. Generally, several types of enemas can be used in different situations. Always check with your doctor to be sure it's safe to use an enema and to find out which kind.

Gastrografin® Enemas

Severe intestinal obstruction is a serious matter that used to be treatable only with surgery. Fortunately, many cases can be treated in the hospital with special enemas. Gastrografin (and several similar products) is a substance that can be used for an enema and has several useful properties. It shows up on radiographs, so the radiologist can see the outline of the bowel to make sure there is not another problem causing intestinal blockage and to ensure the enema is going far enough up into the intestines so that it works. It's very slippery, allowing it to slip by the blockage. It also acts like a sponge, pulling in lots of fluid from the rest of the body to help make the stools stuck in the bowel become more watery and easier to move out.

How they are performed: These enemas always must be done where there is x-ray equipment and a radiologist. This usually means they are done in the hospital. Most children who need them are sick enough to need to be in the hospital anyway.

Undesirable effects: These enemas are somewhat uncomfortable, as is true of any enema, but they can provide prompt relief from the abdominal pain from intestinal blockage. The main danger of this procedure is that so much fluid is pulled into the bowel from the rest of the body that the patient can become dehydrated. For this reason, most doctors will not perform this procedure on an infant unless the baby has an IV line in place, with fluids running in.

Antibloating Medications

Some patients with CF have trouble with abdominal bloating. This may be caused by the thick mucus in the intestines, which can surround little air bubbles and prevents the little bubbles from getting together to make a single bubble that is big enough for a burp. Some drugs containing simethicone (Mylicon®, Silain®) may help dissolve some of that mucus and allow a gentle upward or downward explosion of that air, relieving the pressure and discomfort. These drugs are taken by mouth (tablets or drops) and are very safe.

Liver Medications

Ursodiol (Actigal®), also referred to as ursodeoxycholic acid, is a bile acid that seems to help liquefy the secretions that otherwise block the smallest ducts within the liver and gallbladder. It is taken by mouth and is very safe. Usually, patients with CF liver disease may need to take more vitamins than usual.

Vitamins

These are not really drugs and should be a regular part of the diet. Four vitamins (A, D, E, K) are "fat-soluble," meaning that they dissolve in fat and are absorbed in the body only when fats are absorbed. Thus, patients who have trouble absorbing fats may have low levels of these vitamins. For this reason, most nutrition experts agree that patients with CF should probably receive supplements of these vitamins, at least some of the time. Your physician may periodically check your blood levels of the various vitamins. Some people feel quite well and yet are deficient in several vitamins. For the vitamin E, most preparations you can buy will not work for someone who has trouble absorbing fats, and a form that is partly dissolvable in water needs to be used.

Growth and Appetite Stimulants and Supplements

Hormones

Most of the drugs used to stimulate appetite and growth are anabolic steroids and androgens (male hormones). They are used with increasing frequency but have not been conclusively shown to be safe or effective in patients with CF. These medications include *growth hormone, testosterone,* and *megestrol (Megace®),* actually a female hormone.

How they are taken: These hormones can be given by injection (mostly) or taken by mouth (some).
Undesirable effects: Although the experience with growth hormone and megestrol seems much more benign than the other hormones (mostly the male hormones), it is too early to say with certainty that they are safe and effective. The complications of the male hormones are too numerous to list completely, are worrisome, and can actually result in stopping growth sooner than it would have stopped naturally (as these hormones increase bone growth, they also close the growth plate of the bones—the part of the bones where growth takes place—more quickly than normal). Other undesirable effects include fluid retention, hirsutism (increased hairiness), baldness, various genital disturbances (too big, too little, too excitable, not excitable enough), acne, sleeplessness, liver disease, nausea, ulcer-like symptoms, and finally, disqualification from the Olympics.

If appetite stimulation is all that is needed, your doctor may recommend non-hormonal stimulants. Previously mentioned in the section on *Antihistamines*, cyproheptadine (Periactin®) is an antihistamine that has the potentially beneficial side effect of making you hungry. There are also preparations of appetite stimulants derived from cannabinoids (marijuana) that can be medically prescribed. Dronabinol (Marinol®) is dosed by mouth. Low doses of this medication can have the desired effect of making someone hungry. In larger doses, the side effects can be very similar to the effects of marijuana (confusion, abnormal thinking, paranoia, etc).

Diet Supplements

Many different kinds of diet supplements are available, from vanilla milk shakes and ice cream sundaes to expensive "elemental" (predigested) formulas. These are discussed in Chapter 6. These supplements usually have high calorie contents. They seem to be helpful in some people, whereas in others, the number of calories taken in with the supplements is balanced by the number of calories not eaten in the regular meals. High-calorie recipes (of regular food) can be found in Appendix D of this book. Some CF programs have been successful in helping patients gain weight and height by running nighttime feedings of these dietary supplements through a stomach tube while the patients sleep. Such a program, of course, should never be undertaken without your doctor's knowledge and cooperation.

How they are taken: Some can be sprinkled on top of regular meals, and some can be eaten between meals. Others are designed to be given through a tube (mostly because they taste so bad, but also because they can be given very slowly while the patient sleeps).

Undesirable effects: The supplements may interfere with normal mealtime appetite. The tube feedings require a tube, which can be somewhat uncomfortable and/or inconvenient. Any one of several different kinds of tubes can be used, including a nasogastric tube, which goes through the nose ("naso-") into the stomach ("gastric") and is usually put in each evening and removed in the morning. Another kind of tube is a permanent tube placed by a surgical operation that makes a hole or *stoma* in the wall of the abdomen directly into the stomach (a *gastrostomy* tube) or into the second part of the small intestine, the jejunum (a feeding *jejunostomy* tube). Possible problems from these nighttime feedings include overfilling the stomach.

TRANSPLANT-RELATED DRUGS

Anti-Rejection Drugs

Steroids

(See "*Anti-inflammatory Medications*," page 335, for more on steroids.) Steroids decrease inflammation, and they are important tools in preventing and fighting acute rejection (see Chapter 8).

Antilymphocyte Drugs

Lymphocytes are the white blood cells most responsible for rejection, so specific antilymphocyte drugs have been sought: If you decrease the rejection caused by the lymphocytes without interfering with other white blood cells trying to fight infection, that would be ideal.

Cyclosporine

This is the first very successful antilymphocyte drug used to help treat and prevent rejection.

How it is taken: This drug can be taken intravenously or by mouth. There is currently a formulation that is inhaled, but not readily available since it is still being investigated to see whether it is safe and effective in preventing and/or treating lung transplant rejection.

Undesirable effects: This drug can cause high blood pressure, kidney damage, seizures, shakiness, hairiness, and excessive growth of the gums. Too much may lead to infection.

Tacrolimus (FK-506)

This drug is similar to cyclosporine, but may be a bit more effective.

How it is taken: This drug can be taken intravenously or by mouth.

Undesirable effects: This drug can cause high blood pressure, kidney damage, seizures, shakiness, hairiness, and headache. Too much may lead to infection.

Sirolimus/Everolimus

These drugs are similar to tacrolimus, but are available only in oral form.

Antithymocyte Globulin

Antithymocyte globulin (ATG) is an antibody made by horses and directed against human lymphocytes.

How it is taken: This drug is given intravenously.

Undesirable effects: The drug can cause fever and "flu"-like symptoms, including headache.

OKT3

This is a "bioengineered" antilymphocyte drug.

How it is taken: This drug is given intravenously.

Undesirable effects: The drug can cause fever and "flu-like" symptoms, including headache.

"Antimetabolites"

These drugs interfere with the body's ability to make white blood cells, so there are fewer cells around to reject an organ. (Of course, that also means there are fewer white blood cells to fight infection.)

Azathioprine (Imuran®)

How it is taken: This drug can be given intravenously or by mouth.
Undesirable effects: The main side effect is too much of its desired effect, that is, the white blood cell count getting too low and therefore the body not being able to fight off infection. The platelet count may also go too low, and—since platelets are needed for proper clotting of blood—there can be abnormal bleeding.

Mycophenolate Mofetil (CellCept®)

This drug interferes with DNA production. It is taken orally and has the same undesirable effects as azothioprine. It can also be pretty irritating to the stomach and intestines causing nausea, vomiting, diarrhea, and constipation.

GLOSSARY OF DRUGS

This glossary is a partial list of drugs that can be found under both their generic and trade names. Drugs that are discussed in this appendix contain references to the appropriate section. For example, Pen-Vee K is a form of the antibiotic penicillin, which is discussed under *Lungs: Antibiotics: Penicillins.*

Accolate® (zafirlukast)   A leukotriene-inhibitor anti-inflammatory drug.
Acetylcysteine   A mucolytic (see page 327).
Actigal® (ursodeoxycholic acid)   A bile salt used to treat CF liver disease (see page 348).
acyclovir   An antiviral drug.
ABDEK®   A multivitamin that includes vitamins A, D, E, and K.
ADEK®   A multivitamin that includes vitamins A, D, E, and K.
Adrenalin (epinephrine)   A bronchodilator (see page 328).
Advair®   An inhaled combination of fluticasone (a steroid) and salmeterol, a long-acting bronchodilator) (see page 336)
Advil® (ibuprofen)   An NSAID (see page 337)
Aerobid®   An inhaled steroid (see page 336).
Afinitor® (everolimus)   An anti-rejection drug (see page 350)
Afrin® (oxymetazoline hydrochloride)   A decongestant (see page 341).
albuterol   A beta-agonist bronchodilator (see page 328).
Aldactone® (spironolactone)   A diuretic (see page 342).
Alupent®   A beta-agonist bronchodilator (see page 328).

amantadine   A medication that can help control infection with the influenza virus.

Amcill® (ampicillin)   An antibiotic (see page 330).

amikacin sulfate   An aminoglycoside antibiotic (see page 332).

Amikin®   Amikacin sulfate, an aminoglycoside (see page 332).

aminophylline   A theophylline bronchodilator (see page 328).

amoxicillin   An antibiotic (see page 330).

Amoxil®   Amoxicillin (see page 330).

Amphojel® (aluminum hydroxide gel)   An antacid.

amphotericin   A drug used to fight infection caused by fungi.

ampicillin   An antibiotic (see page 330).

Ancef® (cefazolin sodium)   A cephalosporin antibiotic (see page 331).

Aquamephyton®   A vitamin K preparation (see page 348).

Aquasol A®   A vitamin A preparation (see page 348).

Aquasol E®   A vitamin E preparation (see page 348).

Asbron®   A theophylline bronchodilator (see page 328).

Atgam®   An ATG for fighting organ rejection.

Atrovent® (ipratropium bromide)   A kind of bronchodilator.

Augmentin® (amoxicillin/clavulanate potassium)   An antibiotic (see page 330).

Avazyme® (chymotrypsin)   A digestive enzyme, useful only for digesting protein, and not fat (see page 350).

Axid® (nizatidine)   An antacid (see page 344).

Azactam®   (see aztreonam below).

Azathioprine   An anti-rejection drug (see page 351)

azlocillin   An anti-*Pseudomonas* antibiotic (see page 330).

Azmacort (triamcinolone acetonide)   An inhaled corticosteroid.

aztreonam   An anti-*Pseudomonas* antibiotic (see page 334).

bacampicillin HCl   An ampicillin (see page 330).

Bactrim® (trimethoprim–sulfamethoxazole)   A combination antibiotic (see page 331).

Bactrim DS®   Double-strength Bactrim (see Bactrim).

Basaljel® (aluminum carbonate gel)   An antacid (see page 344).

beclomethasone dipropionate   An inhaled corticosteroid.

Beclovent® (beclomethasone dipropionate)   A corticosteroid (see page 336).

Beconase® (beclomethasone dipropionate)   A nasal steroid spray often used for polyps or nasal allergies (see page 340).

Beepen-VK® (penicillin)   An antibiotic (see page 330).

Benadryl® (diphenhydramine hydrochloride)   An antihistamine (see page 341).

Betapen-VK® (penicillin V potassium)   An antibiotic (see page 330).

Biaxin® (clarithromycin)   A macrolide antibiotic (see page 332).

Bicillin® (penicillin G benzathine)   An injectable (IM) penicillin (see page 330).

Bilezyme® A digestive enzyme combination containing protein-digesting enzymes but no fat-digesting enzymes. Also contains bile salts (see page 343).

bisacodyl A laxative (see page 346).

Boost® A nutritional supplement formula (see page 349).

bran A very rich source of dietary fiber. Taken in pure form, it tastes like rabbit food, but is very effective in helping to prevent constipation (see page 346).

Brethine® (terbutaline sulfate) A beta-agonist bronchodilator (see page 328).

Bricanyl® (terbutaline sulfate) A beta-agonist bronchodilator (see page 328).

budesonide An inhaled steroid.

carbenicillin An anti-*Pseudomonas* antibiotic (see page 330).

Cayston® (inhaled aztreonam) An anti-*Pseudomonas* antibiotic (see page 334).

Ceclor® (cefaclor) A cephalosporin antibiotic (see page 331).

cefaclor A cephalosporin antibiotic (see page 331).

cefadroxil A cephalosporin antibiotic (see page 331).

Cefadyl® (cephapirin sodium) A cephalosporin antibiotic (see page 331).

cefamandole A cephalosporin antibiotic (see page 331).

cefazolin A cephalosporin antibiotic (see page 331).

Cefdinir® A cephalosporin antibiotic (see page 331).

Cefepime® A cephalosporin (see page 331).

Cefobid® A cephalosporin antibiotic with some effect against *Pseudomonas* (see page 331).

cefoperozone A cephalosporin antibiotic with some effect against *Pseudomonas* (see page 331).

cefotaxime A cephalosporin antibiotic (see page 331).

cefoxitin An analog derivative of a cephalosporin antibiotic (see page 331).

cefprozil A cephalosporin antibiotic (see page 331).

ceftazidime An anti-*Pseudomonas* cephalosporin (see page 331).

Ceftin® Cefuroxime.

Cefulac® (lactulose) An anticonstipation medication (see page 346).

cefuroxime A cephalosporin antibiotic (see page 331).

Cefzil® Cefprozil.

Celbenin® (sodium methicillin) An anti-*Staphylococcus* antibiotic (see page 330).

CellCept® (mycophenolate) An anti-rejection drug (see page 351).

Cenalax® An anticonstipation drug (see page 346).

cephalexin A cephalosporin antibiotic (see page 331).

cephaloglycin A cephalosporin antibiotic (see page 331).

cephaloridine A cephalosporin antibiotic (see page 331).

cephalosporins A family of antibiotics (see page 331).

cephalothin A cephalosporin antibiotic (see page 331).

cephapirin A cephalosporin antibiotic (see page 331).

cephradine A cephalosporin antibiotic (see page 331).

chloramphenicol An antibiotic.

Chloromycetin® **(chloramphenicol)**   An antibiotic.

cimetidine   An antacid preparation (see page 344).

Cipro® **(ciprofloxacin)**   A quinolone antibiotic (see page 333).

ciprofloxacin   A quinolone antibiotic (see page 333).

Claforan®   A cephalosporin antibiotic (see page 331).

clarithromycin   A macrolide antibiotic (see page 332).

Cleocin® **(clindamycin)**   An antibiotic.

clindamycin   An antibiotic.

clotrimazole   An antiyeast medication, used for vaginal yeast infections.

cloxacillin   An anti-*Staphylococcus* penicillin (see page 330).

Cloxapen® **(cloxacillin)**   A penicillin.

cod liver oil   A traditional source of vitamins A and D whose main advantage is its bad taste (see page 348).

codeine   A cough suppressant (see page 339).

coffee   A caffeine-containing popular drink. Caffeine is also found in Coca-Cola, Pepsi and in some cases serves as a bronchodilator (see page 328).

Colace® **(docusate sodium)**   A stool softener (see page 346).

colistin   A very potent antibiotic. Usually given inhaled. Given intravenously, it can have severe side effects including headaches and kidney damage.

Coly-Mycin S® **(colistin sulfate)**   An antibiotic.

Cotazym® **(pancrelipase)**   A pancreatic digestive enzyme (see page 343).

Cotazym-B®   A digestive enzyme with bile salts (see page 343).

Cotazym-S®   An enteric-coated pancreatic enzyme (see page 343).

co-trimoxazole   A combination antibiotic (trimethoprim–sulfamethoxazole).

Creon® **(pancreatin)**   An enteric-coated pancreatic enzyme (see page 343).

Criticare®   A nutritional supplement and formula that is very low in fat and includes protein that is predigested.

cromolyn   An inhaled medicine used to prevent bronchospasm.

Cyclosporine®   An anti-rejection drug (see page 350).

Cyproheptadine® **(Periactin®)**   An antihistamine, often used as an appetite stimulant (see page 349).

Decadron® **(dexamethasone)**   A steroid (see page 335).

Declomycin® **(demeclocycline)**   A tetracycline antibiotic (see page 332).

Delatestryl® **(testosterone enanthate)**   A male hormone sometimes used to stimulate growth and appetite (see page 348).

Deltasone® **(prednisone)**   A steroid sometimes used to decrease bronchial inflammation (see page 335).

demeclocycline   A tetracycline antibiotic (see page 332).

Demerol® **[meperidine (pethidine) hydrochloride]**   A narcotic painkiller and sedative.

Depo-Testosterone®   A male hormone (testosterone) in injectable form sometimes used as a growth and appetite stimulant (see page 348).

dexamethasone   A steroid that is sometimes taken by aerosol inhalation (see page 335).

dextromethorphan (DM)   A cough suppressant (see page 339).

Dianabol® (methandrostenolone)   An anabolic and male sex hormone sometimes used as a growth and appetite stimulant (see page 348).

dicloxacillin sodium   An anti-*Staphylococcus* penicillin (see page 330).

digitalis   A drug that strengthens heart contractions (see page 343).

digitoxin   A digitalis drug (see page 343).

digoxin   A digitalis drug (see page 343).

Dilaudid® (hydromorphone hydrochloride)   A narcotic that is occasionally used for pain and for cough suppression.

Dimetane® (brompheniramine maleate)   A combination cough medicine, antihistamine, and decongestant (see page 339).

Dimetapp®   Similar to Dimetane.

diphenhydramine hydrochloride   An antihistamine (see page 341).

disodium cromoglycate   Cromolyn; used in treatment of bronchial asthma.

diuretics   Medications that increase the kidneys' production of urine and thus help rid the body of excess fluid (see page 342).

DNase   A mucolytic (see page 326).

Dorcol® (guaifenesin + phenylpropanolamine hydrochloride + dextromethorphan hydrobromide)   A cough medicine that includes a decongestant and a cough suppressant (see page 339).

doxycycline   A tetracycline antibiotic (see page 332).

Dristan®   A decongestant (see page 339).

Dronabinol®   An appetite stimulant (see page 349).

Dynapen® (dicloxacillin)   An anti-*Staphylococcus* antibiotic (see page 330).

dyphylline   A form of theophylline bronchodilator (see page 328).

E-Mycin®   A macrolide antibiotic (see page 332).

EES® (erythromycin ethylsuccinate)   A macrolide antibiotic (see page 332).

Elixicon® (theophylline)   A theophylline bronchodilator (see page 328).

Elixophyllin®   A form of theophylline bronchodilator (see page 328).

EMLA® cream   A local anesthetic that can be put on the skin to numb a site for IV needle placement.

Ensure®   A calorie supplement (see page 349).

Entolase®   An enteric-coated digestive enzyme (see page 343).

Entolase-HP   An enteric-coated digestive enzyme (see page 343).

enzymes   Catalysts of chemical reactions (see page 343).

ephedrine   Sometimes used as a bronchodilator (see page 328).

epinephrine (adrenalin)   Often used as an emergency bronchodilator, similar in some of its action to the "beta-agonists" (see page 328) but with more effect on the heart (speeds it up).

Erythrocin®   A macrolide antibiotic (see page 332).

erythromycin   The original member of the macrolide family of antibiotics (see page 332).

ethacrynic acid   A diuretic (see page 342).

everolimus   An anti-rejection drug (see page 350).

fiber   An important component of the diet (see page 316).

FK506 (tacrolimus)   An anti-rejection drug (see page 350).

Fleet® enemas   Occasionally used for treating constipation (see page 347).

Flonase® (nasal fluticasone)   A nasal corticosteroid (see page 340).

Flovent® (fluticasone)   An inhaled steroid.

fluticasone   An inhaled or nasal steroid.

formoterol   A long-acting bronchodilator.

Fortaz® (ceftazidime)   A cephalosporin antibiotic (see page 331).

furosemide   A diuretic (see page 342).

ganciclovir   An antiviral agent.

Gantrisin® (sulfisoxazole)   A sulfa antibiotic (see page 331).

Garamycin® (gentamicin)   An aminoglycoside antibiotic (see page 332).

Gastrografin® (meglumine diatrizoate)   A substance that is occasionally used in the hospital for an enema (see page 347).

Gaviscon® (aluminum hydroxide + magnesium carbonate)   An antacid (see page 345).

Gelusil® (aluminum hydroxide + magnesium hydroxide + simethicone)   An antacid (see page 345).

gentamicin   An aminoglycoside antibiotic (see page 332).

GoLYTELY®   A salty liquid that can be drunk in large quantities to "flush out" the intestines (see page 346).

guaifenesin   An expectorant (see page 339, "*Cough Medicines*").

Halotestin® (fluoxymesterone)   A male sex hormone sometimes used for growth and appetite stimulation (see page 348).

heparin   An anticoagulant; that is, a drug that prevents clotting of the blood. This is very useful when used in very small amounts in a needle in a vein. It can keep the blood from clotting up the needle so that the needle can be used for a long time for administration of IV antibiotics.

heparin lock   A needle that is inserted in the vein and periodically rinsed out with heparin solution. This enables the needle to be used for administration of IV antibiotics on an intermittent basis. Once rinsed out, the needle can be plugged up and just taped to the arm without any extra tubing connected to it, leaving the arm free.

Hep-Lock®   The dilute heparin solution used in a heparin lock.

Hexadrol® (dexamethasone)   A steroid sometimes used to decrease bronchial inflammation (see page 335).

Hycodan® (hydrocodone bitartrate)   A combination cough medicine that contains a cough suppressant (see page 339).

Hycotuss® (hydrocodone bitartrate + guaifenesin)   A multi-ingredient cough medicine that includes a cough suppressant (see page 339).

hydrocodone bitartrate   A narcotic sometimes used as a cough suppressant (see page 339).

hydrocortisone   A steroid occasionally used in different forms to decrease bronchial inflammation (see page 335).

Hypersal® (inhaled hypertonic saline)   A mucus clearance agent (see page 327).
ibuprofen   An NSAID (see page 337).
Ilozyme® (pancrelipase)   A pancreatic enzyme (see page 343).
imipenem   An anti-*Pseudomonas* antibiotic (see page 334).
Imuran® (azathioprine)   An anti-rejection drug (see page 351).
Intal®   Cromolyn sodium.
Ipecac®   A medicine used to induce vomiting (used usually after a child has accidentally ingested a poisonous substance).
isoetharine   A bronchodilator drug taken by inhalation (see page 328).
isoproterenol   An inhaled bronchodilator (see page 328).
Isuprel® (isoproterenol)   A bronchodilator taken by inhalation (see page 328).
itraconazole   An antifungal drug.
kanamycin   An aminoglycoside antibiotic (see page 332).
Kantrex® (kanamycin)   An antibiotic (see page 332).
Keflex® (cephalexin)   A cephalosporin antibiotic (see page 331).
Keflin® (cephalothin sodium)   A cephalosporin antibiotic (see page 331).
Kefzol® (cefazolin sodium)   A cephalosporin antibiotic (see page 331).
lactulose   An anticonstipation medication (see page 346).
Lanophyllin®   A form of theophylline bronchodilator (see page 328).
Lanoxin® (digoxin)   A type of digitalis (see page 343).
lansoprazole   A PPI acid suppressor (see page 345).
Larotid® (amoxicillin)   An antibiotic (see page 330).
Lasix® (furosemide)   A diuretic (see page 342).
Ledercillin® (penicillin G procaine)   A form of penicillin (see page 329).
Lincocin® (lincomycin hydrochloride)   An antibiotic.
lincomycin   An antibiotic not commonly used in CF.
Lufyllin® (dyphylline)   A theophylline bronchodilator (see page 328).
Maalox®   An antacid (see page 344).
Marax® (ephedrine sulfate + theophylline + hydroxyzine hydrochloride)   A combination drug including a theophylline bronchodilator (see page 318) and another bronchodilator.
Marinol® (dronabinol)   An appetite stimulant (see page 349).
Maxair® (pirbuterol)   A beta-agonist bronchodilator (see page 328).
Maxipime® (cefepime)   An antibiotic (see page 331).
Medihaler-EPI®   An inhaled form of epinephrine or adrenalin (see page 328).
Medihaler-ISO® (isoproterenol sulfate)   An inhaled bronchodilator with isoproterenol (see page 328).
Medrol®   Methylprednisolone, an oral steroid.
Megace®   megestrol, a female hormone used for stimulating appetite.
megestrol   A female hormone used for stimulating appetite.
Merem   meropenem, an anti-*Pseudomonas* antibiotic.
meropenem   An anti-*Pseudomonas* antibiotic.
Metaprel® (metaproterenol sulfate)   A beta-agonist bronchodilator (see page 328).

metaproterenol sulfate   A beta-agonist bronchodilator (see page 328).

methacycline   A tetracycline antibiotic (see page 332).

methicillin sulfate   An anti-*Staphylococcus* antibiotic (see page 330).

methyltestosterone   A male sex hormone, sometimes used as a growth and appetite stimulant (see page 348).

metoclopramide   A drug that increases the movement of foods through the GI tract and that may decrease gastroesophageal reflux (see page 345).

Mezlin® (mezlocillin)   An anti-*Pseudomonas* antibiotic (see page 330).

milk of magnesia   There are several different preparations: antacids (see page 345) and laxatives, which are used as an anticonstipation preparation (see page 346).

Minocin® (minocycline hydrochloride)   An antibiotic (see page 314).

minocycline   A tetracycline antibiotic (see page 332).

misoprostol   An antacid medication (see page 345).

montelukast   A leukotriene-inhibitor anti-inflammatory drug (see page 337).

Motrin® (ibuprofen)   An NSAID (see page 337).

mucolytics   Chemicals that break up mucus (see page 326).

Mucomyst® (acetylcysteine)   A mucolytic (see page 327).

mycophenolate   An anti-rejection drug (see page 350).

Mycostatin® (nystatin)   A drug that kills yeast infections, which can appear when a patient is taking antibiotics. Mycostatin is occasionally prescribed when a child is taking antibiotics.

Myfortic® (mycophenolate)   An anti-rejection drug (see page 350).

Mylanta® (aluminum hydroxide + magnesium hydroxide + simethicone)   An antacid (see page 347).

Mylicon (simethicone)   An antibloating drug (see page 347).

Nafcil (nafcillin sodium)   An antibiotic.

nafcillin   An anti-*Staphylococcus* antibiotic (see page 330).

Nasacort   A nasal steroid (triamcinolone).

Nasonex   A nasal steroid (mometasone).

Nebcin (tobramycin sulfate)   An aminoglycoside antibiotic (see page 332).

nedocromil   An inhaled anti-inflammatory medication closely related to cromolyn.

neomycin   An antibiotic.

Neoral® (cyclosporine)   An anti-rejection drug (see page 350).

Neo-Synephrine® (phenylephrine hydrochloride)   A decongestant (see page 341).

netilmicin   An aminoglycoside antibiotic (see page 332).

nizatidine   An antacid (see page 344).

Novahistine®   A combination of many ingredients, used for coughs and cold symptoms (see pages 339).

Nutren®   A nutritional supplement formula (see page 349).

nystatin   Used to fight yeast infections, which can appear when a patient is taking antibiotics.

omeprazole   An antacid drug (see page 345).
Omnicef® (cefdinir)   An antibiotic (see page 331).
Omnipen® (ampicillin)   An antibiotic (see page 330).
Orapred®   An oral suspension preparation of the steroid prednisolone.
Organidin® (iodinated glycerol)   An expectorant (see page 339).
oseltamivir   An anti-flu antibiotic (see page 334).
oxacillin   An anti-*Staphylococcus* antibiotic (see page 330).
oxtriphylline   A theophylline bronchodilator (see page 328).
oxytetracycline   A tetracycline antibiotic (see page 332).
palivizumab   A drug to prevent RSV infection.
pancreatin   A digestive enzyme (see page 343).
Pancreaze® (pancrelipase)   An enteric-coated digestive enzyme (see page 343).
pancrelipase   A digestive enzyme (see page 343).
Panmycin® (tetracycline)   An antibiotic (see page 332).
pantoprazole   An antacid (see page 345).
papase   A drug with some enzyme activity (see page 343).
Pediamycin® (erythromycin ethylsuccinate)   A macrolide antibiotic.
Pediapred®   An oral suspension of prednisolone, a steroid.
Pediasure®   A nutritional supplement formula (see page 349).
Pediazole® (erythromycin ethylsuccinate + sulfisoxazole acetyl)   A combination antibiotic that contains erythromycin and a sulfa drug.
penicillin   An antibiotic (see page 329).
Pen-Vee K®   A penicillin antibiotic (see page 329).
phenylephrine hydrochloride   A medication sometimes used in aerosols. It constricts blood vessels and may therefore cut down on swelling in the bronchi, by decreasing the blood flow to the bronchi.
piperacillin sodium   An anti-*Pseudomonas* antibiotic (see page 330).
Pipracil® (piperacillin)   An antibiotic.
pirbuterol   A beta-agonist bronchodilator (see page 328).
Pneumovax®   The so-called "pneumonia vaccine." This is useful for children who have a particular deficiency in their body defenses that enables them to become infected with a germ called *pneumococcus*, such as children with sickle-cell disease. Many physicians feel that it is of no particular value to patients with CF.
Polycillin® (ampicillin)   An antibiotic (see page 330).
Polycose®   A high-calorie diet supplement (see page 349).
Poly-Histine®   A cough and cold preparation (see page 339).
Polymox® (amoxicillin)   An antibiotic (see page 330).
polymyxin B   An antibiotic.
Polymyxin E®   An antibiotic, also known as colistin, that is effective against *Pseudomonas*; however, it is often difficult to tolerate.
prednisolone   A steroid used to decrease inflammation (see page 335).
prednisone   A steroid used to decrease inflammation (see page 335).
Prilosec® (omeprazole)   An antacid drug (see page 345).

Primaxin® (imipenem)   An antibiotic with some activity against *Pseudomonas* (see page 334).

Principen® (ampicillin)   An antibiotic (see page 330).

Prograf® (FK506/tacrolimus)   An anti-rejection drug (see page 350).

Prostaphlin® (oxacillin sodium)   An anti-*Staphylococcus* penicillin antibiotic (see page 330).

Protonix® (pantoprazole)   An antacid (see page 345).

Proventil®   A beta-agonist bronchodilator (see page 328).

prunes   One of the best sources of dietary fiber, especially effective in combating constipation (see page 346).

Pulmicort®   An inhaled form of budesonide, a steroid.

Quibron®   A bronchodilator preparation that contains several different drugs, including theophylline (see page 328) and an expectorant (see page 328).

quinolones   A family of antibiotics (see page 333).

ranitidine   A medication that decreases the stomach's production of acid (see page 344).

Rapamune® (sirolimus)   An anti-rejection drug (see page 350).

Reglan®   Metoclopramide (see page 345).

Rhinocort®   A nasal form of the steroid budesonide.

rimantadine   An anti-influenza drug.

ribavirin   An aerosol medicine that can help control some viral bronchial infections, especially bronchiolitis caused by RSV.

Robitussin® (guaifenesin)   A cough preparation consisting of an expectorant (see page 339).

rofecoxib   An NSAID.

saline   Salt water.

salmeterol   A long-acting inhaled beta-agonist bronchodilator.

Senokot® (senna)   An intestinal stimulant (see page 347).

Serevent® (salmeterol)   A long-acting inhaled bronchodilator.

Silain® (simethicone)   An antibloating drug (see page 347).

sildenafil (Viagra®)   A medication to treat pulmonary hypertension (see page 343).

Singulair® (montelukast)   An anti-inflammatory leukotriene inhibitor.

sirolimus   An anti-rejection drug (see page 350).

Slo-Phyllin Gyrocaps®   A long-lasting theophylline bronchodilator (see page 328).

sodium chloride   Salt.

Somophyllin®   A theophylline preparation (see page 328).

Spectrobid®   A type of penicillin closely related to ampicillin (see page 330).

spironolactone   A diuretic (see page 342).

Sporanox® (itraconazole)   An antifungal drug.

Staphcillin® (sodium methicillin)   An anti-*Staphylococcus* antibiotic (see page 330).

steroids   Very potent drugs that are similar to the chemicals made in the body in the adrenal glands. They are very powerful and can be used safely for a short period of time for some purposes such as decreasing bronchial inflammation (see page 335). They are often used for other purposes, including growth and appetite stimulation (see page 349).

sulfamethoxazole   A sulfa antibiotic (see page 331).

Sulfatrim®   A combination antibiotic trimethoprim–sulfamethoxazole (see page 331).

Sustacal®   A nutritional supplement formula (see page 349).

Sustaire®   A theophylline bronchodilator (see page 328).

Symbicort® (budesonide/formoterol)   An inhaled corticosteroid/long-acting bronchodilator combination (see page 336).

Synagis® (palivizumab)   A drug to prevent RSV infection (see page 335).

tacrolimus   An anti-rejection drug (see page 350).

Tagamet® (cimetidine)   An antacid drug (see page 344).

Tamiflu® (oseltamivir)   An anti-flu antibiotic (see page 334).

Tazidime   ceftazidime.

Tegopen® (cloxacillin sodium)   An anti-*Staphylococcus* penicillin (see page 330).

terbutaline sulfate   A beta-agonist bronchodilator (see page 328).

Terramycin® (oxytetracycline)   A tetracycline antibiotic (see page 332).

testionate   A male steroid hormone used for growth and appetite stimulation (see page 348).

testosterone   The primary male hormone (see page 348).

tetracycline   An antibiotic family (see page 332).

Theo-Dur®   A theophylline bronchodilator (see page 328).

Theolair®   A theophylline bronchodilator (see page 328).

theophylline   A family of bronchodilators (see page 328).

ticarcillin   An anti-*Pseudomonas* penicillin (see page 330).

Tigacyl® (tigecycline)   An antibiotic (see page 332).

tigecycline   An antibiotic (see page 332).

Tilade®   Nedocromil.

Timentin®   An anti-*Pseudomonas* and anti-*Staphylococcus* antibiotic (see page 331).

TOBI® (inhaled tobramycin)   An inhaled anti-*Pseudomonas* antibiotic (see page 332).

tobramycin   An aminoglycoside antibiotic (see page 332).

Tornalate® (methanesulfonate)   A beta-agonist bronchodilator (see page 328).

triamcinolone   An inhaled steroid (see page 335).

Triaminic® (phenylpropanolamine hydrochloride + pheniramine maleate + pyrilamine maleate)   A cold preparation (see page 339).

trimethoprim   An antibiotic usually found in combination with a sulfa drug (see page 331).

Tussionex®   A cough mixture including an antihistamine; a narcotic cough suppressant (see page 339).

Ultrase®   A pancreatic enzyme supplement (see page 343).

Vancenase® (beclomethasone dipropionate)   A nasal steroid spray (see page 340).

Vantin®   A cephalosporin antibiotic (see page 331).

Veetid B-Cillin® (penicillin)   An antibiotic (see page 329).

Velosef®   A cephalosporin antibiotic (see page 331).

Ventolin® (albuterol sulfate)   A beta-agonist bronchodilator (see page 328).

Vfend® (voriconazole)   An anti-fungal antibiotic (see page 335).

Viagra® (sildenafil)   A medication to treat pulmonary hypertension (see page 343).

Vibramycin®   A tetracycline antibiotic (see page 332).

Viokase® (pancreatin)   A digestive enzyme (see page 343).

Vioxx® (rofecoxib)   An NSAID.

Vipep®   A nutritional supplement formula (see page 349).

Virazole® (see ribavirin).

Vital®   A nutritional supplement formula (see page 349).

Vivonex®   A nutritional supplement formula (see page 349).

voriconazole   An anti-fungal antibiotic (see page 335).

Winstrol® (stanozolol)   A sex steroid hormone (see page 348).

Wycillin (penicillin)   An antibiotic (see page 329).

zafirlukast   A leukotriene-inhibitor anti-inflammatory drug.

Zantac® (ranitidine)   Helps to decrease the stomach's production of acid (see page 344).

Zenpepp® (pancrelipase)   An enteric-coated digestive enzyme (see page 343).

zymase   A digestive enzyme (see page 343).

Zyrtec® (cetirizine)   An antihistamine.

Zyvox® (lenezolid)   An antibiotic.

Airway Clearance Techniques

POSTURAL DRAINAGE TECHNIQUES

Infants

The doctor will decide what positions your child will need for chest physical therapy (CPT) and how often to do the therapy. Schedule it before or at least 1 hour after eating. Figures C.1–C.9 show the different lobes to be treated (shaded in grey) and the areas to be percussed (dark ovals).

1. To make percussion more comfortable, your child should wear a thin layer of clothing such as a shirt or you may use a blanket or towel over the skin. Do not percuss on bare skin.
2. Place your child on a padded surface, using blankets or pillows for positioning and support. Use the checked positions.
3. Percuss each area rhythmically and vigorously. For small children, use a CPT cup (below, left). For older children use cupped hands (below, right).

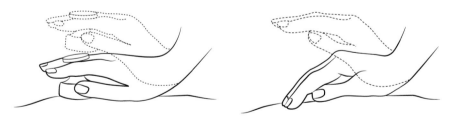

4. Percuss only over the ribs. Avoid percussing over the spine, breastbone, stomach, lower ribs, and lower back to prevent injury to body organs.

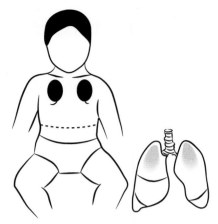

FIGURE C.1. **Right and left upper lobes – apical segments.** Place child in an upright position with back supported. Percuss just below the collarbones.

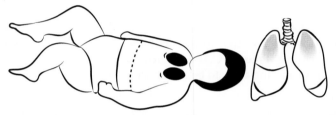

FIGURE C.2. **Right and left upper lobes – anterior segments.** Place child on the back. Percuss between the collarbone and nipple on both sides.

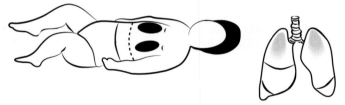

FIGURE C.3. **Right and left lower lobes – anterior segments.** Place child on the back. Percuss both sides just below the nipple and above the lower ribs. This position is commonly avoided in small infants (<4–6 months of age).

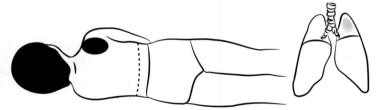

FIGURE C.4. **Right upper lobe – posterior segment.** Place child on the left side. Percuss on the top part of the right shoulder blade.

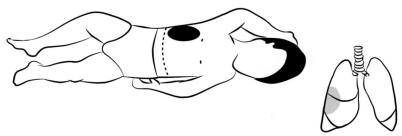

FIGURE C.5. Right lower lobe – lateral segment. Place child on the left side. Percuss below the right armpit and above the lower ribs.

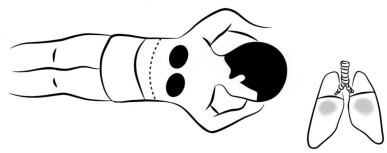

FIGURE C.6. Right and left lower lobes – superior segments. Place child on the abdomen (belly). Percuss on the bottom of, and just below, the shoulder blades.

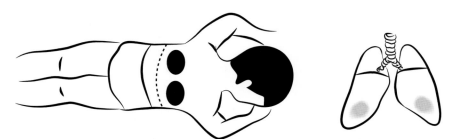

FIGURE C.7. Right and left lower lobes – basal segments. Place child on the abdomen (belly). Percuss below the shoulder blades and above the lower ribs.

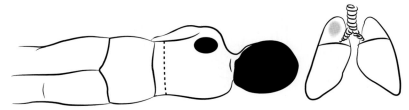

FIGURE C.8. Left upper lobe – posterior segment. Place child on the right side. Percuss on the top part of the left shoulder blade.

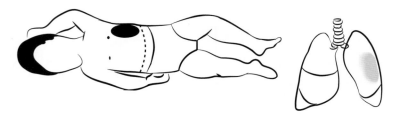

FIGURE C.9. Left lower lobe – lateral segment. Place child on the right side. Percuss below the left armpit and above the lower ribs.

Toddlers

Figures C.10–C.18 show the different lobes to be treated (shaded in grey) and the areas to be percussed (dark ovals). The following points will be helpful in performing postural drainage (PD).

- Clap 1 minute for each position—cough, repeat once (2 minutes total per position).
- Each session should last a maximum of 30 to 40 minutes.
- Always do treatment sessions before meals.
- Two to three sessions per day are usually recommended.

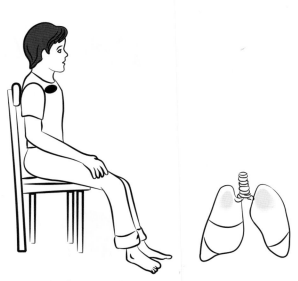

FIGURE C.10. Right and left upper lobes – apical segments. Child is sitting up with back supported. Percuss just below the collarbones.

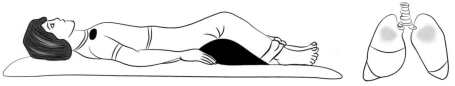

FIGURE C.11. Right and left upper lobes – anterior segments. Child lies on the back with a pillow under the knees. Percuss between the collarbone and nipple on both sides.

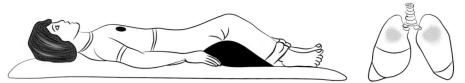

FIGURE C.12. Right and left lower lobes – anterior segments. Child lies on the back with a pillow under the knees. Percuss both sides just below the nipple and above the lower ribs.

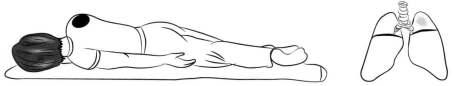

FIGURE C.13. Right upper lobe – posterior segment. Child lies on left side with a pillow under the left armpit. Have child lean forward at a 45° angle against the pillow. Percuss on the top part of the right shoulder blade.

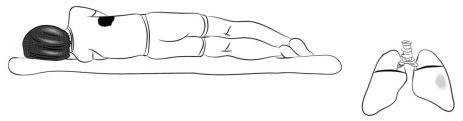

FIGURE C.14. Right lower lobe – lateral segment. Child lies on the left side with a pillow under the left lower ribs and hip. Percuss below the right armpit and above the lower ribs.

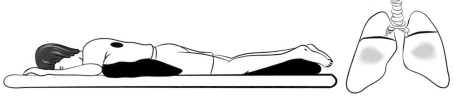

FIGURE C.15. Right and left lower lobes – superior segments. Child lies with pillows under the abdomen (belly) and legs. Percuss on the bottom of, and just below, the shoulder blades.

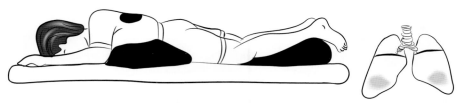

FIGURE C.16. Right and left lower lobes – basal segments. Child lies with pillows under abdomen (belly) and legs. Percuss below the shoulder blades and above the lower ribs.

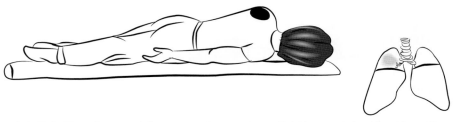

FIGURE C.17. Left upper lobe – posterior segment. Child lies on right side with a pillow under the right armpit. Have child lean forward at a 45° angle against the pillow. Percuss on the top part of the left shoulder blade.

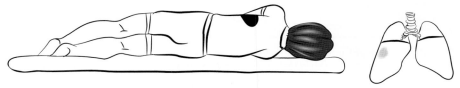

FIGURE C.18. Left lower lobe – lateral segment. Child lies on the right side with a pillow under the right lower ribs and hip. Percuss below the left armpit and above the lower ribs.

Other Considerations

Children may become frightened initially when given PD. As this treatment is very important, you should be encouraged not to apologize or sympathize for having to give this form of treatment. Children should understand, to the best of their ability, why the treatment is being done and accept it as part of the daily routine. Children should be encouraged to talk and sing, as this helps them to breathe. Children should not be offered rewards for future treatments. The drainage should be done with as little fuss as possible.

Your child does not need to dislike the time spent in physical therapy. You can make this time a pleasant, quiet opportunity to spend in conversation, or you can provide entertainment by playing records or tapes, or by doing drainage in front of the television.

Percussion is less tiring if you keep your arms relaxed and do the movement with your wrists. If your child has trouble with a position (poor color, hard time breathing, fighting it), sit him or her up until breathing returns to normal, and try again. If you have tried a position three times and your child still has trouble, go on to the next position. If you cannot give the full therapy again at the next session, call the doctor.

FLUTTER TECHNIQUE

The flutter technique has been very successful for children, adolescents, and adults and is done independently A simple piece of equipment is needed, namely, the Flutter® device (Figure C.19).

The device (as you may recall from Chapter 3) is a handheld device, small enough to carry around in your pocket, that looks a little like a kazoo. It has a stainless-steel ball in it that vibrates up and down (flutters, you might say) as you blow into the tube. The vibrations are transmitted backward down through the patient's mouth into the trachea and bronchi, where they shake the mucus free from the bronchial walls.

Instructions for its use are as follows:

- Sit with your back straight and head slightly tilted back so that your throat and windpipe are wide open. Some patients prefer to place their elbows on a table to help keep them from slouching.
- Hold the Flutter® so that the stem is parallel to the floor (this places the cone at a slight angle, enabling the ball to flutter and roll). You'll then try slightly different positions and see which gives you the most vibrating sensation in your chest.
- The inhalation step (breath in) is very important. Take in as big a breath as possible. Then *hold* that breath for at least 2 to 3 seconds.
- Then, at the end of the breath-hold, place the Flutter® in your mouth and begin to exhale at a constant speed. You should *not* breathe out as fast as you can, but try different speeds of blowing out, and see which speed makes the most fluttering feeling in your chest and helps you clear mucus best. While you're

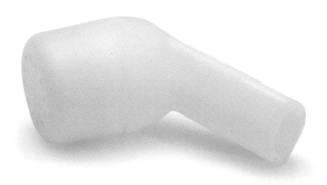

FIGURE C.19. The Flutter (Scandipharm)

blowing out, keep your cheeks flat (don't let the vibrations be wasted on your cheeks; instead you want them to go to your lungs). While you're learning, you might hold your cheeks lightly with your other hand to keep them from vibrating.

■ Exhale as much air as possible. Really squeeze it out to help clean those small airways. This is a maximum effort (remember, not maximum hard blast, but maximum long breath out).

■ Leave the Flutter® in your mouth and take in another big breath (through your nose) and repeat the whole Flutter® breath several times.

■ Now, remove the Flutter®, take in a big breath, hold it for 2 to 3 seconds, and "huff" out a breath, holding your mouth and throat open, and cough.

aCAPELLA®

The acapella is another handheld device that provides both oscillation of the mucus in the airways and positive pressure to help push open the airways (Figure C.20). To use the acapella®, assume a comfortable position, sitting up straight with good posture. You may rest elbows on a tabletop to aid in comfort and positioning. First-time users should have acapella Choice® dial set at lowest setting by rotating dial counterclockwise all the way to number 1 on the dial. Then, inhale through the nose to a volume beyond a normal breath, but without filling the lungs completely, and hold breath for 2 to 3 seconds. Place the acapella Choice® in the mouth with a good seal and exhale normally at a constant speed. Exhalation should last 3 to 4 seconds and a vibrating sensation should be felt in the chest. If exhalation cannot be maintained for this long, rotate dial on the device until sufficient exhalation time is achieved or until vibrating sensation is the strongest. Repeat for 10

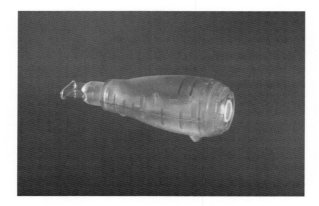

FIGURE C.20. acapella (Smiths Medical)

to 20 breaths to loosen mucus, depending on doctor's prescription, and then cough or perform huff coughing to expel mucus.

QUAKE®

Like the acapella and Flutter®, the Quake® also provides oscillation and positive pressure to the airways (Figure C.21). The speed of the oscillations from the Quake, however, is provided by turning a "crank" rather than from the force of air from the lungs. This may benefit patients with severely reduced lung function.

Before starting, take two or three easy breaths with your abdominal muscles (tummy breathing) and then one slow, deep breath in, starting as an easy "tummy" breath, and hold it for 3 to 4 seconds, and then breathe out easily. Then take another deep breath and do either three little coughs or one big "huff" cough. This will clear out any loose mucus in your throat and lungs. Next, place the mouthpiece in your mouth, with lips tight around it. Try to keep your cheeks from "puffing." While turning the handle (at approximately one to two rotations per second), take an easy, big breath in (starting with abdominal muscles) and hold your breath for 3 to 5 seconds before breathing out (with abdominal muscles) with a little force into the Quake®, continuing to turn the handle. Breathe in bigger than normal, but not as big as with pulmonary function tests (PFTs) and breathe out slightly longer than normal, but not as long as with PFTs. Adjust the speed of your breaths in and out and also the speed of the handle rotations to get the vibrating sensation that seems to loosen your secretions the best. Repeat this for three to six breaths. These are the "loosening breaths." Try not to cough yet. Next, breathe in slowly, through the Quake®, as deep as you can, hold for 3 seconds, and then breathe out hard and long (as with PFTS) using your abdominal muscles. Continue to turn the handle while doing these bigger breaths. Repeat this two more times. Then take the mouthpiece from your mouth and try to cough (again, a big breath with three little coughs or one big "huff" cough). Repeat until you feel that all the loosened mucus has been cleared. Repeat these steps for a total of 20 minutes.

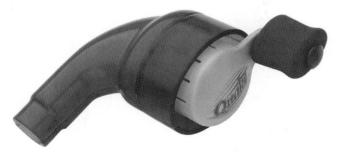

FIGURE C.21. Quake® (Thayer Medical)

HIGH FREQUENCY CHEST COMPRESSION VESTS

The vests also have been successful for many children, adolescents, and adults (Figures C.22–C.24). It allows older children and adults to be independent in their airway clearance. The devices are not easily portable and are very expensive. The instructions are as follows:

- Be sure that your vest fits properly.
- It's fine to do bronchodilator, saline, or steroid aerosols during vest treatments.
- It's probably wise to delay antibiotic aerosol treatments until after the vest treatment (to avoid coughing the antibiotic right out, before it's had a chance to work in the lower airways).

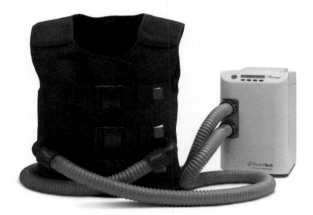

FIGURE C.22. InCourage vest system (Respirtech, Minneapolis, MN)

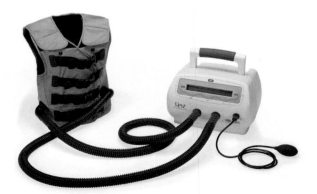

FIGURE C.23. The Vest model105a (Hill Rom)

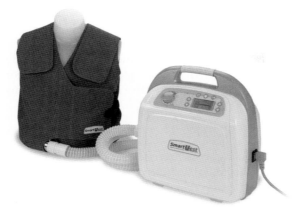

FIGURE C.24. Smart Vest (ElectroMed)

- Stop to cough and clear airways every 5 to 10 minutes.
- Use a pressure setting as high as is comfortable. It is preferable to use several different frequencies (some devices change the frequency automatically or can be programmed to change frequency, others require you to change the frequency with a dial).

OTHER TECHNIQUES

The following techniques are used more in Europe than in North America. What follows is just a brief description of each.

Positive Expiratory Pressure Mask

For the PEP (positive expiratory pressure) mask technique, the patient breathes through a special mask that has an exhale valve that requires some air pressure to open. It is thought that this expiratory pressure is transmitted back down the airways and helps to prop them open during the exhalation, allowing mucus to be pushed out along with the air (remember that usually during exhalation, the airways tend to narrow a little bit, so this keeps them open wider than they would normally be).

Active Cycle of Breathing

This technique has three phases, breathing control (quiet breathing), thoracic expansion (deep breaths in), and forced expiration or huffs (quick, strong—but never violent—breaths out, with the mouth and throat open).

Autogenic Drainage

Autogenic drainage involves a series of breaths controlled so that some are done with very little air in the lungs, some with a medium amount, and some with the lungs filled almost to capacity. This technique requires instruction by someone very skilled in its use before it can be effective in mobilizing mucus.

Exercise

Many people believe that vigorous exercise may be helpful to loosen mucus and to keep bronchi clear. Certainly, hard exercise, laughing, or crying often result in a coughing spell that brings up mucus, even in people who do not raise mucus during the traditional PD treatments. Since there is not yet any scientific evidence that exercise can successfully replace the time-honored PD treatments, it is best to encourage patients to be very active and to do their treatments. (Exercise is discussed at greater length in Chapter 10.)

Some High Calorie Recipes

PASTA POT

By Stefani Czekaj

> 2 lb ground beef
> 2 medium onions, chopped
> 1 clove garlic, minced
> 1 (14 oz) jar spaghetti sauce
> 1 (16 oz) can stewed tomatoes
> 3 oz canned or fresh mushrooms
> 8 oz shell or spring macaroni
> 3 cups sour cream
> 8 oz provolone cheese, shredded
> 8 oz mozzarella cheese, shredded

Cook beef in skillet; drain excess fat. Add onions, garlic, spaghetti sauce, stewed tomatoes, and mushrooms. Simmer 20 minutes. Meanwhile, cook macaroni according to package directions; drain and rinse in cold water.

Pour shells into deep casserole, cover with tomato meat sauce. Spread sour cream over sauce and add provolone cheese. Top with mozzarella cheese. Cover casserole and bake at 350°F for 35 to 40 minutes. Uncover and bake until cheese melts and browns.

> Yield: 10 servings
> 1 serving: 613 calories

Note: For higher calories use cheeses made with whole milk.

FETTUCCINE ALFREDO

By Kevin Helmick

> 1 (8 oz) package fettuccine, uncooked
> ½ cup melted butter
> ¾ cup grated Parmesan cheese

375

4 tbsp half and half
salt and pepper

Cook pasta according to package directions; drain well. In warm serving dish combine butter, cheese, half and half, salt, and pepper. Add pasta to mixture. Gently toss to coat all fettuccine. Top with Parmesan cheese.

Yield: 4 servings
1 cup: 450 calories

SPINACH PASTA

By Peggy Tommarello

½ cup vegetable oil
1 tbsp butter
1 tsp salt
1 tsp basil
2 cloves garlic, halved
1 package frozen spinach, cooked
½ lb small shells, cooked and drained
1 (6 oz) can grated Parmesan cheese

Sauté first five ingredients; add cooked spinach. Mix well. Sauté for 7 to 10 minutes. Add cooked pasta and then the Parmesan cheese. Stir until pasta is coated; heat thoroughly. Serve hot.

Yield: 6 servings
1 serving: 363 calories

VEGETABLE PIZZA

2 packages crescent rolls
2 (8 oz) packages cream cheese, softened
1 cup mayonnaise
2 tsp onion powder
2 tsp dry dill, crumbled
2 cups chopped broccoli
2 cups chopped cauliflower
1 green pepper, chopped
2 tomatoes, diced and drained
2 medium carrots, shredded

Unroll and pat crescent rolls onto a cookie sheet to make crust. Bake at 350°F until light, golden brown. Cool. Combine the cream cheese, mayonnaise, onion powder, and dill. Spread over cooled crust. Top with the broccoli, cauliflower, green pepper, and tomatoes. Place shredded carrots on top. Cut in small triangles to serve.

Yield: 12 servings
1/12 recipe: 272 calories

SHRIMP SPREAD

    8 oz cream cheese, softened
    1 small onion, diced
    ¼ cup mayonnaise
    1 (6 oz) can mini-shrimp
    ½ tbsp lemon juice
    ¼ tsp garlic powder
    ½ tbsp Worcestershire sauce
    ¾ cup cocktail sauce

Mix all ingredients except cocktail sauce. Refrigerate for at least 1 hour. When ready to serve, mound cheese mixture in middle of plate. Pour cocktail sauce over the mound of cheese. Serve with a favorite cracker. (Crabmeat can be substituted for the shrimp.)

    Yield: 24 servings
    1/24 recipe: 60 calories

ARTICHOKE PIZZAZZ

By Karen Ketyer

    1 (14 oz) can artichoke hearts, drained and chopped
    1 cup grated Parmesan cheese
    1 cup shredded mozzarella cheese
    1 cup mayonnaise
    2 tbsp chopped green onion
    1 dash garlic powder

Combine all ingredients and put in a 1½ quart casserole dish or quiche pan. Bake at 350°F, for 25 to 30 minutes. Serve hot with a sturdy cracker.

    Yield: 1 quart
    1/20 recipe: 88 calories

PEANUT BUTTER ROUND-UPS

By Amanda Ogden

    1 cup shortening
    1 cup granulated sugar
    1 cup brown sugar, firmly packed
    2 eggs
    1 cup peanut butter
    2 cups all-purpose flour
    ½ teaspoon salt
    2 tsp baking soda
    1 cup quick rolled oats

Mix the ingredients one at a time in order of recipe; mix well. Place a teaspoonful of mixture for each ball on cookie sheet. Press with fork. Bake at 350°F for 10 to 12 minutes.

Yield: 6 dozen balls
1 ball: 85 calories

LEMON BARS

By Louise Bauer

1 cup (2 sticks) butter
2 cups all-purpose flour
3 tbsp granulated sugar
2 (8 oz) packages cream cheese
2 cups powdered sugar
2 small packages lemon pudding and pie filling (not instant)
1 medium container Cool Whip
chopped nuts

Combine butter, flour, and sugar like a pie dough. Pat into bottom of jelly-roll pan or cookie sheet. Bake at 325°F for 15 minutes. Cool.

Blend cream cheese and powdered sugar with electric mixer. Spread on cooled crust.

Cook pudding according to package directions. Spread on top of cream cheese layer. Let gel. Cover with Cool Whip and sprinkle with chopped nuts, if desired. Cut into bars to serve.

Yield: 24 bars
1 bar: 260 calories

MILKY WAY CAKE

By David Orenstein

1 lb of Milky Way bars
1 cup buttermilk (or plain yogurt)
3 sticks butter
½ tsp baking soda
4 eggs
2 tsp vanilla
2½ cups flour
½ cup chopped nuts
2 cups granulated sugar
2 cups powdered sugar

Melt about 11 oz of the candy bars and one stick butter in double boiler until smooth; set aside. Cream granulated sugar and one stick butter add eggs one at a time, beat until smooth; add flour, buttermilk (or yogurt), and baking soda. Add Milky Way mix, 2 tsp vanilla, and nuts. Bake in greased and floured bundt pan or angel food pan for 1 hour 20 minutes at 325°F.

Frosting: Melt remaining candy bars (about 5 oz) and the other stick of butter in double boiler until smooth, add little vanilla and powdered sugar until desired thickness, add a little milk if necessary. This cake should be stored in the fridge, but it probably won't need to be stored long!

Yield: 12 servings
1 serving: 705 calories

ORENSTEIN FAMILY BROWNIES

*By Florence, Jacob, Herbert, and David Orenstein
and Miriam Sumner*

4 1-oz cubes unsweetened baking chocolate
1 cup butter
3 eggs
2 cups sugar
1 cup flour
1 cup chopped walnuts
½ tsp vanilla (optional)
(raisin lovers can add ½ to 1 cup raisins)

Preheat oven to 350°F. Grease large flat cookie pan (about 10 × 15 inches) with closed ends.

Melt chocolate and butter in double boiler over hot water, add sugar, then eggs, flour, and walnuts (and vanilla and raisins, if you're using them). Spread in pan. Bake 20 to 30 minutes.

Yield: 24 pieces
1 brownie: 175 calories, but no one can eat one.

GERMAN APPLE PIE

By Michelle Gruskos

1 cup flour
1 cup sugar
¾ cup melted butter
1 egg
½ cup finely chopped walnuts
½ cup raisins
enough sliced apples to fill 9-inch pie pan
cinnamon mixture (1 tbsp sugar + 1 tsp cinnamon)

Preheat oven to 350°F. Fill pie pan with sliced apples. Sprinkle cinnamon mixture over. Mix all other ingredients in bowl and spread over apples. Bake at 350°F for 45 minutes.

Yield: 6 big pieces
1 piece: 387 calories

STICKY DATE PUDDING

By Jenny Cooper, Sydney, Australia

6 oz dates, stoned and chopped
1 tsp baking soda
10 oz boiling water
4 tbsp butter
6 oz caster (very fine) sugar
2 eggs
6 oz flour
½ tsp vanilla

Sauce:

14 oz brown sugar
1 cup thick cream
9 oz butter
1 vanilla bean, split

Preheat oven to 350°F and butter a 7-inch square cake tin. Mix dates and baking soda. Pour water over dates/soda, and leave to stand. Cream butter and sugar, then add eggs, one at a time, beating well after each. Fold flour in gently, then stir in date mixture and vanilla and pour into prepared tin. Bake in center of oven for 30 to 40 minutes until cooked when tested with toothpick.

Sauce: Bring all ingredients to a boil. Reduce heat and simmer for 5 minutes. Remove vanilla bean. Pour a little sauce over warm pudding and return to oven for 2 to 3 minutes so that sauce soaks in. Cut pudding into squares and pour extra sauce over.

Yield: 6 pieces
1 piece: 980 calories!!

SWEET AND SOUR STRAWBERRY DESSERT

By Judy Fulton

1 qt fresh strawberries
8 oz sour cream
1 cup firmly packed brown sugar

Wash and hull strawberries. Dry and slice. Mix brown sugar and sour cream and top strawberries.

Yield: 6 servings
1 serving: approximately 240 calories

PEANUT BUTTER BANANA SHAKE

By Tonya Boyer

1 small banana, chunked
1½ cups whole milk

¼ cup smooth peanut butter
2 tsp granulated sugar
½ tsp vanilla extract

Combine all ingredients in blender and mix until smooth and frothy.

Yield: 2 drinks
1 drink: 350 calories

SCOTCHEROOS

By Renee Exler

1 cup light corn syrup
1 cup granulated sugar
1 cup peanut butter
6 cups Rice Krispy cereal
1 cup semi-sweet chocolate chips
1 cup butterscotch morsels

Cook corn syrup and sugar over medium heat in saucepan until sugar is dissolved; stir frequently. When mixture starts to boil, remove from heat and stir in peanut butter; mix well. Add Rice Krispy cereal; stir until well coated. Press mixture into buttered 9 × 13 × 2-inch pan. Set aside.

Melt chocolate chips and butterscotch morsels over low heat; stirring constantly. Spread over cereal mixture. Allow to cool, then cut into 1 × 2-inch squares.

Yield: 24 squares
1 × 2-inch square: 96 calories

CHEESECAKE SQUARES

By Amanda Ogden

1 (14 oz) can sweetened condensed milk
½ cup lemon juice or two to three lemons squeezed
1 tbsp grated lemon rind
⅔ cup shortening
1 cup brown sugar, firmly packed
1¾ cups all-purpose flour
1 tsp salt
1½ cups quick-cooking oats

Blend milk, lemon juice, and lemon rind with electric mixer until thick; set aside. Mix together shortening and sugar. Combine flour and other dry ingredients. Blend into shortening mixture. Blend in rolled oats. Place half of the oats mixture into a 9 × 13 × 2-inch pan and press and flatten down. Spread the lemon mixture over the oats mixture. Cover with remaining oat mixture, patting lightly. Bake at 375°F for 25 to 30 minutes. Cool and cut into bars.

Yield: 24 squares
1 square: 203 calories

HEATH BARS

By Jane Strange

> 50 to 60 soda crackers
> ¼ cup butter, melted
> 1 cup (2 sticks) butter
> 1 cup dark brown sugar, firmly packed
> 1 (12 oz) package milk chocolate chips
> 1 cup chopped nuts

Line large cookie sheet with tin foil; spread melted butter. Place the crackers on buttered cookie sheet.

In medium saucepan cook sugar and 1 cup butter until dissolved; stirring constantly. Allow sugar and butter to boil. Pour mixture over crackers. Bake at 375°F for 7 minutes. Remove from oven and sprinkle with chocolate chips. As the chips melt, spread to smooth out. Sprinkle with nuts. Place in refrigerator to cool. Cut into bars to serve.

> Yield: 24 bars
> 1 bar: 236 calories

KID PLEASIN' CHOCOLATE MOUSSE

> 1 (6 oz) package chocolate instant pudding mix
> 3 cups cold whole milk
> 1 cup frozen whipped topping, thawed
> 12 cream-filled chocolate sandwich cookies, crumbled
> 8 cream-filled chocolate sandwich cookies, whole

Combine pudding mix and milk in a small mixing bowl; beat at low speed in an electric mixer until blended. Beat at low speed an additional 2 minutes. Fold in ½ cup whipped topping and cookie crumbs. Spoon mousse into eight (6 oz) dessert dishes. Cover and chill.

Garnish each serving with a drop of remaining whipped topping and a whole cookie just before serving.

> Yield: 8 (6 oz) servings
> ⅛ recipe: 276 calories

MIRACLE PUDDING

By Brenda McCullen

> 2 small packages chocolate instant pudding mix
> 1 (14 oz) can sweetened condensed milk
> 1 large container Cool Whip

Prepare pudding according to package directions. Combine remaining ingredients with pudding and mix well. Refrigerate until chilled. Any flavor pudding may be used.

Yield: 8 servings
⅛ recipe: 513 calories

PUPPY CHOW

By Brenda McCullen

1 stick (½ cup) butter
1 (12 oz) package chocolate chips
½ cup peanut butter
8 cups Rice Chex or Crispix cereal
2 cups powdered sugar

Melt the first three ingredients in a medium saucepan. Place the cereal in a large plastic container and add the melted mixture. Shake sealed container until all the cereal is coated. Add the powdered sugar.

Yield: 12 servings
1/12 recipe: 500 calories

FRUIT PIZZA

By Clare Jean Haury

1 package yellow cake mix
¼ cup water
¼ cup margarine, softened
2 eggs
¼ cup packed brown sugar
½ cup pecans, chopped
2 packages Dream Whip
fresh fruit

Grease and flour two 12-inch pizza pans. Combine half the cake mix and all other ingredients except the pecans, fruit, and Dream Whip. Mix well. Add remaining cake mix and mix well. Fold in pecans. Divide evenly between the two pans and spread to the edges. Bake at 350°F for 15 to 20 minutes. Cool. Prepare Dream Whip according to directions on package. Top each cake with one package of Dream Whip and add sliced fresh fruit to decorate.

Yield: 12 servings
1/12 recipe: 350 calories

ADDITIONAL RECIPES

Additional recipes can be found in two cystic fibrosis cookbooks:

Cooking Up Calories from the Antonio J. and Janet Palumbo Cystic Fibrosis Center at Children's Hospital of Pittsburgh, **by Judy Fulton, M.P.H, R.D., L.D.N,** CF Dietitian, and **Amy Wengryn,** CF parent

A Way of Life—a cookbook written for an individual with cystic fibrosis, **by Mary Marcus, M.S., R.D., et al.**—can be ordered from Lulu by going to the following webpage:

http://www.lulu.com/content/2482231

The History of Cystic Fibrosis

Some highlights in the history of cystic fibrosis are as follows:

1705   A book of folk philosophy states that a salty taste means that a child is bewitched.

1857   The Almanac of Children's Songs and Games from Switzerland quotes from Middle Ages: "Woe is the child who tastes salty from a kiss on the brow, for he is hexed, and soon must die."

1938   Andersen first describes cystic fibrosis (CF), calling it cystic fibrosis of the pancreas.

1946   di Sant'Agnese and Andersen report using antibiotics to treat CF lung infection.

1953   di Sant'Agnese and colleagues describe the sweat abnormality in CF.

1955   First review of use of pancreatic enzymes.

1959   Gibson and Cook describe a safe and accurate way to do sweat testing.

1964   Doershuk, Matthews, and colleagues describe a modern comprehensive treatment program.

1978   First use of enteric-coated pancreatic enzymes.

1981–1983   Description by Knowles and colleagues and Quinton and coworkers of electrolyte transport abnormalities.

1989   Tsui, Riordan, and Collins discover *CF* gene.

1990   Correction of chloride transport defect in CF cells in culture by adenovirus-mediated gene transfer.

1992   First trials of gene transfer in living people with CF.

1993   FDA approves DNase, the first drug developed specifically for CF.

1997   Establishment of Therapeutics Development Network (TDN) in United States by Cystic Fibrosis Foundation.

2008   VX-770, a twice-a-day oral pill, is shown to correct the underlying molecular defect in CF.

2009   Virtually all states and the District of Columbia require newborns to be screened for CF.

Modified from Taussig LM. *Cystic fibrosis.* New York: Thieme-Stratton, 1984.

Bibliography and Resources

SUGGESTED READING

General—Textbooks

Allen JL, Rubenstein RC, Panitch HB, eds. *Cystic fibrosis.* Lung Biology in Health & Disease Series (Volume 242). London: Informa Healthcare, 2010. *An excellent up-to-date, comprehensive text on cystic fibrosis (CF), with contributions by many of the world's experts.*

Davis PB, ed. *Cystic fibrosis.* New York: Marcel Dekker, Inc., 1993. *An excellent text.*

Doershuk CF. *Cystic fibrosis in the 20th century.* Cleveland, OH: AM Publishing, 2001. *A fascinating look at the history of CF and CF science and care from the very personal viewpoints of many of he people who lived and made the history*

Hodson ME, Geddes DM, eds. *Cystic fibrosis.* London: Chapman & Hall Medical, 1995. *A comprehensive text on CF; an excellent resource.*

Orenstein DM, Rosenstein BJ, Stern RC. *Cystic fibrosis: medical care.* Philadelphia, PA: Lippincott Williams & Wilkins, 2000. General overview, also aimed at professional audience.

Orenstein DM, Stern RC, eds. *Treatment of the hospitalized cystic fibrosis patient.* New York: Marcel Dekker, Inc., 1998. *In-depth medical detail, aimed at physician audience; actually covers more than just hospitalized patients.*

Yankaskas JR, Knowles MR, eds. *Cystic fibrosis in adults.* Philadelphia, PA: Lippincott–Raven Publishers, 1999. *Excellent medical text, with in depth coverage of all aspects of CF medical care for adults.*

General—Journal Articles

Davis PB, Drumm M, Konstan MW. Cystic fibrosis: state of the art. *Am J Resp Crit Care Med* 1996;154:1229–1256.

Gawande A. The bell curve: what happens when patients find out how good their doctors really are? *The New Yorker.* December 6, 2004.

Of Historical Interest

Andersen DH. Cystic fibrosis of the pancreas and its relation to celiac disease: a clinical and pathologic study. *Am J Dis Child* 1938;356:344–395. *The earliest description of CF as a single entity.*

di Sant'Agnese PA, Darling RC, Perera GA, et al. Abnormal electrolyte composition of sweat in cystic fibrosis of the pancreas: clinical significance and relationship of the disease. *Pediatrics* 1953;12:549–563. *Original description of the high salt content in CF sweat.*

Doershuk CF, Matthews LW, Tucker AS, et al. A five-year clinical evaluation of a therapeutic program for patients with cystic fibrosis. *J Pediatr* 1964;65:677–693. *The first paper to show the benefit of a comprehensive treatment program for patients with CF.*

Drumm ML, Pope HA, Cliff WH, et al. Correction of the cystic fibrosis defect *in vitro* by retrovirus-mediated gene transfer. *Cell* 1990;62:1227–1233.

Gibson LE, Cooke RE. A test for concentration of electrolytes in sweat in cystic fibrosis of the pancreas utilizing pilocarpine by iontophoresis. *Pediatrics* 1959;23:545–549. *Landmark report detailing a laboratory method for collection and analysis of CF sweat.*

Knowles M, Gatzy J, Boucher R. Increased bioelectric potential difference across respiratory epithelia in cystic fibrosis. *N Engl J Med* 1981;305:1489–1495. *The first of the papers to elucidate the problem with electrolyte transport across mucous membranes in CF.*

Quinton PM, Bijman J. Higher bioelectric potentials due to decreased chloride absorption in the sweat glands of patients with cystic fibrosis. *N Engl J Med* 1983;308:1185–1189. *Initial publication demonstrating that the problem in nose and respiratory tree also existed in sweat glands, and that it was primarily a problem with chloride not being able to pass through mucous membranes.*

Rich DP, Anderson MP, Gregory RJ, et al. Expression of cystic fibrosis transmembrane conductance regulator corrects defective chloride channel regulation in cystic fibrosis airway epithelial cell. *Nature* 1990;347:358–363.

Rommens JM, Iannuzzi MC, Kerem BS, et al. Identification of the cystic fibrosis gene: chromosome walking and jumping. *Science* 1989;245:1059–1065. *Landmark paper announcing discovery and cloning of CF gene by Drs. Lap-Chee Tsui, Francis Collins, and Jack Riordan (and their colleagues), from Toronto and Michigan.*

These last two papers appeared almost simultaneously and showed that the CF cell defect could be cured in the laboratory with gene transfer.

For Classroom Teachers

Young A. *Cystic fibrosis in the classroom.* Distributed via Scandipharm (Birmingham, AL). *Superb introduction to CF for teachers who have a student with CF in their classes.*

"WEBLIOGRAPHY": SOME SELECTED SITES ON THE WORLD WIDE WEB

(To the reader, Surfer: BEWARE!! Sites may change; content of some sites you might find in a Google search may vary from superb to wacko!)

Web Site	Sponsor/Comments
http://www.cff.org	Cystic Fibrosis Foundation/*Probably the best single site; up-to-date, reliable*
http://www.cftrust.org.uk/	The United Kingdom's CF Trust site
http://www.cfww.org	Cystic Fibrosis Worldwide/*A very good site with international flavor*
http://personal.nbnet.nb.ca/ normap/CF.htm	Norma Kennedy Plourde, a Canadian woman with cystic fibrosis/*This site is excellent, with many useful links to other helpful sites*
http://www.cfvoice.com	*Information and games for children, teens, and adults on a variety of CF topics*

Cystic Fibrosis Care Centers in the United States

ALASKA

Providence Alaska Medical Center
Anchorage, AK 99519
Program type: Affiliate
Directors: Dion Roberts, M.D., Elizabeth
  Galloway, M.D.
(907) 212-4824

ALABAMA

University of Alabama at Birmingham
  (UAB)
Birmingham, AL 35233
Program type: Adult
Directors: Kevin Leon, M.D.,
  Randall K. Young, M.D.
(205) 934-5400

The Children's Hospital/UAB
Birmingham, AL 35233
Pediatric Program Director:
  Hector H. Gutierrez, M.D.,
  Wynton Hoover, M.D.
(205) 558-2402

USA Children's Medical Center
Mobile, AL 36640
Center Director
Lawrence J. Sindel, M.D., B.S.
(251) 343-6848

ARKANSAS

University of Arkansas for Medical Sciences
Little Rock, AR 72205
Program type: Adult:
Director: Paula Anderson, M.D.
(501) 296-1170

Arkansas Children's Hospital
Little Rock, AR 72202
Pediatric Program Director:
  John L. Carroll, M.D., Gulnur Com, M.D.
(501) 364-4000

ARIZONA

Phoenix Children's Hospital
Phoenix, AZ 85016
Program type: Adult
Director: Gerald D. Gong, M.D.
(602) 546-0985

Phoenix Children's Hospital
Phoenix, AZ 85016
Pediatric Program Director:
  Peggy Radford, M.D.
(602) 546-0985

Tucson CF Center
Tucson, AZ 85724
Center Directors:

Wayne J. Morgan, M.D., C.M.,
  Cori Daines, M.D.
(520) 694-9988

CALIFORNIA

USC Keck School of Medicine
Los Angeles, CA 90033
Program type: Adult
Director: Adudpa Pursh Rao, M.D.
(323) 442-8330

Children's Hospital of Los Angeles
Los Angeles, CA 90027
Pediatric Program Director:
  Arnold C.G. Platzker, M.D.
(323) 361-4545

California Pacific Medical Center
San Francisco, CA 94115
Program type: Adult
Director: Christopher Brown, M.D.
(415) 923-3421

Children's Hospital at Oakland
Oakland, CA 94609
Pediatric Program Director:
  Karen A. Hardy, M.D.
(510) 428-3314

University of California at San
  Francisco
San Francisco, CA 94143
Program type: Adult
Director: Mary Ellen Kleinhenz, M.D.
(415) 353-2961

University of California at San Francisco
San Francisco, CA 94143
Pediatric Program Director:
  Dennis W. Nielson, M.D., Ph.D.
(415) 353-7337

University of California at Davis
  Medical Center
Sacramento, CA 95817
Program type: Adult

Directors: Brian Morrissey, M.D.,
  Carroll Cross, M.D.
(916) 734-4200

University of California at Davis Medical
  Center
Sacramento, CA 95817
Pediatric Program Director:
  Ruth McDonald, M.D.
(916) 734-3112

Kaiser Permanente Medical Care Program
Oakland, CA 94611
Program type: Adult
Director: Bryon Quick, M.D.
(510) 752-6555

Kaiser Permanente Medical Care Program
Oakland, CA 94611
Pediatric Program Director:
  Gregory F. Shay, M.D.
(510) 752-7098

Long Beach Memorial Medical Center
Long Beach, CA 90801
Program type: Adult
Director: Jeffrey Riker, M.D.
(562) 933-8740

Miller Children's at Long Beach Memorial
  Medical Center
Long Beach, CA 90801
Pediatric Program Director:
  Eliezer Nussbaum, M.D., Terry Chin,
  M.D., Ph.D.
(562) 933-8567

University of California San Diego
  Medical Center-Thornton
La Jolla, CA 92037
Program type: Adult
Director: Douglas J. Conrad, M.D.
(858) 657-7073

Rady Children's Hospital San Diego/
  University of California San Diego
San Diego, CA 92123

Pediatric Program Director:
  Mark S. Pian, M.D.
(858) 966-5846

Stanford University
Palo Alto, CA 94305
Program type: Adult
Director: David Weill, M.D.
(650) 497-8841

Stanford University Medical Center
Palo Alto, CA 94304
Pediatric Program Director:
  Carlos E. Milla, M.D.
(650) 497-8841

Sutter Medical Center
Sacramento, CA 95817
Center Director:
  Bradley E. Chipps, M.D.
(916) 733-7032

Loma Linda University Medical
  Center
Loma Linda, CA 92350
Program type: Affiliate
Directors: Yvonne Fanous, M.D.,
  Henry Opsimos, M.D.
(909) 835-1808

Kaiser Permanente Los Angeles Medical
  Center
Los Angeles, CA 90027
Program type: Affiliate
Directors: Muhammad Saeed, M.D.,
  Tina Chou, M.D.
(323) 783-6118

Children's Hospital Central California
Madera, CA 93638
Program type: Affiliate
Director: Reddy Sudhakar, M.D., Ph.D.
(559) 353-5550

Children's Hospital of Orange County
Orange, CA 92868
Program type: Affiliate

Director: Bruce Nickerson, M.D.
(714) 532-7983

Naval Medical Center San Diego—FOR
  MILITARY PERSONNEL ONLY
San Diego, CA 92134
Program type: Affiliate
Director: Henry Wojtczak, M.D.
(619) 532-6896

Pediatric Diagnostic Center
Ventura, CA 93003
Program type: Affiliate
Director: Chris Landon, M.D.
(805) 641-4490

East Bay UCSF—Outreach Clinic
Pleasanton, CA 94143
Program type: Outreach
Director: Nancy C. Lewis, M.D.
(925) 598-3500

California Pacific Medical Center—
  Outreach Clinic
San Francisco, CA 94143
Program type: Outreach
Director: Christopher Brown, M.D.
(510) 428-3305

COLORADO

National Jewish Health
Denver, CO 80206
Program type: Adult
Director: Jerry A. Nick, M.D., B.S.
(303) 398-1178

The Children's Hospital Denver
Aurora, CO 80045
Pediatric Program Director:
  Frank J. Accurso, M.D.
(720) 777-6181

Memorial Hospital—Outreach Program
Colorado Springs, CO 80903
Program type: Outreach
(719) 365-2244

CONNECTICUT

Yale University School of Medicine
New Haven, CT 6520
Program type: Adult
Director: John McArdle, M.D.
(203) 785-4198

Yale University School of Medicine
New Haven, CT 6520
Pediatric Program Director:
   Marie E. Egan, M.D.
(203) 785-4081

Central Connecticut Cystic Fibrosis Center
Hartford, CT 6107
Program type: Adult
Director: Rick F. Knauft, M.D.
(860) 547-1876

Central Connecticut Cystic Fibrosis
   Center
Hartford, CT 6102
Pediatric Program Director:
   Craig D. Lapin, M.D.
(860) 545-9440

DISTRICT OF COLUMBIA

Children's National Medical Center
Washington, DC 20010
Program type: Adult
Director: Peter Levit, M.D.
(202) 476-2128

Children's National Medical Center
Washington, DC 20010
Pediatric Program Director:
   Anastassios Koumbourlis, M.D., M.P.H.
(202) 476-2128

DELAWARE

Alfred I. duPont Hospital
   for Children
Wilmington, DE 19899
Center Director: Aaron Chidekel, M.D.
(302) 651-6400

FLORIDA

University of Florida
Gainesville, FL 32610
Program type: Adult
Director: Veena B. Antony, M.D.
(352) 273-8735

University of Florida
Gainesville, FL 32610
Pediatric Program Director:
   Pamela M. Schuler, M.D.
(352) 273-8380

University of Miami Adult CF Center
Miami, FL 33136
Program type: Adult
Director: Matthias Salathe, M.D.
(305) 243-6387

University of Miami
Miami, FL 33136
Pediatric Program Director:
   Annabelle Quizon, M.D.,
   Andrew R.A. Colin, M.D.
(305) 243-6162

Nemours Children's Clinic–Jacksonville
Jacksonville, FL 32207
Center Directors:
Bonnie B. Hudak, M.D.,
   David Schaeffer, M.D.
(904) 697-3788

Tampa General Hospital
Tampa, FL 33606
Program type: Adult
Director: Mark Rolfe, M.D.
(813) 844-4634

All Children's Hospital
St. Petersburg, FL 33701
Pediatric Program Director:
   Magdalen Gondor, M.D.
(727) 767-4146

Central Florida Pulmonary Group
Orlando, FL 32803

Program type: Adult
Directors: Francisco Calimano, M.D.,
  Daniel Layish, M.D.
(407) 841-1100

Nemours Children's Clinic—Orlando
Orlando, FL 32806
Pediatric Program Director:
  David E. Geller, M.D., Jeffery Joeb, M.D
(407) 650-7270

Florida Pediatric Pulmonology/Children's
  Hospital of Southwest Florida
Ft. Myers, FL 33908
Program type: Affiliate
Director: Luis A. Faverio, M.D., F.A.A.P.
(239) 466-1243

Joe DiMaggio Children's Hospital
Hollywood, FL 33021
Program type: Affiliate
Directors: Morton Schwartzman, M.D.,
  Juan Martinez, M.D.
(954) 265-6333

Miami Children's Hospital
Miami, FL 33155
Program type: Affiliate
Director: Maria E. Franco, M.D.
(305) 662-8380

Nemours Children's Clinic—Pensacola
Pensacola, FL 32504
Program type: Affiliate
Director: Kristin Van Hook, M.D.
(850) 505-4785

University of South Florida
Tampa, FL 33606
Program type: Affiliate
Director: Bruce M. Schnapf, D.O.
(813) 259-8767

St. Mary's Medical Center
West Palm Beach, FL 33407
Program type: Affiliate
Director: Maurice Cruz, M.D.
(561) 840-6065

Sarasota Clinic—Outreach Clinic
Sarasota, FL 34238
Program type: Outreach
(727) 892-4146

Tampa Clinic–Outreach Clinic
Tampa, FL 33612
Program type: Outreach
(727) 892-4146

GEORGIA

Emory University
Atlanta, GA 30322
Program type: Adult
Director: Viranuj Sueblinvong, M.D.
(404) 778-3261

Emory University
Atlanta, GA 30322
Pediatric Program Director:
  Michael Schechter, M.D., Daniel B.
  Caplan, M.D.
(404) 727-5728

Medical College of Georgia
Augusta, GA 30912
Program type: Adult
Director: Caralee Forseen, M.D.
(706) 721-4658

Medical College of Georgia
Augusta, GA 30912
Pediatric Program Director:
  Kathleen McKie, M.D.
(706) 721-2390

Children's Healthcare of Atlanta at
  Scottish Rite
Atlanta, GA 30342
Program type: Affiliate
Directors: Peter H. Scott, M.D.,
  Kevin Kirchner, M.D.
(404) 785-2898

HAWAII

Tripler Army Medical Center—FOR
  MILITARY PERSONNEL ONLY

Honolulu, HI 96859
Program type: Affiliate
Director: Jane E. Gross, M.D., Ph.D.
(808) 433-6434

IOWA

Blank Children's Health Center
Des Moines, IA 50309
Center Director: Ricardo Flores, M.D.
(515) 241-6548

University of Iowa
Iowa City, IA 52242
Program type: Adult
Director: Douglas Hornick, M.D.
(319) 356-8133

University of Iowa
Iowa City, IA 52242
Pediatric Program Director:
  Miles Weinberger, M.D.,
  Richard Ahrens, M.D.
(319) 356-2229

Mary Greeley Hospital–McFarland Clinic
Ames, IA 50010
Program type: Affiliate
Director: Edward Nassif, M.D.
(515) 239-4482

IDAHO

Saint Luke's Cystic Fibrosis Center of Idaho
Boise, ID 83712
Program type: Affiliate
Director: Henry R. Thompson, M.D.
(208) 381-7092

ILLINOIS

Northwestern University
Chicago, IL 60611
Program type: Adult
Director: Manu Jain, M.D.
(773) 880-4382

Children's Memorial Hospital
  Northwestern University

Chicago, IL 60614
Pediatric Program Director:
  Susanna A. McColley, M.D.
(773) 880-4382

Rush University Medical Center
Chicago, IL 60612
Program type: Adult
Director: Robert A. Balk, M.D.
(312) 942-6744

Rush University Medical Center
Chicago, IL 60612
Pediatric Program Director:
  Girish Sharma, M.D.,
  John Lloyd-Still, M.D.
(312) 563-2270

Lutheran General Hospital
Niles, IL 60714
Program type: Adult
Director: Arvey M. Stone, M.D.
(847) 759-4770

Lutheran General Children's Hospital CF
  Center
Park Ridge, IL 60068
Pediatric Program Director:
  Gabriel Aljadeff, M.D.
(847) 318-9330

University of Chicago
Chicago, IL 60637
Program type: Adult
Director: Edward Naureckas, M.D.
(773) 702-9660

University of Chicago
Chicago, IL 60637
Pediatric Program Director:
  Lucille A. Lester, M.D.
(773) 702-6169

Saint Francis Medical Center
Peoria, IL 61603
Program type: Adult
Director: W. Anthony Sauder, M.D.
(309) 624-6565

Saint Francis Medical Center
Peoria, IL 61603
Pediatric Program Director:
  Jalayne M. Lapke, M.D., F.A.A.P
(309) 624-6565

Loyola University Medical Center
Maywood, IL 60153
Program type: Adult
Director: Sean M. Forsythe, M.D.
(708) 327-9134

Loyola University Medical Center
Maywood, IL 60153
Pediatric Program Director:
  Charles Dumont, M.D.
(708) 327-9134

Advocate Hope Children's Hospital
Oak Lawn, IL 60453
Program type: Affiliate
Director: Javeed Akhter, M.D.
(708) 684-5810

Southern Illinois University School of
  Medicine
Springfield, IL 62794
Program type: Affiliate
Directors: Mark Johnson, M.D.,
  Joseph Henkle, M.D.
(217) 545-5864

Carle Clinic Association
Urbana, IL 61801
Program type: Affiliate
Director: Donald Davison, M.D.
(217) 383-3100

INDIANA

Indiana University
Indianapolis, IN 46202
Program type: Adult
Director: Aruna Sannuti, M.D., B.S.
(317) 278-3267

Riley Hospital for Children,
  Indiana University Medical Center

Indianapolis, IN 46202
Pediatric Program Director:
  Michelle S. Howenstine, M.D.
(317) 274-7208

Lutheran Children's Hospital
Ft. Wayne, IN 46804
Program type: Affiliate
Director: Pushpom Z. James, M.D.
(260) 435-7123

Saint Joseph Regional Medical Center
South Bend, IN 46617
Program type: Affiliate
Director: James B. Harris III, M.D.
(574) 335-6240

Deaconess Hospital–Outreach Clinic
Evansville, IN 47747
Program type: Outreach
(812) 858-3131

KANSAS

Via Christi–St. Francis Campus
Wichita, KS 67206
Program type: Adult
Director: Daniel C. Doornbos, M.D.
(316) 858-3463

Via Christi–Saint Francis Campus
Wichita, KS 67218
Pediatric Program Director:
  C. Maria Riva, M.D.
(316) 858-3463

University of Kansas Medical Center
Kansas City, KS 66160
Program type: Adult
Directors: Frank Quijano, M.D.,
  Steven Stites, M.D.
(913) 588-6045

University of Kansas Medical Center
Kansas City, KS 66160
Pediatric Program Director:
  Mitzi Scotten, M.D.
(913) 588-6224

KENTUCKY

University of Louisville
Louisville, KY 40202
Program type: Adult
Director: Rodney J. Folz, M.D., Ph.D.
(502) 584-8563

University of Louisville
Louisville, KY 40202
Pediatric Program Director:
  Nemr S. Eid, M.D.
(502) 629-8830

University of Kentucky
Lexington, KY 40536
Program type: Adult
Director: Michael I. Anstead, M.D.
(859) 257-5536

University of Kentucky
Lexington, KY 40536
Pediatric Program Director:
  Jamshed F. Kanga, M.D.
(859) 323-6211

LOUISIANA

Tulane University
New Orleans, LA 70112
Program type: Adult
Director: Dean B. Ellithorpe, M.D.
(504) 988-5800

Tulane University
New Orleans, LA 70112
Pediatric Program Director:
  Scott H. Davis, M.D.
(504) 988-5300

Louisiana State University Health
  Sciences Center
Shreveport, LA 71130
Pediatric Program Director:
  Kimberly L. Jones, M.D.
(318) 675-6094

Louisiana State University Health
  Sciences Center
Shreveport, LA 71130
Program type: Adult
Director: Kimberly L. Jones, M.D.
(318) 675-6094

MASSACHUSETTS

Children's Hospital Boston
Boston, MA 2115
Program type: Adult
Director: Ahmet Uluer, D.O.
(617) 355-1900

Children's Hospital Boston
Boston, MA 2115
Pediatric Program Director:
  Henry L. Dorkin, M.D.
(617) 355-7881

UMass Memorial Health Care–
  Pediatric Pulmonary, Asthma and CF
  Center
Worcester, MA 1655
Center Director: Brian P. O'ullivan, M.D.
(508) 856-4155

Massachusetts General Hospital
Boston, MA 2114
Program type: Adult
Director: Leonard Sicilian, M.D.
(617) 724-0520

Massachusetts General Hospital
Boston, MA 2114
Pediatric Program Director:
  Allen Lapey, M.D.
(617) 726-8707

Baystate Medical Center
Springfield, MA 1199
Center Director:
  Robert A. Kaslovsky, M.D.
(413) 794-0815

Tufts Medical Center
Boston, MA 2111

Program type: Affiliate
Director: William F. Yee, M.D.
(617) 636-7917

MARYLAND

Johns Hopkins Adult CF Program
Baltimore, MD 21205
Program type: Adult
Director: Michael P. Boyle, M.D., F.C.C.P.
(410) 502-7044

The Johns Hopkins University
Baltimore, MD 21287
Pediatric Program Director:
  Peter J. Mogayzel Jr., M.D., Ph.D.,
  Pamela L. Zeitlin, M.D., Ph.D.
(410) 955-2795

National Institutes of Health
Bethesda, MD 20892
Program type: Adult
Directors: Milica S. Chernick, M.D.,
  James E. Balow, M.D.
(301) 496-6821

National Naval Medical Center—
  FOR MILITARY PERSONNEL ONLY
Bethesda, MD 20889
Program type: Affiliate
Director: Andrew J. Lipton, M.D.,
  M.P.H., T.M.
(301) 295-4919

MAINE

Maine Medical Center
Portland, ME 4102
Program type: Adult
Director: Jonathan Zuckerman, M.D.
(207) 828-1122

Maine Medical Partners Pediatric
  Specialty Care
Portland, ME 4102
Pediatric Program Director:
  Anne Marie Cairns, D.O.
(207) 662-5522

Eastern Maine Medical Center
Bangor, ME 4401
Program type: Affiliate
Director: Thomas Lever, M.D.
(207) 973-7559

MICHIGAN

Wayne State University Harper University
  Hospital
Detroit, MI 48201
Program type: Adult
Directors: Dana G. Kissner, M.D.,
  Ayman Soubani, M.D.
(313) 745-9151

Children's Hospital of Michigan
Detroit, MI 48201
Pediatric Program Director:
  Ibrahim Abdulhamid, M.D.
(313) 745-5541

Michigan State University—Kalamazoo
  Center for Medical Studies
Center Director:
  Kalamazoo, MI 49008
Douglas Homnick, M.D., M.P.H.
(269) 337-6433

Helen DeVos Women and Children's Center
Grand Rapids, MI 49503
Program type: Adult
Director: Stephen Fitch, M.D.
(616) 391-2125

Grand Rapids CF Center
Grand Rapids, MI 49503
Pediatric Program Director:
  John Schuen, M.D.
(616) 391-2125

Michigan State University CF
  Center—Lansing
Lansing, MI 48912
Center Director:Myrtha
  Gregoire-Bottex, M.D.
(517) 364-5440

University of Michigan Health System
Ann Arbor, MI 48109
Program type: Adult
Director: Richard H. Simon, M.D.
(734) 647-9342

University of Michigan Health System
Ann Arbor, MI 48109
Pediatric Program Director:
  Samya Nasr, M.D.
(734) 936-4185

Hurley Children's Clinic at Mott
Children's Health Center Outreach
  Program
Flint, MI 48503
Program type: Outreach
Director: Cem Demirci, M.D.
(810) 257-9344

MINNESOTA

University of Minnesota
Minneapolis, MN 55455
Program type: Adult
Director: Jordan Dunitz, M.D.
(612) 625-5995

University of Minnesota
Minneapolis, MN 55455
Pediatric Program Director:
  Warren Regelmann, M.D.
(612) 625-5995
Children's Hospitals and Clinics
Minneapolis, MN 55404
Program type: Affiliate
Director: John McNamara, M.D.
(612) 813-3300

MISSOURI

The Children's Mercy Hospital—
  University of Missouri at Kansas City
Kansas City, MO 64108
Pediatric Program Director:
  Philip Black, M.D.
(816) 983-6490

Washington University School of
  Medicine
St. Louis, MO 63110
Program type: Adult
Director: Daniel Rosenbluth, M.D.
(314) 454-8640

St. Louis Children's Hospital Washington
  University School of Medicine
St. Louis, MO 63110
Pediatric Program Director:
  Thomas Ferkol Jr., M.D.
(314) 454-2694

University of Missouri
Columbia, MO 65212
Program type: Adult
Director: Melissa Kouba, M.D.
(573) 882-6978

Children's Hospital University of Missouri
  Health Sciences Center
Columbia, MO 65212
Pediatric Program Director:
  James Acton, M.D.
(573) 882-6921

Saint Louis University Medical Center
St. Louis, MO 63110
Program type: Adult
Director: Ravi P. Nayak, M.D.
(314) 977-6190

Cardinal Glennon Children's Medical
  Center (St. Louis University)
St. Louis, MO 63104
Pediatric Program Director:
  Blakeslee E. Noyes, B.A., M.D.,
  Gary Albers, M.D.
(314) 268-4107

Southeast Missouri Hospital–Outreach
  Clinic
Cape Girardeau, MO 63701
Program type: Outreach
Director: Connie Fenton, R.N., B.S.N.
(573) 882-6978

St. John's Speciality Clinic–Outreach
  Clinic
Springfield, MO 65804
Program type: Outreach
Contact: Connie Fenton, R.N., B.S.N.
(573) 882-6978

MISSISSIPPI

University of Mississippi Medical Center
Jackson, MS 39216
Program type: Adult
Director: Suzanne Miller, M.D.
(601) 815-1145

University of Mississippi Medical Center
Jackson, MS 39216
Pediatric Program Director:
  Joe Donaldson, M.D. (Interim)
(601) 984-5205

MONTANA

Saint Vincent's–Outreach Program
Billings, MT 59101
Program type: Outreach
(406) 237-4280

Great Falls–Outreach Clinic
Great Falls, MT 59401
Program type: Outreach
(406) 771-3388

NORTH CAROLINA

Duke University Medical Center
Durham, NC 27710
Program type: Adult
Director: Peter S. Kussin, M.D.
(919) 668-7630

Duke University Medical Center
Durham, NC 27710
Pediatric Program Director:
  Judith Voynow, M.D.,
  Thomas Miles Murphy, M.D.
(919) 681-3364

University of North Carolina at
  Chapel Hill
Chapel Hill, NC 27599
Program type: Adult
Directors: Michael R. Knowles, M.D.,
  James R. Yankaskas, M.D.
(919) 966-7933

University of North Carolina at
  Chapel Hill
Chapel Hill, NC 27599
Pediatric Program Director:
  Margaret W. Leigh, M.D.,
  George Retsch-Bogart, M.D.
(919) 966-1401

Wake Forest University Baptist Medical
  Center
Winston-Salem, NC 27157
Program type: Adult
Director: John Conforti, D.O.
(336) 713-4500

Wake Forest University Baptist Medical
  Center
Winston-Salem, NC 27157
Pediatric Program Director:
  Karl H. Karlson Jr., M.D.
(336) 713-4500

Mission Children's Clinic
Asheville, NC 28803
Program type: Affiliate
Director: Bruce K. Bacot, M.D.
(828) 213-1740

Asthma & Allergy Specialists, PA
Charlotte, NC 28277
Program type: Affiliate
Directors: William Ashe, M.D.,
  Hugh R. Black, M.D.
(704) 341-9600

NORTH DAKOTA

St. Alexius Heart and Lung Clinic
Bismarck, ND 58502

Pediatric Program Director:
  Carla Zacher, M.D., F.A.A.P.
(701) 530-7500

St. Alexius Heart and Lung Clinic
Bismarck, ND 58502
Program type: Adult
Director: James A. Hughes, M.D.
(701) 530-7500

MeritCare Medical Center
Fargo, ND 58102
Program type: Affiliate
Director: Stephen Tinguely, M.D.
(701) 234-6600

NEBRASKA

University of Nebraska Medical Center
Omaha, NE 68198
Program type: Adult
Director: Peter J. Murphy, M.D.
(402) 559-9101

University of Nebraska Medical Center
Omaha, NE 68198
Pediatric Program Director:
  John L. Colombo, M.D.
(402) 559-6275

NEW HAMPSHIRE

Dartmouth Hitchcock Medical Center
Lebanon, NH 3756
Pediatric Program Director:
  H. Worth Parker, M.D.
(603) 653-9884

Dartmouth Hitchcock Medical Center
Lebanon, NH 3756
Pediatric Program Director:
  Pamela Hofley, M.D.
(603) 653-9884

NEW JERSEY

Bristol-Myers Squibb Children's
  Hospital at Robert Wood Johnson
  University Hospital

New Brunswick, NJ 9801
Program type: Adult
Director: William Sexauer, M.D.
(732) 235-6511

Bristol-Myers Squibb Children's Hospital
  at Robert Wood Johnson University
  Hospital
New Brunswick, NJ 9801
Pediatric Program Director:
  Thomas F. Scanlin, M.D.
(732) 235-5210

Monmouth Medical Center
Long Branch, NJ 7724
Program type: Adult
Director: Doantrang Du, M.D.
(732) 222-4474

Monmouth Medical Center
Long Branch, NJ 7740
Pediatric Program Director:
  Robert L. Zanni, M.D.
(732) 222-4474

Morristown Memorial Hospital
Morristown, NJ 7962
Program type: Adult
Directors: Stanley B. Fiel, M.D.,
  Frederic Scoopo, M.D.
(973) 971-4103

Goryeb Children's Hospital of Atlantic
  Health System
Morristown, NJ 7962
Pediatric Program Director:
  Arthur B. Atlas, M.D.
(973) 971-4142

Saint Barnabas Medical Center
Livingston, NJ 7039
Program type: Affiliate
Director: Dorothy S. Bisberg, M.D.
(973) 322-7600

St. Joseph's Children's Hospital
Paterson, NJ 7503
Program type: Affiliate

Director: Roberto V. Nachajon, M.D.
(973) 754-2550

NEW MEXICO

University of New Mexico School of
 Medicine
Albuquerque, NM 87131
Program type: Adult
Director: Diane Goade, M.D.
(505) 272-4992

University of New Mexico School of
 Medicine
Albuquerque, NM 87131
Pediatric Program Director:
 Lea Davies, M.D.
(505) 272-6633

NEVADA

Adult Cystic Fibrosis Center
Las Vegas, NV 89107
Program type: Adult
Director: Angelica Honsberg, M.D.
(702) 598-4411

University of Nevada School of Medicine
 Children's Lung Specialists
Las Vegas, NV 89107
Pediatric Program Director:
 Craig T. Nakamura, M.D.
(702) 598-4411

Renown Regional Medical Center
 Children's Hospital
Reno, NV 89503
Program type: Affiliate
Director: Sonia Budhecha, M.D.
(775) 785-6522

NEW YORK

Albany Medical College
Albany, NY 12208
Program type: Adult
Director: Jonathan M. Rosen, M.D.
(518) 262-5196

Albany Medical College
Albany, NY 12208
Pediatric Program Director:
 Paul G. Comber, M.D., Ph.D.
(518) 262-6880

Women and Children's Hospital of
 Buffalo
Buffalo, NY 14222
Program type: Adult
Director: Michael Aronica, M.D., M.P.H.
(716) 878-7524

Women and Children's Hospital of
 Buffalo
Buffalo, NY 14222
Pediatric Program Director:
 Drucy Borowitz, M.D.
(716) 878-7524

Columbia University, Adult Cystic Fibrosis
 Program
New York City, NY 10032
Program type: Adult
Director: Emily DiMango, M.D.
(212) 305-0290

Children's Hospital of New York Columbia
 University
New York City, NY 10032
Pediatric Program Director:
 Lynne M. Quittell, M.D.
(212) 305-5122

University of Rochester Medical Center,
 Strong Memorial Hospital
Rochester, NY 14642
Program type: Adult
Director: Robert Horowitz, M.D.
(585) 654-5432

University of Rochester Medical Center,
 Strong Memorial Hospital
Rochester, NY 14642
Pediatric Program Director:
 Karen Z. Voter, M.D.,
 Clement L. Ren, M.D.
(585) 275-2464

University Medical Center at Stony Brook
Stony Brook, NY 11794
Center Director:
  Catherine Kier, M.D.
(631) 444-8340

Long Island Jewish Medical Center
New Hyde Park, NY 11040
Program type: Adult
Director: Rubin I. Cohen, M.D.
(516) 465-5400

The Steven & Alexandra Cohen Children's
  Medical Center of New York
Great Neck, NY 11021
Pediatric Program Director:
  Joan K. DeCelie-Germana, M.D.
(516) 622-5280

New York Medical College/Westchester
  Medical Center
Valhalla, NY 10595
Program type: Adult
Director: Caren Behar, M.D.
(914) 493-7585

The Children's Hospital at Westchester
  Medical Center/New York Medical
  College
Valhalla, NY 10595
Pediatric Program Director:
  Allen J. Dozor, M.D.
(914) 493-7585

SUNY Upstate Medical University
Syracuse, NY 13210
Program type: Adult
Director: James Sexton, M.D.
(315) 464-6323

SUNY Upstate Medical University
Syracuse, NY 13210
Pediatric Program Director:
  Ran D. Anbar, M.D.
(315) 464-6323

Mount Sinai School of Medicine
New York City, NY 10029

Program type: Affiliate
Directors: Richard J. Bonforte, M.D.,
  Andrew Ting, M.D.
(212) 241-7788

Samaritan Medical Center and Child &
  Adolescent Health Associates
Watertown, NY 13601
Program type: Affiliate
Director: Ronald Perciaccante, M.D.
(315) 785-4046

Good Samaritan Hospital
West Islip, NY 11795
Program type: Affiliate
Director: Louis Guida Jr., M.D.
(631) 321-2100

OHIO

University Hospitals Case Medical
  Center/Rainbow Babies and
  Children's Hospital
Cleveland, OH 44106
Program type: Adult
Director: Steven D. Strausbaugh, M.D.,
  F.C.C.P.
(216) 844-7700

University Hospitals Case Medical
  Center/Rainbow Babies and
  Children's Hospital
Cleveland, OH 44106
Pediatric Program Director:
  Michael W. Konstan, M.D.
(216) 844-7700

Nationwide Children's Hospital
Columbus, OH 43205
Program type: Adult
Director: John Heintz, M.D.
(614) 722-4766

Nationwide Children's Hospital
Columbus, OH 43205
Pediatric Program Director:
  Karen S. McCoy, M.D.
(614) 722-4766

Children's Hospital Medical Center of
  Akron
Akron, OH 44308
Program type: Adult
Director: Titus Sheers, M.D.
(330) 543-3249

Children's Hospital Medical Center of
  Akron
Akron, OH 44308
Pediatric Program Director:
  Nathan C. Kraynack, M.D.
(330) 543-3249

Wright State University School of Medicine
Dayton, OH 45404
Program type: Adult
Director: Gary M. Onady, M.D., Ph.D.
(937) 641-3440

The Children's Medical Center of Dayton
Dayton, OH 45404
Pediatric Program Director:
  Robert J. Fink, M.D.
(937) 641-3440

University of Cincinnati Medical Center
Cincinnati, OH 45267
Program type: Adult
Director: Patricia M. Joseph, M.D.
(513) 475-8523

Cincinnati Children's Hospital Medical
  Center
Cincinnati, OH 45229
Pediatric Program Director:
  Raouf Amin, M.D.
(513) 636-6771

Northwest Ohio Cystic Fibrosis Center
Toledo, OH 43606
Program type: Adult
Director: Jeffrey Lewis, M.D.
(419) 291-2207

Northwest Ohio Cystic Fibrosis Center–
  Pediatric Program
Toledo, OH 43606

Pediatric Program Director:
  Pierre A. Vauthy, M.D.
(419) 291-2207

OKLAHOMA

Oklahoma Cystic Fibrosis Center–Adult
  Program
Oklahoma City, OK 73104
Program type: Adult
Director: Kellie Jones, M.D.
(405) 271-6390

Oklahoma Cystic Fibrosis Center
Oklahoma City, OK 73104
Pediatric Program Director:
  James Royall, M.D.
(405) 271-6390

Oklahoma Cystic Fibrosis Center—Tulsa
Tulsa, OK 74129
Program type: Affiliate
Director: James Royall, M.D. (Interim)
(918) 660-3679

OREGON

Oregon Health Sciences University
Portland, OR 97201
Program type: Adult
Director: Gopal Allada, M.D.
(503) 494-1620

Oregon Health Sciences University
Portland, OR 97201
Pediatric Program Director:
  Michael Wall, M.D.
(503) 494-8023

Kaiser Permanente Northwest Region
Portland, OR 97227
Program type: Affiliate
Director: Richard C. Cohen, M.D.
(503) 331-5877

PENNSYLVANIA

University of Pennsylvania Hospital
Philadelphia, PA 19104

Program type: Adult
Director: Denis Hadjiliadis, M.D., M.H.S.
(215) 662-8766

Children's Hospital of Philadelphia
  University of Pennsylvania
Philadelphia, PA 19104
Pediatric Program Director:
  Ronald Rubenstein, M.D., Ph.D.
(215) 590-3749

Drexel University of Medicine,
  Hahnemann University Hospital
Philadelphia, PA 19129
Program type: Adult
Director: Jeffrey Hoag, M.D.,
  M.S., F.C.C.P.
(215) 762-7581

Drexel University College of Medicine,
  St. Christopher's Hospital for
  Children
Philadelphia, PA 19134
Pediatric Program Director:
  Laurie Varlotta, M.D.
(215) 427-5183

University of Pittsburgh School of
  Medicine
Pittsburgh, PA 15213
Program type: Adult
Directors: Joel H. Weinberg, M.D., Joseph
  M. Pilewski, M.D.
(412) 648-6161

Children's Hospital of Pittsburgh of
  UPMC—University of Pittsburgh
Pittsburgh, PA 15213
Pediatric Program Director: David M.
  Orenstein, M.D., Daniel Weiner, M.D.
(412) 692-5661

Hershey Medical Center Pennsylvania
  State University
Hershey, PA 17033
Program type: Adult
Director: Robert L. Vender, M.D.
(717) 531-6525

Hershey Medical Center Pennsylvania
  State University
Hershey, PA 17033
Pediatric Program Director:
  Gavin R. Graff, M.D., W. Stuart
  Warren, M.D.
(717) 531-5338

Lehigh Valley Hospital & Health Network
Bethlehem, PA 18017
Program type: Affiliate
Directors: Robert W. Miller, M.D.,
  Dharmesh Suratwala, M.D., M.B.B.A.
(484) 884-3333

Geisinger Medical Center
Danville, PA 17822
Program type: Affiliate
Director: Carlos Perez, M.D.
(570) 271-7910

Saint Luke's Hospital–Outreach Clinic
Bethlehem, PA 18017
Program type: Outreach
Director: Laurie Varlotta, M.D.
(610) 954-4975

RHODE ISLAND

Brown University Medical School
Providence, RI 2903
Program type: Adult
Director: Walter Donat, M.D.
(401) 444-6540

Brown University Medical School Rhode
  Island Hospital Cystic Fibrosis Center
Providence, RI 2903
Pediatric Program Director:
  Mary Ann Passero, M.D.
(401) 444-6540

SOUTH CAROLINA

University of South Carolina
Columbia, SC 29203
Center Director: Daniel C. Brown, M.D.
(803) 434-2505

Medical University of South Carolina
Charleston, SC 29425
Program type: Adult
Director: Patrick A. Flume, M.D.
(843) 792-0729

Medical University of South Carolina
Charleston, SC 29403
Pediatric Program Director:
  Isabel Virella-Lowell, M.D.
(843) 876-1555

Children's Respiratory Center
Greenville, SC 29605
Program type: Affiliate
Director: Jane Vance Gwinn, M.D.
(864) 220-8000

SOUTH DAKOTA

Sanford USD Medical Center
Sioux Falls, SD 57117
Program type: Adult
Directors: Susan Rohr, M.D.,
  David Thomas, M.D.
(605) 312-1000

Sanford USD Medical Center
Sioux Falls, SD 57117
Pediatric Program Director:
  James Wallace, M.D.
(605) 312-1000

TENNESSEE

University of Tennessee Adult CF Program
Memphis, TN 38104
Program type: Adult
Director: Amado Freire, M.D., M.P.H.
(901) 545-6969

University of Tennessee HSC Le Bonheur
  Children's Medical Center
Memphis, TN 38103
Pediatric Program Director:
  Dennis C. Stokes, M.D.
(901) 287-5222

Vanderbilt University Medical Center
Nashville, TN 37232
Program type: Adult
Director: Bonnie S. Slovis, M.D.
(615) 322-2386

Vanderbilt Children's Hospital
  Vanderbilt University Medical
  Center
Nashville, TN 37232
Pediatric Program Director:
  Elizabeth Perkett, M.D.
(615) 343-7617

T.C. Thompson Children's Hospital
Chattanooga, TN 37403
Program type: Affiliate
Director: Joel C. Ledbetter, M.D.
(423) 778-6501

East Tennessee Children's Hospital
Knoxville, TN 37916
Program type: Affiliate
Director: John Rogers, M.D.,
  Eduardo Riff, M.D.
(865) 637-8481

TEXAS

Baylor College of Medicine/
  Baylor Clinic/The Methodist
  Hospital
Houston, TX 77030
Program type: Adult
Director: Marcia Katz, M.D.
(713) 798-2500

Baylor College of Medicine/
  Texas Children's Hospital
Houston, TX 77030
Pediatric Program Director:
  Christopher M. Oermann, M.D.,
  Peter Hiatt, M.D.
(832) 822-2778

St. Paul Medical Center
Dallas, TX 75235

Program type: Adult
Director: Randall L. Rosenblatt,
  M.D., B.A.
(214) 456-2361

Children's Medical Center of Dallas
Dallas, TX 75235
Pediatric Program Director:
  Claude B. Prestidge, M.D.
(214) 456-2361

Cook Children's Medical Center
Fort Worth, TX 76104
Program type: Adult
Directors: John Burk, M.D.,
  Steven Q. Davis, M.D., M.S., F.C.C.P.
(682) 885-6299

Texas Tech University Health Sciences
  Center
Lubbock, TX 79430
Program type: Affiliate
Director: Adaobi Kanu, M.D.
(806) 743-7337

Cook Children's Medical Center
Fort Worth, TX 76104
Pediatric Program Director:
  James C. Cunningham, M.D.,
  Nancy L. Dambro, M.D.
(682) 885-6299

Tri-Services Military Cystic Fibrosis
  Center—FOR MILITARY
  PERSONNEL ONLY
Fort Sam Houston, TX 78234
Program type: Affiliate
Director: Catherine Shoff, M.D.
(210) 916-4927

Tri-Services Military Cystic Fibrosis
  Center—FOR MILITARY
  PERSONNEL ONLY
Fort Sam Houston, TX 78234
Pediatric Program Director:
  John M. Palmer, M.D.
(210) 916-4927

Christus Santa Rosa Children's
  Hospital
San Antonio, TX 78207
Program type: Adult
Director: Peter Fornos, M.D.
(210) 704-4100

Christus Santa Rosa Children's Hospital
San Antonio, TX 78207
Pediatric Program Director:
  Donna Beth Willey-Courand, M.D.
(210) 704-4100

Dell Children's Medical Center of Central
  Texas
Austin, TX 78723
Program type: Affiliate
Directors: Bennie McWilliams, M.D.,
  Allan Frank, M.D.
(512) 324-8264

Allergy Alliance of the Permian Basin
Midland, TX 79701
Program type: Affiliate
Director: John D. Bray, M.D.
(432) 561-8183

Children's Hospital at Scott & White
Temple, TX 76508
Program type: Affiliate
Director: John Saito, M.D.
(254) 724-3227

University of Texas Health Center at
  Tyler
Tyler, TX 75708
Program type: Affiliate
Director: Rodolfo Amaro, M.D.
(903) 877-7777

Texas Tech University Health Sciences
  Center–Outreach Clinic
Amarillo, TX 79106
Program type: Outreach
Directors: James C. Cunningham, M.D.,
  Maynard Dyson, M.D.
(806) 354-5437

UTAH

Intermountain Cystic Fibrosis Center
University of Utah Health Sciences
Center
Salt Lake City, UT 84132
Program type: Adult
Directors: Ted G. Liou, M.D.,
Holly Carveth, M.D.
(801) 585-2804

Intermountain Cystic Fibrosis Center
University of Utah Health Sciences Center
Salt Lake City, UT 84132
Pediatric Program Director:
Barbara Chatfield, M.D.
(801) 662-1765

VIRGINIA

University of Virginia
Charlottesville, VA 22908
Program type: Adult
Director: Mark K. Robbins, M.D.
(434) 924-9687

University of Virginia
Pediatric Program Director:
Charlottesville, VA 22908
Deborah K. Froh, M.D.
(434) 924-2250

Virginia Commonwealth University
Richmond, VA 23235
Center Director: H. Joel Schmidt, M.D.
(804) 828-2982

Children's Hospital of the King's
Daughters
Norfolk, VA 23507
Program type: Adult
Director: Ignacio Ripoll, M.D.
(757) 668-7137

Children's Hospital of the King's Daughters
Eastern Virginia Medical School
Norfolk, VA 23507

Pediatric Program Director:
Cynthia A. Epstein, M.D.
(757) 668-7137

Pediatric Lung Center Inova Fairfax
Hospital
Fairfax, VA 22031
Program type: Affiliate
Director: John Osborn, M.D.
(703) 289-1410

Naval Medical Center, Portsmouth—
FOR MILITARY PERSONNEL ONLY
Portsmouth, VA 23708
Program type: Affiliate
Director: Rees Lee, M.D.
(757) 953-2955

VERMONT

Fletcher Allen Health Care
Burlington, VT 5401
Program type: Adult
Director: Laurie A. Whittaker, M.D.
(802) 847-1158

Vermont Children's Hospital
Burlington, VT 5401
Pediatric Program Director:
Thomas Lahiri, M.D.
(802) 847-8600

WASHINGTON

University of Washington Medical
Center
Seattle, WA 98195
Program type: Adult
Director: Moira L. Aitken, M.D.
(206) 598-4615

Pediatric Pulmonary and CF Clinic
Spokane, WA 99210
Program type: Affiliate
Director: Michael M. McCarthy, M.D.
(509) 474-6960

Seattle Children's Hospital
Seattle, WA 98105
Pediatric Program Director: Ronald L.
  Gibson, M.D., Ph.D.
(206) 987-2024

Madigan Army Medical Center—FOR
  MILITARY PERSONNEL ONLY
Tacoma, WA 98431
Program type: Affiliate
Director: Donald Moffitt, M.D.
(253) 968-1878

Mary Bridge Children's Health Center
Tacoma, WA 98405
Program type: Affiliate
Directors: Lawrence A. Larson, D.O.,
  David H. Ricker, M.D.
(253) 403-3131

WISCONSIN

University of Wisconsin
Madison, WI 53792
Program type: Adult
Director: Guillermo A. doPico, M.D.
(608) 263-7203

University of Wisconsin
Madison, WI 53792
Pediatric Program Director: Michael J.
  Rock, M.D.
(608) 263-6420

Froedtert & Medical College of
  Wisconsin
Milwaukee, WI 53201
Program type: Adult
Director: Julie A. Biller, M.D.
(414) 805-9401

Children's Hospital of Wisconsin
  Froedtert & Medical College of
  Wisconsin

Milwaukee, WI 53201
Pediatric Program Director:
  Diana Quintero, M.D.
(414) 266-6730

Saint Vincent's Hospital
Green Bay, WI 54301
Program type: Affiliate
Director: Peter Holzwarth, M.D.
(920) 433-8508

Gundersen Lutheran Medical Center
La Crosse, WI 54601
Program type: Affiliate
Director: Todd Mahr, M.D.
(608) 775-5848

Marshfield Clinic
Marshfield, WI 54449
Program type: Affiliate
Director: Bradley J. Sullivan, M.D.
(715) 387-5251

WEST VIRGINIA

West Virginia University CF Center
Morgantown, WV 26505
Pediatric Program Director: Kathryn S.
  Moffett, M.D.
(304) 293-1227

West Virginia University Charleston
  Division
Charleston, WV 25302
Program type: Affiliate
Director: Raheel Khan, M.D., F.A.A.P.
(304) 388-1552

County Health Department–Outreach
  Program
Casper, WY 82601
Program type: Outreach
(307) 235-9340

Cystic Fibrosis Care Centers Worldwide

ARGENTINA

Ciudad de Buenos Aires
Centro Nacional de Genetica Medica
Dpto. Genética Experimental
Av. Las Heras 2670–4º Piso
1425 Ciudad de Buenos Aires
pivetta@genes.gov.ar
54.11.48012326/54.11.48092000
  (int. 2163)

Ciudad de Buenos Aires
Hospital "Maria Ferrer"
Finochietto 849
1272 Ciudad de Buenos Aires
54.11.43071445
(Contact Person: Dr. Enrique)

Ciudad de Buenos Aires
Hospital de Niños "Ricardo Gutierrez"
Unidad No. 3
Sánchez de Bustamante 1399
1425 Ciudad de Buenos Aires
54.11.49629212/54.11.49629229/
  54.11.49629232

Ciudad de Buenos Aires
Hospital de Pediatria "Dr. Pedro de
  Elizalde"
Av. Montes de Oca 40
1270 Ciudad de Buenos Aires
(54)11.43074788/11.43075553/
  11.43075842

Ciudad de Buenos Aires
Hospital de Pediatria
  "Prof. Dr. Juan Garrahan"
Combate de los Pozos 1881
1245 Ciudad de Buenos Aires
54.11.49431455

Buenos Aires
La Plata
Hospital de Niños "Sor Maria Ludovica"
Calle 14 entre 65 y 66
1900 La Plata (Pcia. Buenos Aires)
54.0221.4210448

Córdoba
Hospital de Niños
Corrientes 643
5000 Córdoba
(Contact Person: Dr. Carlos Rezzónico)

Mendoza
Hospital "Emilio Civit"
Parque Gral. San Martín
5300 Mendoza

Neuquén
Hospital de Neuquén
Buenos Aires 353
8400 Neuquén

Santa Fe
Granadero Baigorria
Hospital Escuela "Eva Perón"

Ruta 11s/No
2152 Granadero Baigorria
54.0341.4710940

Santa Fe
Rosario
Hospital Provincial "Del Centenario"
Urquiza 3101
2000 Rosario (Pcia. Santa Fe)
54.0341.4307320

Santa Fe
Rosario
Hospital de Niños "Víctor J. Vilela"
Virasoro 1855
2000 Rosario (Pcia. Santa Fe)
54.0341.4808125

Santa Fe
Hospital "J.B. Iturraspe"
Boulevard Pellegrini 3551
3000 Santa Fe

Santa Fe
Hospital de Niños "Dr. O. Alassia"
Mendoza 4551
3000 Santa Fe

AUSTRALIA

Ibn Al-Haytham Hospital
962.6.5516823
(Contact Person:
   Dr. M. Rawashdeh Amman)

Adelaide
The Royal Adelaide Hospital CF
   Adult Clinic
275 North Terrace
Adelaide SA 5000
61.8.82225132/61.8.82225957
(Contact Person: Dr. Hugh Greville)
Adult: Yes

Bundaberg
Bundaberg Base Hospital
Bundaberg
QLD 4760

61.7.41520699
(Contact Person: Dr. J. Williams/
   Dr. C. Ryan)

Cairns
Flecker House
5 Upward Street
Cairns
QLD 4870
61.7.40515430/61.7.40310686
(Contact Person: Dr. R. Messer)

Cairns
Flecker House
130 Abbott Street
Cairns
QLD 4870
61.7.40314095/61.7.40518411
(Contact Person: Dr. G. Simpson)

Camperdown
Cystic Fibrosis Adult Clinic
Royal Prince Alfred Hospital
Missenden Road
Camperdown, NSW 2050
61.2.95157427/61.2.95158196
(Contact Person: Prof. Peter Bye)

Chermside
The Prince Charles Hospital
Rode Road
Chermside
QLD 4032
61.7.33508406/61.7.33508510
(Contact Person: Dr. Scott Bell)
Adult: Yes

Clayton
Monash Medical Centre
Department of Paediatric Respiratory
   Medicine
Monash Medical Centre
Locked Bag 29
Clayton, VIC 3168
61.3.95942045/61.3.95945415
(Contact Person: Dr. David Armstrong/
   Dr. Peter Solin)

Gosford
Gosford District Hospital Cystic Fibrosis
  Clinic
Holden Street
Gosford NSW 2250
61.2.43245077/61.2.43250629
(Contact Person: Dr. J. Pendergast)

Herston
Royal Brisbane Hospital
Herston
QLD 4006
61.7.32538111/61.7.32571765
(Contact Person: Dr. I. Brown)

Herston
Royal Children's Hospital
Herston Road
Herston
QLD 4006
61.7.36365270/61.7.36361958
(Contact Person: Dr. Paul Francis)

Hobart
Royal Hobart Hospital
48 Liverpool Street
Hobart
TAS 7000
61.3.62228475/61.3.62228951
(Contact Person: Dr. Ian Stewart/
  Dr. Colin Sherrington)

Launceston
Launceston General Hospital
Charles Street
Launceston, TAS 7250
61.3.63327111/61.3.63327577
(Contact Person: Dr. J. Markos)

Mackay
Mackay Base Hospital
Mackay, QLD 4740
61.7.49686000
(Contact Person: Dr. M. Williams)

Nedlands
Sir Charles Gairdner Hospital Adult CF
  Clinic

Verdun Street
Nedlands, WA 6009
61.8.93463251/61.8.93463606
(Contact Person: Dr. Gerard Ryan)
Adult: Yes

New Lambton Heights
Dr. D. Cooper/Dr. Peter Gibson
Lookout Road
New Lambton Heights
NSW 2305
61.2.49213676/61.2.49213599
(Contact Person: John Hunter Children's
  Hospital)

North Adelaide
Dr. James Martin
King William Road
North Adelaide, SA 5006
61.8.82047234/61.8.82047050
(Contact Person: Women's & Children's
  Hospital)

Parkville
Royal Children's Hospital
Flemington Road
Parkville, VIC 3052
61.3.93455844/61.3.93491289
(Contact Person: Dr. Phil Robinson)

Perth
Princess Margaret Hospital for Children
G.P.O. Box D184
Perth, WA 6001
61.8.93408830/61.8.93408983
(Contact Person: Dr. Barry Clements)

Prahran
The Alfred Hospital CF Adult Clinic
Commercial Road
Prahran, VIC 3181
61.3.92763476/61.3.92763434
(Contact Person: Prof. John Wilson)

Randwick
Prince of Wales Hospital
High Street
Randwick, NSW 2131

61.2.93824631/61.2.93824627
(Contact Person: Dr. Frank Maccioni)
Adult: Yes

Randwick
The Sydney Children's Hospital Cystic
  Fibrosis Clinic
High Street
Randwick, NSW 2131
61.2.93821477/61.2.93821580
(Contact Person: Dr. John Morton)

Rockhampton
Rockhampton Base Hospital
Rockhampton, QLD 4700
61.7.49206211
(Contact Person: Dr. L. Gray)

South Brisbane
Mater Children's Hospital
Raymond Terrace
South Brisbane, QLD 4101
61.7.38394870/61.7.38401178/
  61.7.38328201
(Contact Person: Dr. Ian Robertson/
  Dr. Simon Bowler)

Southport
Allamanda Medical Centre
Suite 5, 25 Spendelove Avenue
Southport, QLD 4215
61.7.55327755/61.7.55329413
(Contact Person: Dr. Darrell Price)
Children: Yes

Southport
Gold Coast Hospital
Nerang Street
Southport, QLD 4215
61.7.55718649/61.7.55718996
(Contact Person: Dr. Iain Feather)

Townsville
Townsville Base Hospital
Townsville, QLD 4810
61.7.47819211
(Contact Person: Dr. W. Frischmann/
  Dr. P. Ryan)

Westmead
Cystic Fibrosis Adult Clinic Westmead
  Hospital
Hawkesbury Road
Westmead, NSW 2145
61.2.98456797/61.2.98457286
(Contact Person: Dr. Peter Middleton)

Westmead
New Children's Hospital
Department of Respiratory Medicine
New Children's Hospital
Hawkesbury Road
Westmead, NSW 2145
61.2.98453395/61.2.98453396
(Contact Person: Dr. Peter Cooper)

BELGIUM

Antwerpen
CF Clinic St. Vincentiusziekenhuis
St. Vincentiusstraat 20
2018 Antwerpen
32 3 285 20 00/Fax: 32 3 285 28 85
(Contact Person: Dr. L. van Schil)
Adult: Yes

Bruxelles
CF Clinic Hôpital Erasme ULB
Route de Lennik 808
1070 Bruxelles
+32 2 526 39 85/+32 2 555 44 14
(Contact Person: Dr. Cnoop)
Adult: Yes

Bruxelles
CF Clinic Hôpital Universitaire des
  Enfants Reine Fabiola
Place Van Gehuchten
1020 Bruxelles
+32 2 477 21 11/+32 2 477 32 78
(Contact Person: Dr. Casimir)
Children: Yes

Bruxelles
CF Clinic U.C.L. Saint-Luc
Avenue Hippocrate 10
1200 Bruxelles

32.2.7641385/32.2.7648911
(Contact Person: Dr. Lebecque)

Bruxelles
CF Clinic UZ Brussel
Laarbeeklaan 101
1090 Bruxelles
32 2 477 41 11/Fax: 32 2 477 58 00
(Contact Person: Prof. Dr. A. Malfroot)
Children: Yes
Adult: Yes

De Haan
Rehabilitation centre Zeepreventorium
Koninklijke Baan 5
8420 de Haan
32 59 23 39 11/32 59 23 40 57
(Contact Person: Dr. H. Franckx)

Edegem
CF Clinic UZ Antwerpen
Wilrijkstraat 10
2650 Edegem
32.3.8213537/32.3.8291194
(Contact Person: Prof. Kristine Desager)
Children: Yes

Gent
CF Clinic UZ Gent
De Pintelaan 185
9000 Gent
32.9.2402111/32.9.2403875
(Contact Person: Prof. Dr. Robberecht/
Prof. F. DE Baets)

Leuven
CF Clinic UZ Gasthuisberg
Herestraat 49
3000 Leuven
32.16.332211/32.16.343842
(Contact Person: Prof. Dr. C. de Boeck/
Prof Lebecque)
Children: Yes
Adult: Yes

Liege
CF Clinic CHR de la Citadelle
bld. du 12è de Ligne 1

4000 Liege
32 41 25 61 11/Fax: 32 41 26 47 47
(Contact Person: Dr. Leclercq)

Pulderbos
Rehabilitation Centre
Revalidatiecentrum Voor
Kinderen en Jongeren
Reebergenlaan 4
2240 Pulderbos
32.3.4843600/32.3.4845770
(Contact Person: Dr. Schuddinck)
Children: Yes

CANADA

Calgary
Alberta Children CF Clinic
Lisa Semple
1820 Richmond Road S.W., Calgary,
AB T2T 5C7
1.403.2097319/1.403. 2297647
Children: Yes

Calgary
Southern Alberta Adult CF Clinic
TBA University of Calgary Medical
Clinic–Area 6
Foothills Hospital
1403–29 Street N.W.
Calgary, AB T2N 2T9
1.403.6704365/1.403.2702772
Adult: Yes

Edmonton
University of Alberta Hospitals
112 Street and 84th Avenue
7–109 Clinical Sciences Building
Edmonton, AB T6G 2B7
1.780.4076745/1.780.4073112
(Contact Person: Joan Tabak)

Vancouver
B.C. Children
4480 Oak Street
Vancouver, BC V6 H 3V4
1.604.8752146/1.604.8752349
(Contact Person: Anna Gravelle)

Vancouver
St. Paul's Hospital
1081 Burrard Street
Vancouver, BC V6Z 1Y6
1.604.8068522/1.604.8068122
(Contact Person: Janet Hopkins)

Victoria
Victoria General Hospital
35 Helmcken Road
Victoria, BC V8Z 6R5
1.250.7274187/1.250.7274223/
  1.250.7274221
(Contact Person: Eleanor Shambrook/
  Sharon Wiltse)

Winnipeg
Children's Hospital of Winnipeg
840 Sherbrook Street
Winnipeg, MB R3A 1S1
1.204.7872401/1.204.7871944
(Contact Person: Marilyn Lowe)

Winnipeg
Health Science Centre
810 Sherbrook Street
Winnipeg, MB R3A 1R8
1.204.7871521/1.204.7872420
(Contact Person: Tamara Wells)

Saint john
Saint John Regional Hospital
P.O. Box 2100
Saint John, NB E2L 4L2
1.506.6486793/1.506.6486060
(Contact Person: Diana Peacock)

The Janeway Child Health Centre
Elizabeth Sheppard
710 Newfoundland Drive
St. John's, NB A1A 1R8
1.709.7784389/1.709.7784333
(Contact Person: St. John)

Halifax
IWK Grace Health Centre
5850 University Avenue
Halifax, NS B3J 3G9

1.902.4288219/1.902.4283223
(Contact Person: Paula Barrett)

Halifax
Queen Elizabeth II Health Sciences
  Centre
1796 Robie Street
Halifax, NS B3H 3A7
1.902.4734147/1.902.4736202
(Contact Person: Fran Gosse)

Hamilton
Hamilton Health Sciences
  Corporation
Mcmaster Campus Department
  of Pediatrics
1200 Main Street West, Room 3F18
Hamilton, ON L8N 3Z5
1.905.5212100/1.905.5273086/
  1.905.5212654
(Contact Person: Rosamund Hennessey)

Kingston
Hotel dieu Hospital
166 Brock Street
Kingston, ON K7L 5G2
1.613.5443400/1.613.5448320
(Contact Person: Darlene McCulloch)

Kitchener
Kitchener-Waterloo Health Centre of
  Grand River Hospital
835 King Street West
Kitchener, ON N2G 1G3
1.519.7494300/1.519.7492622/
  1.519. 7494317
(Contact Person: Joy Geiger)

London
Children's Hospital of Western Ontario
London Health Sciences Centre
London, ON N6A 4G5
1.519.6858500 ext. 52692/
  1.519.6858130
(Contact Person: Elizabeth Hunter)

Ottawa
Children's Hospital of Eastern Ontario

401 Smyth Road
Ottawa, ON K1H 8L1
1.613.7372214/1.613.7384832
(Contact Person: Anne Smith)

Ottawa
Ottawa General Hospital
501 Smyth Road
Ottawa, ON K1H 8L6
1.613.7378198/1.613.7396266
(Contact Person: Kathleen Devecseri)

Sudbury
Laurentian Hospital
41 Chemin Du Lac Ramsey
Sudbury, ON P3E 5J1
1.705.5222200/1.705.5223263/
  1.705.5237089
(Contact Person: Charlene Piche)

Toronto
St. Michael's Hospital
30 Bond Street
Toronto, ON M5B 1W8
1.416.8645409/1.416. 8645651
(Contact Person: Anna Tsang)

Toronto
The Hospital for Sick Children
555 University Avenue
Toronto, ON M5G 1×8
1.416.8135826/1.416.8136246
(Contact Person: Louise Taylor)

Windsor
Hotel Dieu Grace Hospital
1030 Ouellette Avenue
Windsor, ON N9A 1E1
1.519.9734431/1.519.2589918
(Contact Person: Dagmar Ray)

Québec
Chicoutimi
Hôpital de Chicoutimi
C.P. 5006
Chicoutimi (Québec) G7H 5H6
1.418.5411037/1.418. 5411134
(Contact Person: Suzanne Mignault)

Québec
Fleurimont
Centre Universitaire de Santé
  de L'Estrie
3001 12E Av. Nord
Fleurimont (Québec) J1H 5N4
1.819.3461110/1.819.3412820/
  1.819.8206454
(Contact Person: Marguerite Plante)

Québec
Gatineau
Centre Hospitalier de Gatineau
909 Boul. de la Vérendrye Ouest
C.P. 2000
Gatineau (Québec) J8P 7H2
1.819.5618195/1.819.5618390
(Contact Person: Thérèse Faucher)

Québec
Hull
Centre Hospitalier Régional de
  L'Outaouais
116 Boul. Lionel Émond
Hull (Québec) J8Y 1W7
1.819.5956053/1.819.5951582
(Contact Person: Denise Lévesque)

Québec
Montréal
Centre Hospitalier Thoracique de
  Montréal
3650 Rue Saint-Urbain
Montréal (Québec) H2X 2P4
1.514.8495201/1.514.8495280/
  1.514. 8432076
(Contact Person: France Paquet)

Québec
Montréal
Hôpital de Montréal Pour
  Enfants
2300 Rue Tupper
Montréal (Québec) H3H 1P3
1.514.9344400/1.514.9342643/
  1.514.9344364
(Contact Person: Jackie Townshend)
Children: Yes

Québec
Montréal
Hôpital Sainte-Justine
3175 Chemin de la Côte-Ste-Catherine
Montréal (Québec) H3T 1C5
1.514.3454724/1.514.3454804
(Contact Person: Diane Dupont)

Québec
Montréal
Hôtel-Dieu de Montréal
Service de Pneumologie
Hôtel-Dieu de Montréal
3840 Rue Saint-Urbain
Montréal (Québec) H2W 1T8
1.514.8432670/1.514.8432769
(Contact Person: Jocelyne Lavallée)

Québec
Rimouski
Centre Hospitalier Régional
  de Rimouski
150 Av. Rouleau
Rimouski (Québec) G5L 5T1
1.418.7248561/1.418.7248615
(Contact Person: Francine Raymond)

Québec
Rouyn-Noranda
Centre Hospitalier Rouyn-Noranda
4 9E Rue
Rouyn-Noranda (Québec) J9X 2B2
1.819.7620995/1.819.7976837
(Contact Person: Louise Boucher)

Québec
Ste-Foy
Centre Hospitalier de L'Universite Laval
2705 Boul. Sir Wilfrid-Laurier
Ste-Foy (Québec) G1V 4G2
1.418.6564141/1.418.6567730/
  1.418.6542137
(Contact Person: Manon Roussin)

Regina
Regina General Hospital
1440–14th Avenue
Regina, SK S4P 0W5

1.306.7664289/1.306.7664946
(Contact Person: Marlene Hall)

Saskatoon
University Hospital
Saskatoon, SK S7N 0×0
1.306.9668120/1.306.9753767
(Contact Person: Cathy Turtle)

CUBA

Ciudad de La Habana
Hospital Pediatr. Doc. "Juan M Marquez"
Comisión Cubana de Fibrosis Quistica
Ave. 31 esq. 76
Marianao, CP 11400
Ciudad de La Habana

CZECH REPUBLIC

Bratislava
Nutarch
Podunajske Biskupice
Krajinska 101
825 56 Bratislava
421.2.40 251 155/421.2.40 251 566
(Contact Person: MUDr. Jaroslava Orosova/
  MUDr. Hana Kayserova/
  MUDr. Branislav Drugda/
  MUDr. Branislav REMIS)

Brno
Pediatric Department
Cernopolni 9
662 63 Brno
420.5.4512562/420.5.4512245
(Contact Person: Dr. Alena Holcikova)

Ceske Budejovice
Pediatric Department ILF
B. Nemcove 54
370 87 Ceske Budejovice
420.38.7878737
(Contact Person: Dr. Ivana Sekyrova)

Hradec Kralove
Pediatric Department University Hospital
University Hospital

500 36 Hradec Kralove
420.49.583.3433
(Contact Person: Dr. Hubert Vanicek)

Labem Bukov
Department TRN ILF Masaryk Hospital
401 13 USTI nad Labem Bukov
420.47.5682325
(Contact Person: Dr. Ivana Tumova)

Litvinov
Pediatric Department
Tylova 2067
436 01 Litvinov
420.35.6173486
(Contact Person: Dr. Jiri Biolek)

Motol
2nd Pediatric Department University
  Hospital Motol
V Uvalu 84
150 18 Praha 5—Motol
420.2.24432269/420.2.24432253/
  420.2.24432220
(Contact Person: Dr. Vera Vavrova/
  Dr. Jana Bartosova)

Olomouc
Pediatric Department University Hospital
I.P. Pavlova 6
775 20 Olomouc
420.68.5853560/420.68.5852929/
  420.68.5853559
(Contact Person: Dr. Antonin Kolek)

Ostrava
Pediatric Department ILF
Syllabove 19
703 86 Ostrava
420.69.6924378
(Contact Person: Dr. Jaroslava Hubova)

Pzen
University Hospital
Pediatric Department University Hospital
Dr. E. Benese 13
305 99 Pzen
420.19.7402916

(Contact Person: Dr. Helena
  Honomichlova)

Zlin
Bata Hospital
Pediatric Department Bata Hospital
Havlickovo n. 600
760 01 Zlin
420.67.7552019/420.67.7552913
(Contact Person: Dr. Lenka Toukalkova)

DENMARK

Aarhus
Cystic Fibrosis Center Aarhus
Department of Pediatrics A
Skejby Sygehus Brendstrupgaardsvej 100
DK-8200 Aarhus
45.8949.6740/45.8949.6023
(Contact Person: Prof. P.O. Schiotz)
Children: Yes

Copenhagen
Cystic Fibrosis Center Copenhagen
Department of Pediatrics GGK-5003
  Rigshospitalet
Blegdamsvej 9
DK-2100 Copenhagen
45.3545.4832/45.3545.5006/
  45.3545.6717
(Contact Person: Dr. Christian Koch)

FINLAND

Helsinki
Helsinki University Hospital
Hospital for Children and Adolescents
Stenbäckinkatu 11
FIN-00290 Helsinki
erkki.savilahti@hus.fi/merja.kajosaari
  @hus.fi
+358 9 4711
www.hus.fi
(Contact Person: Dr. Erkki Savilahti/
  Dr. Merja Kajosaari)

Karkku
Hoikka Resource Centre

International Physiotherapy Group for
  Cystic Fibrosis—Pulmonary Association
Hoikka Resource Centre
Hoikantie 15
FIN 38100 Karkku
leena.jokinen@hoikkacentre.fi
+358 3 5121273/+358 3 5121220
www.hengitysliitto.fi/www.hoikkacentre.fi
(Contact Person: Leena Jokinen)

FRANCE

Aix en Provence
CHG d'Aix en Provence
Service de Pédiatrie
13616 Aix en Provence Cedex 1
d.theveniau@ch-aix.fr
33.4.42335031/33.4.42335185
(Contact Person: Dr. Dominique Théveniau)

Amiens
CHU Nord
Srvce Pédiatrie I—Unité Pneumo. Infantile
Place Victor Pauchet
80054 Amiens Cedex
33.3.22668260/33.3.22668483
(Contact Person: Dr. Jean-Claude Pautard)

Angers
CHU—Centre Robert Debré
4 Rue Larrey
49033 Angers Cedex 01
jlginies@pediatrie.net
33.2.41354987/33.2.41354173
(Contact Person: Prof. Jean-Louis Giniès)

Besançon
Hôpital Saint Jacques
Service de Pédiatrie
2 place Saint-Jacques
25030 Besançon Cedex
33.3.81218143/33.3.81218830
(Contact Person: Dr. Marie-Laure Dalphin)
Children: Yes

Bordeaux
CHU—Groupe Pellegrin
Hôpital des Enfants

Place Amélie Raba Léon
33076 Bordeaux
Cedex
bordeaux1@eunet.mail.fr
33.5.57.970505/33.5.57.970500
(Contact Person: Dr. Michaël Fayon)

Bordeaux
Centre Muco Adulte Aquitaine
17 Rue de Rivière
33000 Bordeaux
domblide@infonie.fr
33.5.56.443451/33.5.56.793226
(Contact Person: Dr. Philippe Domblides)
Adult: Yes

Boulogne
Centre de Pneumologie de l'Enfant
104 avenue Victor Hugo
92100 Boulogne
resppanif@yahoo.com
33.1.46999898/33.1.46999897
(Contact Person: Dr. Bertrand Delaisi)
Children: Yes

Brest
CHU—Hôpital Augustin Morvan Péd.
Service de Pédiatrie Marfan
5 avenue Foch—BP 824
29609 Brest Cedex
33.2.98223659/33.2.98223494
(Contact Person: Dr. Jean-Marie Lefur)
Children: Yes

Brive
Centre Hospitalier Général de Brive
Service de Pédiatrie
Boulevard du Dr Verlhac—BP 432
19100 Brive Cedex
33.5.55926043/33.5.55926189
(Contact Person: Dr. Philippe Gautry)
Children: Yes

Caen
CHU Clémenceau
Service de Pédiatrie A
avenue Georges Clémenceau
14033 Caen Cedex

33.2.31272594/33.2.31272655
(Contact Person: Prof. Jean-François
  Duhamel)
Children: Yes

Clermont Ferrand
Hôtel Dieu—Pavillon Hacquart
Pédiatrie A
avenue Vercingétorix—BP 69
63003 Clermont Ferrand Cedex
alabbé@chu-clermontferrand.fr
33.4.73750027/33.4.73354172
(Contact Person: Prof. André Labbé)
Children: Yes

Créteil
Centre Intercommunal de Créteil
Service de Pédiatrie
40 avenue de Verdun
94010 Créteil Cedex
33.1.45175420/33.1.45175426
(Contact Person: Prof. Philippe Reinert)

Dax
CHG de Dax
Service de Pédiatrie
Boulevard Yves du Manoir—BP 323
40107 Dax Cedex
33.5.58914976/33.5.58913996
(Contact Person: Dr. Richard Barbier)
Children: Yes

Dijon
Hôpital d'Enfants du Bocage
Service de Pédiatrie 1
21034 Dijon Cedex
frederichuet@chu-dijon.fr
33.3.80293415/33.3.80293803
(Contact Person: Prof. Frédéric Huet)
Children: Yes

Dunkerque
CHG de Dunkerque
Srvce de Pédiatrie et Médecine de l'ados
59385 Dunkerque Cedex 01
33.3.28285693/33.3.28285936
(Contact Person: Dr. Guy-André Loeuille)
Children: Yes

Elbeuf
CHG des Feugrais
Service de Pédiatrie
Rue du Dr Villers—BP 346
76503 Elbeuf Cedex
33.2.32963540/33.2.35873687
(Contact Person: Dr. Kamel Lashinat)

Giens
Hôpital Renée Sabran
Unité de soins pour mucoviscidose
Boulevard Edouard Herriot
83406 Giens Cedex
33.4.94381740/33.4.94381887
(Contact Person: Dr. Jean-Pierre
  Chazalette)

Grenoble
CHU de Grenoble
Service de Pneumologie—Centre Muco
BP 217x
38043 Grenoble Cedex 9
isabelle.pin@ujf-grenoble.fr
33.4.76768732/33.4.76765617
(Contact Person: Dr. Isabelle Pin)

Grenoble
CHU de Grenoble-Péd.
Département de Pédiatrie—
  Centre Muco
BP 217
38043 Grenoble Cedex 9
isabelle.pin@ujf-grenoble.fr
33.4.76765469/33.4.76765830
(Contact Person: Dr. Isabelle Pin)

La Roche sur Yon
CHD Les Oudairies
Service de Pédiatrie
85025 La Roche sur Yon
33.2.51446201/33.2.51446298
(Contact Person: Dr. Pierre Blanchard)

Le Chesnay
Hôpital André Mignot
Service de Pédiatrie
177 Rue de Versailles
78157 Le Chesnay Cedex

pediatrie@ch-versailles.fr
33.1.39638944/33.1.39639396
(Contact Person: Dr. Pierre Foucaud)

Le Havre
C.H. du Havre—Hôpital de Jour
Service de Pédiatrie
55 bis Rue Gustave Flaubert—BP 24
76600 Le Havre
bleluyer@hps.tm.fr
33.2.32733630/33.2.32733636
(Contact Person: Dr. Bernard Le Luyer)
Children: Yes

Lens
Centre Hospitalier de Lens
Service de Pédiatrie
99 route de la Bassée
62307 Lens
ismedical1@ch-lens.fr
33.3.21691105/33.3.21691534
(Contact Person: Dr. Anne Sardet)
Children: Yes

Lille
H. Calmette—Clinique Maladies Respirat.
Service de Pneumo. Immuno-Allergologie
Unité EFR
59037 Lille Cedex
bwallaert@nordnet.fr
33.3.20445036/33.3.20446693
(Contact Person: Prof. Benoît Wallaert)

Lille
Hôpital Jeanne de Flandres
Clinique de Pédiatrie Gastroentérologie—
  Mucoviscidose
59037 Lille Cedex
dturck@chru-lille.fr
33.3.20446885/33.3.20446134
(Contact Person: Prof. Dominique Turck)

Lille
Hôpital Saint Antoine
Service de Pédiatrie
329 Boulevard Victor Hugo—BP 255
59019 Lille Cedex
hsa.pediatrie@nordnet.fr

33.3.20783114/33.3.20783195
(Contact Person: Dr. Manuëla Scalbert)
Children: Yes

Limoges
CHU Dupuytren
Service de Pédiatrie 1
2 avenue Martin Luther-King
87042 Limoges Cedex
delumley@unilim.fr
33.5.55056801/33.5.55056795
(Contact Person: Prof. Lionel de Lumley)
Children: Yes

Lisieux
CHG Robert Bisson
Service de Pédiatrie
4 Rue Roger Aini
14100 Lisieux
eckart14@aol.com
33.2.31613213/33.2.31613318
(Contact Person: Dr. Marcel Guillot)

Marseille
Hôpital Sainte Marguerite
Service de Chirurgie Thoracique
270 Boulevard Sainte-Marguerite
13274 Marseille Cedex 9
33.4.91744619/33.4.91744590
(Contact Person: Dr. Martine
  Reynaud-Gaubert)
Adult: Yes

Marseille
Hôpital d'Enfants de la Timone
Service de Pédiatrie
13385 Marseille Cedex 5
jsarles@ap-hm.fr
33.4.91386743/33.4.91386736
(Contact Person: Prof. Jacques Sarles)
Children: Yes

Montpellier
Hôpital Arnaud de Villeneuve
Service de Pédiatrie II
371 Avenue du Doyen Gaston Giraud
34090 Montpellier Cedex 5
d-rieu@chu-montpellier.fr

33.4.67336571/33.4.67547148
(Contact Person: Prof. Daniel Rieu)
Children: Yes

Nantes
Hôpital G. et R. Laënnec
Unité de Transplantation Thoracique
BP 1005
44093 Nantes Cedex 01
haloun.alain@chu-nantes.fr
33.2.40165092/33.2.40165092
(Contact Person: Dr. Alain Haloun)

Nantes
Hôpital Mère-Enfant
Service de Pédiatrie médicale
Quai Moncousu
44093 Nantes Cedex 01
vdavid@chu-nantes.fr
33.2.40083172/33.2.40083483
(Contact Person: Dr. Valérie David)

Nice
Hôpital l'Archet
Service de Pédiatrie
06003 Nice Cedex
33.4.92036073/33.4.93447178
(Contact Person: Prof. Marc Albertini)
Children: Yes

Palavas
Institut Saint Pierre
Service de Pédiatrie
Rue Giniez Mares
34250 Palavas Les Flots
33.4.67077558/33.4.67680990
(Contact Person: Dr. Bernard Rolin)
Children: Yes

Paris
H. Necker Enfants Malades Pneumo.
Service Pneumo. Allergo.
 Pédiatrique
149 Rue de Sèvres
75730 Paris Cedex 15
pneumo.allergo@nck.ap-hop-paris.fr
33.1.44484942/33.1.44381740
(Contact Person: Prof. Pierre Scheinmann)

Paris
H. Necker Enfants Malades Péd.
Unité de Pédiatrie Générale
149 Rue de Sèvres
75743 Paris Cedex 15
33.1.44494882/33.1.47833226
(Contact Person: Prof. Gérard Lenoir)
Children: Yes

Paris
Hôpital Cochin
Service de Pneumologie
27 Rue du Faubourg
 Saint-Jacques
75014 Paris
dominique.hubert@cch.ap-hop-paris.fr
33.1.58412372/33.1.46338253
(Contact Person: Dr. Dominique Hubert)

Paris
Hôpital Robert Debré
Gastroentérologie Pédiatrique
48 Boulevard Sérurier
75019 Paris
jean.navarro@rdb.ap-hop-paris.fr
33.1.40034788/33.1.40032353
(Contact Person: Prof. Jean Navarro)
Children: Yes

Paris
Hôpital Trousseau
Service Pédiatrique/Pneumo.
 de l'Enfant
75571 Paris Cedex 12
annick.clement@trs.ap-hop-paris.fr
33.1.44736668/33.1.44736718
(Contact Person: Prof. Annick Clément)
Children: Yes

Pessac
Hôpital du Haut-Lévêque
Service de Chirurgie Thoracique
 Maison du Haut-Lévêque
Avenue de Magellan
33604 Pessac Cedex
claire.dromer@chu-aquitaine.fr
33.5.56.555051/33.5.56.555021
(Contact Person: Dr. Claire Dromer)

Pierre Bénite
C.H. Lyon Sud
Srvce Médecine Interne—Bât
  1K Giraud
165 Chemin du Grand Revoyet
69495 Pierre Bénite Cedex
isabelle.durieu@chu-lyon.fr
33.4.78861354/33.4.78863264
(Contact Person: Dr. Isabelle Durieu)
Adult: Yes

Pierre Bénite
CH Lyon Sud
Service de Pédiatrie—Unité
  Pneumologie
165 Chemin du Grand Revoyet 69495
  Pierre Bénite Cedex
33.4.78861557/33.4.78865724
(Contact Person: Prof. Gabriel Bellon)
Children: Yes

Poitiers
CHU—La Milètrie
Service de Pédiatrie
350 Avenue Jacques Coeur—BP 577
86021 Poitiers Cedex
d.oriot@chu.univ-poitiers.fr
33.5.49.444390/33.5.49443820
(Contact Person: Dr. Catherine Gambert)
Children: Yes

Reims
CHU—American Memorial Hospital
Service de Pédiatrie A
47 Rue Cognacq-Jay
51092 Reims Cedex
mabely@chu-reims.fr
33.3.26787007/33.3.26788262
(Contact Person: Dr. Michel Abely)
Children: Yes

Rennes
CHRU—Hôpital Sud—for adults
Pneumologie Adultes—Centre de Soins
  Muco.
16 Boulevard de Bulgarie—BP 56129
35056 Rennes Cedex 2
benoit.desrues@chu-rennes.fr

33.2.23302764/33.2.23302766
(Contact Person:
  Prof. Benoît Desrues)

Rennes
CHRU—Hôpital Sud—Péd.
Annexe Pédiatrique—Centre de Soins
  de Muco.
16 Boulevard de Bulgarie—BP 56129
35056 Rennes Cedex 2
hop-ren@mail.eunet.fr
33.2.99266756/33.2.23302764
(Contact Person: Prof. Michel Roussey)
Children: Yes

Roscoff
Centre Hélio Marin—Clinique
  "Mucoviscidose"
Presqu'île de Perharidy
29684 Roscoff Cedex
admissions@chm-roscoff.fr
33.2.98293916/33.2.98293424
(Contact Person: Dr. Gilles Rault)

Rouen
CHU—Hôpital Charles Nicolle—for
  adults
Clinique Pneumologique
1 Rue de Germont
76031 Rouen Cedex
dominique@chu-rouen.fr
33.2.32888247/33.2.32888240
(Contact Person:
  Dr. Stéphane Dominique)

Rouen
CHU—Hôpital Charles Nicolle Péd.
Service de Pédiatrie
1 Rue de Germont
76031 Rouen Cedex
Olivier.Mouterde@chu-rouen.fr
33.2.32888216/33.2.32888188
(Contact Person: Dr. Olivier Mouterde)
Children: Yes

Saint Denis
Hôpital d'Enfants
Service de Pédiatrie

Hôpital d'Enfants
97476 Saint Denis Cedex
hop.enfants@guetali.fr
33.0.262908700/33.0.262908710
(Contact Person:
    Dr. Jean-François Lesure)
Children: Yes

Saint Nazaire
CHR de Saint Nazaire
Service de Pédiatrie
Boulevard Laënnec—BP 414
44606 Saint Nazaire Cedex
33.2.40906100/33.2.40905201
(Contact Person: Dr. Georges Picherot)

Saint Pierre
Hôpital de Saint Pierre
Service de Pédiatrie
Le Tampon 350
97448 Saint Pierre Cedex
michel.renouil@wanadoo.fr
33.0.262359143/33.0.262359234
(Contact Person: Dr. Michel Renouil)
Children: Yes

Saintes
Centre Hospitalier de Saintes
Service de Pédiatrie
9 place du 11 novembre—BP 326
17108 Saintes Cedex
33.5.46927676/33.5.46927791
(Contact Person: Dr. Marc Besson-Léaud)

Strasbourg
Hôpital de Hautepierre
Service de Pédiatrie 2
avenue Molière
67098 Strasbourg Cedex
leonard-donato@chru-strasbourg.fr
33.3.88.127785/33.3.88.127132
(Contact Person: Dr. Lionel Donato)

Strasbourg
Hôpital de Hautepierre—Centre de Soins
    adultes
Service de Pneumologie
Hôpital de Hautepierre

Avenue Molière
67098 Strasbourg Cedex
romain.kessler@chru-strasbourg.fr
33.3.88.116768/33.3.88.127827
(Contact Person: Dr. Romain Kessler)
Adult: Yes

Suresnes
Hôpital Foch—Pneumo.
Service de Pneumologie 40 Rue
    worth—BP 36
92151 Suresnes Cedex
i.caubarrere@hopital-foch.org
33.1.46252635/33.1.42043281
(Contact Person: Prof. Isabelle Caubarrère)

Toulouse
CHU Purpan—Hôpital des Enfants
Maladies respirat. et Allerg. de l'Enfant
31026 Toulouse Cedex 3
bremont.f@chu-toulouse.fr
33.5.34558586/33.5.34558589
(Contact Person: Dr. François Brémont)
Children: Yes

Toulouse
CHU de Rangueil—Pneumo
Service de Pneumologie-Allergologie
Avenue du Pr Jean Poulhès
31403 Toulouse Cedex 4
MURRIS.M@chu-toulouse.fr
33.5.61322771/33.5.61322957
(Contact Person: Dr. Marlène Murris-Espin)

Toulouse
Mucozenne
Pneumologie et Allergologie de l'Enfant
31000 Toulouse
michelpiot@yahoo.fr
33.5.61526436/33.5.61331174
(Contact Person:
    Dr. Bernard Sablayrolles)
Children: Yes

Tours
CHU Bretonneau
Service de Pneumologie Adultes
Unité Muco. Fonction.—2Bd Tonnellé

37044 Tours Cedex 1
eb@med.univ-tours.fr
33.2.47476936/33.2.2.47473882
(Contact Person: Dr. Françoise Varaigne)
Adult: Yes

Tours
CHU Clocheville
Service de Pédiatrie R
49 Boulevard Béranger
37044 Tours Cedex
33.2.47474747/33.2.47664370
(Contact Person: Prof. Jean-Claude Rolland)
Children: Yes

Valenciennes
Centre Hospitalier de Valenciennes
Service de Pédiatrie
Avenue Desandrouins
59322 Valenciennes Cedex
33.3.27143026/33.3.27143462
(Contact Person: Dr. Elisabeth Tassin)

Vandoeuvre-lès-Nancy
Hôpitaux de Brabois Pneumo.
Service de Pneumologie A
Rue du Morvan
54511 Vandoeuvre Les Nancy Cedex
p.scheid@chu-nancy.fr
33.3.83153400/33.3.83153564
(Contact Person: Dr. Philippe Scheid)

Vandoeuvre-lès-Nancy
Hôpitaux de Brabois Pédiat.
Srvce Pédiatrie 3 & Génétique Clinique
54511 Vandoeuvre les Nancy Cedex
m.vidailhet@chu-nancy.fr
33.3.83154747/33.3.83154647
(Contact Person: Dr. Jocelyne Derelle)
Children: Yes

Vannes
Centre Hospitalier Prosper Chubert
Service de Pédiatrie
Boulevard du Général Guillaudot
56017 Vannes Cedex
33.2.97014160/33.2.2.97014369
(Contact Person: Dr. Valérie Moisan-Petit)

Voiron
CH de Voiron
Service de Pédiatrie
38500 Voiron
33.4.76671416/33.4.76671597
(Contact Person: Dr. Jean-Pierre Gout)

ISRAEL

Tel Hashomer
Safra Children Hospital, Sheba
    Medical Center
Derekh shiba 2, Ramat Gan
ori.efrati@sheba.health.gov.il
03-5305012
(Contact Person: Dr. Ori Efrati)

Jerusalem
Hadassah University Hospital,
    Mount Scopus
Shderot Churchill, Jerusalem
kerem@hadassah.org.il
02-5845326
(Contact Person: Prof. Eitan Kerem)

Haifa
Caramel Medical Center
Mikhal 7, Haifa
rivlin_joseph@clalit.org.il
04-8250367
(Contact Person: Dr. Yosef Rivlin)

Rambam Medical Center
Ha Aliya Ha Shniya 8, Haifa
L_bentur@rambam.health.gov.il
04-8542784
 (Contact Person: Prof. Leah Bentur)

Petach Tikva
Atara Grub Moshe Leib Schneider
    Children's Medical Center
Kaplan 14, Petakh Tikva
Hannah@hotmail.com
03-9253654
(Contact Person: Prof. Hanna Blau)

Beer Sheva
Soroka Medical Center

Shderot David Ben Gurion Be'er-Sheva
michaa@bgumail.bgu.ac.il
6400624 – 08
(Contact Person: Dr. Micha Aviram)

ITALY

Abruzzo
Teramo
Ospedale di Teramo
C.R.R. Divisione di Pediatria
Ospedale di Teramo
Teramo
Abruzzo
39.861.4291
(Contact Person: Dr. Paolo Moretti)

Basillicata
Potenza
Ospedale di Villa
S.R.R.—Attivita di Supporto presso
Divisione Pediatrica
Ospedale di Villa
85100 Potenza
Basillicata
39.975.352845/39.975.312111 (int. 236)
(Contact Person: Dr. Rosaria Abate/
  Dr. Donatello Salvatore)

Calabria
Catanzaro
Ospedale di Soverato
C.R.R. Attivita di Supporto presso
Divisione Pediatrica
Ospedale di Soverato
88100 Catanzaro
39.967.539111

Campania
Napoli
II Facolta di Medicina
C.R.R. Clinica Pediatrica della II Facolta
  di Medicina
Via Pansini 5
80100 Napoli
Campania
39.81.7463273/39.81.7463500
(Contact Person: Prof. Giorgio de Ritis)

Emilia
Parma
C.R.R. Centro di Fisiopatologia
  Respiratoria Infantile
Universita di Parma
Via Gramsci 14
43100 Parma
39.521.991198/39.521.290461/
  39.521.290458
(Contact Person: Prof. Augusta Battistini)

Friuli Venezia Giulia
Trieste
Instituto per Infanzia Burlo Garofolo
C.R.R. Divisione Pediatria
Istria 65
34100 Trieste
Friuli Venezia Giulia
39.40.3785111/39.40.3785210
(Contact Person: Dott.ssa Brevella Giglio)

Lazio
Roma
C.R.R. Servizio fibrosi Cistica e Fisioterapia
  Instituto clinica Pediatrica
Policlinico Umberto I
Viale Regina Elena 312
00100 Roma
Lazio
39.6.497891 (int. 289)/39.6.4454898
(Contact Person: Prof. Mariano Antonelli)

Lazio
Roma
Centro di Diagnosi e Terapia della
  Fibrosis Cistica
Divisione Pediatrica di
  Gastroenterologia Ospedale
  Bambino Gesu
Piazza S. Onofrio 4
00100 Roma
Lazio
39.6.66859.2330/39.6.66859.2296
(Contact Person: Dr. Massimo Castro/
  Dr. Lucidi)

Liguria
Genova

C.R.R. Centro Regionale per le Malattie
  Endocrine e Metaboliche dell'Eta
  Evolutive
Sez. Fibrosis Cistica Clinica Pediatrica 1a
  Instituto G. Gaslini
16100 Genova
Liguria
39.10.387496/39.10.5636366/
  39.10.3776590
(Contact Person: Prof. Cesare Romano)

Lombardia
Milano
C.R.R. IIa Clinicica Pediatrica
  de Marchi Instituti Clinici
  di Perfezionamento
  di Milano
Via della Commenda 9
20100 Milano
Lombardia
39.2.55111043/39.2.57992456/
  39.2.55195341
(Contact Person: Prof. Annamaria Giunta)

Marche
Ancona
Ospedale dei Bambini g. Salesi
C.R.R. Centro Fibrosi Cistica
Divisione di Pediatria e Neonatologia
Ospedale dei Bambini g. Salesi
Via Corridoni, 11
60123 Ancona
Marche
39.71.5962351/39.71.5962354
(Contact Person: Prof. Guiseppe Caramia/
  Dr. Rolando Gagliardini)

Piemonte
Orbassano
Clinica Universitaria Tisiologica Reg.
  Gonzole Ospedale S. Luigi
C.R.R. Settore Adulti: Centro Fibrosi
  Cistica Reparto Pneumologia
10043 Orbassano (TO)
Piemonte—Valle D'Aosta
39.11.9026432/39.11.9038674/
  39.11.9038639

Piemonte
Torino
Ospedale Infantile Regina Margherita
C.R.R. Settore minori: Centro
  Dipartimentale Clinico-Ospedaliero
  per la Fibrosi Cistica
Ospedale Infantile Regina Margherita
Piazza Polonia 94
10100 Torino
Piemonte—Valle d'Aosta
39.11.69227247/39.11.69227267/
  39.11.69227765
(Contact Person: Prof. Nicoletta Ansaldi/
  Prof. Domenico Castello)

Puglia
Acquaviva Delle Fonti
Ospedale di Acquaviva Delle Fonti
Attivita di Supporto presso
Divisione Pediatrica
Ospedale di Acquaviva Delle Fonti (BA)
Puglia
39.80.760374
(Contact Person: Dr. Nicole D'Andrea)

Puglia
Bari
C.R.R. Servizio di Prevenzione e Cura
  della Mucoviscidosi
Clinica Pediatrica IIa—Policlinico
Piazza Giulio Cesare
70100 Bari
Puglia
39.80.5527527/39.80.278911
(Contact Person: Prof. Nicola Rigillo)

Puglia
Cerignola
Attivita di Supporto presso
Divisione Pediatrica
Ospedale di Cerignola (FG)
Puglia
39.885.419111
(Contact Person: Dr. Luigi Ratclif)

Puglia
San Giovanni Rotondo
Ospedale di San Giovanni Rotondo

Attivita di Supporto Presso
Divisione Pediatrica Ospedale di San
  Giovanni Rotondo (FG)
Puglia
39.882.853721/39.882.853621
(Contact Person: Dr. Germano Pio Ercolino)

Romagna
Cesena
Ospedale M. Bufalini
C.R.R. Centro per la Fibrosi Cistica
  Divisione di Pediatria e Patologia
  Neonatale
Ospedale M. Bufalini
ULSS n. 39
47023 Cesena (FO)
Romagna
39.547.352837.302322
(Contact Person: Prof. Giancarlo Biasini/
  Dr. Angelo Miano)

Sardegna
Cagliari
Ospedale G. Brotzu
C.R.R Divisione di Pediatria
Ospedale G. Brotzu
ULSS n. 21
Via Peretti 09100 Cagliari
Sardegna
39.70.539551/39.70.541468/
  39.70.539682
(Contact Person: Prof. Mario Silvetti)

Sicilia
Messina
C.R.R. Instituto Clinica Pediatrica
Policlinico Universitario
98100 Messina
Sicilia
39.90.2935007/39.90.2935007
(Contact Person: Prof. Giuseppe Magazzu)

Sicilia
Palermo
Ospedale dei Bambini G. de Cristina
C.R.R. Servizio per la Diagnosi e Cura
  della Fibrosi Cistica
Ospedale dei Bambini G. de Cristina

Piazza Porta Montalto
90100 Palermo
Sicilia
39.91.6666074/39.91.6666226
(Contact Person: Prof. Vincenzo Balsamo)

Toscana
Firenze
Centro Regionale Toscano per la
  Fibrosi Cistica
Dipartimento di Pediatria Ospedale Meyer
Via L. Giodano 13
50100 Firenze
Toscana
39.55.56621/39.55.570380
(Contact Person: Prof. Lore Marianelli)

Toscana
Grosseto
Ospedale di Grosseto
Attivita di Supporto Presso
Divisione Pediatrica Ospedale di Grosseto
39.564.485329
(Contact Person: Dr. Adalberto Campagna)

Toscana
Livorno
Ospedale di Livorno
Attivita di Supporto Presso
Divisione Pediatrica Ospedale di Livorno
Toscana
39.586.418111
(Contact Person: Dr. Maria Vittoria Perez)

Trentino Alto Adige
Bolzano
Ospedale di Bolzano
Attivita di Supporto Presso
Divisione Pediatrica
Ospedale di Bolzano
Trentino Alto Adige
39.471.908111
(Contact Person: Dr. Lydia Pescolderung)

Umbria
Gualdo Tadino
C.R.R. Servizio Supporto Fibrosi Cistica
  e Fisioterapia

Ospedale Calai—Divisione di Pediatria
06023 Gualdo Tadino (PG)
Umbria
39.75.9109301
(Contact Person: Dr. Angelo Cosimi)

Veneto
Verona
C.R.R. Centro Regionale Veneto di Ricerca
Prevenzione Riabilitazione ed
  Insegnamento per la Fibrosi Cistica
Ospedale Civile Maggiore
Piazzale Stefani 1
37100 Verona
Veneto
39.45.8072370/39.45.8072042
(Contact Person: Prof. B.H. Assael)

JORDAN

Irbid
The Medical School
University of Science & Technology
P.O. Box 3030
Irbid
(Contact Person: Dr. M. Rawashdeh)

THE NETHERLANDS

Alkmaar
Medisch Centrum Alkmaar—for adults/
  children
Wilhelminalaan 12
1800 AM Alkmaar
31.72.5484444/31.72.5482179

Amsterdam
AMC/Emma Kinderziekenhuis—for
  children
Meibergdreef 9
1105 AZ Amsterdam
31.20.5669111/31.20.5664440

Amsterdam
Ac. Medisch Centrum (AMC)—for adults
Meibergdreef 9
1105 AZ Amsterdam
31.20.5669111/31.20.5664440

Amsterdam
Academisch Ziekenhuis VU—for adults–
  children
De Boelelaan 1117
1007 MB Amsterdam
31.20.4444444/31.20.4444645

Den Haag
Juliana Kinderziekenhuis—children's
  hospital
Sportlaan 600
2566MJ Den Haag
31.70.3127200/31.70.3126161

Den Haag
Ziekenhuis Leijenburg—for adults
Leyweg 275
2504 LN Den Haag
31.70.3592000/31.70.3595040

Groningen
Ac. Ziekenhuis Groningen (AZG)—for
  adults/children
Hanzeplein 1
9700 RB Groningen
31.50.3619111/31.50.3614351

Maastricht
Ac. Ziekenhuis Maastricht (AZM)—for
  children
P. Debyelaan 25
6202 AZ Maastricht
31.43.3876543/31.43.3878787

Rotterdam
AZR/Sophia Kinderziekenhuis—
  for children
Dr. Molewaterplein 60
3000 CB Rotterdam
31.10.4636363/31.10.4636800

Rotterdam
Ac. Ziekenhuis Rotterdam (AZR)—for
  adults
Dr. Molewaterplein 40
3000 CA Rotterdam
31.10.4639222/31.10.4635305

Utrecht
UMC/Wilhelmina Kinderziekenhuis—for
  children
Lundlaan 6
3508 AB Utrecht
31.30.2504000

Utrecht
Universitair Medisch Centrum (UMC)—
  for adults
Heidelberglaan 100
3508GA Utrecht
31.30.2509111

NEW ZEALAND

Auckland
Green Lane Hospital
Dr. John Kolbe
Private Bag
Auckland 3
64.9.6389919/64.9.6383896

Auckland
Starship Children's Hospital
Dr. Alison W Wesley
Private Bag 92024
Auckland
64.9.3074949/64.9.3076480/64.9.3074913
Children: Yes

Christchurch
Christchurch Hospital
Department of Paediatrics
Private Bag 4710
Christchurch
64.3.3640734/64.3.3640919
(Contact Person: Dr. Philip Pattemore)
Children: Yes

Christchurch
Christchurch Hospital
Private Bag 4710
Christchurch
64.3.3640919
(Contact Person: Dr. Peter Thornley,
  Respiratory Physician)

Dunedin
Dunedin Hospital
Private Bag 1921
Dunedin
64.3.4740999/
  64.3.4747623
(Contact Person:
  Dr. Christopher Hewitt)

Hamilton
Waikato Hospital
Private Bag 3200
Hamilton
64.7.8398899
(Contact Person: Dr. David Graham)

Hamilton
Waikato Hospital
Private Bag 3200
Hamilton
64.7.8398899
(Contact Person: Dr. Graeme Mills)

Wellington South
Capital Coast Healthcare
Private Bag 7902
Wellington South
64.4.3855999/64.4.43855856
(Contact Person: Dr. Alan Farrell)

Wellington South
Capital Coast Healthcare
Private Bag 7902
Wellington South
64.4.3855999/64.4.3855856
(Contact Person:
  Dr. David Jones)

NORWAY

Oslo
Ullevål Hospital
Department of Pediatrics
0407 Oslo
47.23.01.5591
(Contact Person:
  Olav Trond Storrosten, M.D.)

ROMANIA

Alba—Iulia
County Hospital Pediatric Department
Revolutiei Avenue 23
2500 Alba—Iulia
(Contact Person: Dr. Mihaela Mînascurta)

Baia—Mare
County Hospital Pediatric Department
Cosbuc Street 31
4800 Baia—Mare
40.62.426031/40.62.426859
(Contact Person: Dr. Nelia Munteanu)

Brasov
County Hospital Pediatric Department
Nicopole Street 45
2200 Brasov
40.68.415130
(Contact Person: Dr. Laura Dracea)
Children: Yes

Cluj—Napoca
Clinic I Paediatrics University of Medicine
  and Pharmacy Cluj—Napoca
Motilor Street 68
3400 Cluj—Napoca
40.64.197706/40.64.192446
(Contact Person:
  Prof. Dr. Paula Grigorescu—Sido)

Craiova
County Hospital Clinic II
Paediatrics Faculty of Medicine Craiova
Maresal Antonescu Street 60
1100 Craiova
40.51.132498
(Contact Person: Dr. Eva Nemes)

Deva
County Hospital
New Born Department
22 Decembrie Street
2700 Deva
40.54.215050
(Contact Person: Dr. Camelia Balas)

Iasi
Children's Hospital Clinic III
  Pediatrics
Vasile Lupu Street 62
6600 Iasi
40.32.175740/40.32.177309
(Contact Person: Prof. Dr. Dan Moraru)

Oradea
Children's Hospital
Ostasilor Street 12
3700 Oradea
40.59.441844/40.59.442687
(Contact Person: Dr. Rodica Mihalceanu)

Timisoara
Clinic II Paediatrics University of
  Medicine and Pharmacy
Paltinis Street 1–3
1900 Timisoara
40.56.194529/40.56.194529
(Contact Person: Prof. Dr. Ioan Popa)

SLOVAK REPUBLIC

Banská Bystrica
Nemocnica F.D. Roosevelta
974 00 Banska Bystrica
421.48.441.3375
(Contact Person: Dr. Adriana Zigova)

Kosice
FNsP Kosice
Trieda SNP 1
040 11 Kosice
421.55.640 4137/421.55.640 4151
(Contact Person: Dr. Anna Feketeova)

SOUTH AFRICA

Cape Town
Groote Schuur (Cape Town)
  Adult CF Clinic
Cape Town
27.21.4044369
(Contact Person: Prof Paul Will)
Adult: Yes

Cape Town
Red Cross Children's Hospital
Klipfontein Road, Rondebosch, 7700
27.21.6585111
(Contact Person: Prof. John Ireland/
    Dr. Tony Westwood)

Durban
Addington Hospital (Durban)—CF Clinic
Durban
27.31.3322111
(Contact Person: Dr. Graham Ducasse)

Durban
St Augustine's Medical Centre
Chelmsford Road.
Durban 4001
27.31.2010215
(Contact Person: Dr. Jonathan Egner)

Johannesburg
Johannesburg Hospital—adult respiratory
    clinic
Private Bag X39
Johannesburg, 2000
27.11.4884911/27.11.4883496
    (page no. 1025)
(Contact Person: Dr. Mervyn Mer)

Johannesburg
Johannesburg Hospital—Paediatric CF
    Clinic
Private Bag X39
Johannesburg, 2000
27.11.4883983
(Contact Person: Dr. Susan Klugman)
Children: Yes

Johannesburg
Sandton Clinic
Cnr Main Road & Peter Place, Bryanston,
    Johannesburg, 2021
27.11.706 6060
(Contact Person: Dr. Dave Richard)

Port Elizabeth
Port Elizabeth Greenacres Hospital

Port Elizabeth 6045
27.41.3633900
(Contact Person: Dr. Paul Gebers)

Pretoria
Steve Biko Academic Hospital—CF Clinic
c/o Voortrekkers Road and Malan Street,
Capital Park, Pretoria
27.12.354 6244/27.12.3541564
(Contact Person: Dr. Fanie Naude)

SPAIN

Algeciras
Hospital Punta de Europa
Ctra. de Getafe s/n
11207 Algeciras
Cádiz
956580420
(Contact Person:
    Dr. Julio Guerrero Vázquez)

Almeria
Hospital Torrecardenas
Pasaje Torrecardenas s/n
04009 Almeria
Almeria
951212100
(Contact Person: Dr. Morales Ferrer)

Barcelona
Hospital Principes D Espanyo
Feria Llarga s/n
08950 Esplugues de Llobregat
Barcelona
933357011
(Contact Person:
    Dr. Federico Manresa Presas)

Barcelona
Hospital de Terrasa
Ctra. Torrebonica
08221 Terrasa
Barcelona
937310007
(Contact Person:
    Dr. Socorro Uriz Urzainqui)

Fuentesnuevas
Hospital de Ponferrada
C/de la Dehesa s/n
24411 Fuentesnuevas
Ponferrada (León)
987455200

La Linea de la Concepción
Hospital La Linea de la Concepción
Cmenendez Pelayo 103
11300 La Linea de la Concepción
956175550

Madrid
Hospital Severo Ochoa
Av. de Orellana s/n
28911 Leganes
Madrid
916944811
(Contact Person: Dr. Gonzalez Alvarez)

Motril
Hospital Santa Ana
Ctra. Antigua de Granada s/n
18600 Motril
Granada
958603506
(Contact Person: Dr. Eduardo Ortega Paez)

Pozoblanco
Hospital Valle de Pedroches
Av. de la Constitución s/n
14400 Pozoblanco
Córdoba
957771511
(Contact Person: Dr. Juan Amor Truejos)

Ubeda
Hospital San Juan de la Cruz
Ctra. de Linares Km. 1
23400 Ubeda
953797100
(Contact Person: Dr. Antonio Torres Torres)

Alicante
Alcoy
Hospital Virgen de los Lirios
Poligono de Caramanxel s/n

03800 Alcoy
Alicante
966527400/966527448
(Contact Person: Dr. Fernando Clemente)

Alicante
Hospital Clinico San Juan
Ctra. Alicante-Valencia s/n
03550 San Juan de Alicante
Alicante
965938700/965908652
(Contact Person: Dr. Mercedes Juste)

Alicante
Hospital General de Alicante
Maestro Alonso 109
03010 Alicante
Alicante
965908300/965245971
(Contact Person: Dr. Juan Gonzalez Perab)

Alicante
Elche
Hospital General de Elche
Partida Huertos y Molinos s/n
03071 Elche
Alicante
966606000/966606108
(Contact Person: Dr. Jesus Garde Garde)

Alicante
Elda
Hospital General de Elda
Ctra. Elda-Sax s/n
03600 Elda
Alicante
966989000
(Contact Person: Dr. Isabel Ortin Septien)

Alicante
Villajoyosa
Hospital Comarcal La Vilajolosa
Partida Galandu 5
03570 Villajoyosa
Alicante
966859200/966859300
(Contact Person:
   Dr. Amparo Gomez Granell)

Badajoz
Hospital Infanta Cristina
Ctra. Madrid-Lisboa s/n
06080 Badajoz
Badajoz
924218100
(Contact Person: Dr. Antonio Serrano)

Barcelona
Hospital Vall dHebron
(Contact Person: Dr. Nicolas Cobos)
Passeig Vall dHebron s/n
08023 Barcelona
Barcelona
934893170

Barcelona
Esplugues de Llobregat
Hospital Sant Joan de Deu
P§ Sant Joan de Deu 2
08950 Esplugues de Llobregat
Barcelona
932804000
(Contact Person: Dr. Jose Luis Seculi)

Barcelona
Sabadell
Hospital Nen Jesus
Bonaigua 31
08208 Sabadell
Barcelona
937237358
(Contact Person:
    Dr. Oscar Asensio de la Cruz)

Bilbao
Infantil de Cruces
Pl. Barrio de Cruces
48903 Bilbao
Bilbao
944850086
(Contact Person: Dr. Carlos Vazquez)

Cadiz
Hospital Puerta del Mar
Av. Ana de Villa 21
11009 Cadiz

Cadiz
956242100
(Contact Person: Dr. Mena/
    Dr. Antonio Alienza)

Castellón
Hospital General de Castellón
Av. Benicasim s/n
12004 Castellón
Castellón
964200100/964252345
(Contact Person: Dr. Eduardo Bues)

Castellón
Vinaroz
Hospital de Vinaroz
Av. Gil de Atrocillo s/n
12005 Vinaroz
Castellón
964400032/964400736
(Contact Person: Dr. Rabasco)

Cáceres
Hospital San Pedro Alcantara
Av. de Millan Astray
    s/n 10003 Cáceres
Cáceres
927256200/927256202
(Contact Person: Dr. Lopez)

Cádiz
Jerez de la Frontera
Hospital de Jerez
Ctra. de Circunvalación s/n
11407 Jerez de la Frontera
Cádiz
956358000
(Contact Person: Dr. Garcia Chesa)

Cádiz
San Fernando
Hospital Naval San Carlos
Capitan Conforto s/n
11100 San Fernando
Cádiz
956599000
(Contact Person:
    Dr. Juan M. García-Cubillana)

Córdoba
Hospital Reina Sofia
Av. Menendez Pidal s/n
14004 Córdoba
Córdoba
957217000
(Contact Person: Dr. Vaquero)

Granada
Hospital Virgen de las Nieves
Av. Constitución 100
18012 Granada
Granada
958241100
(Contact Person: Dr. Valenzuela)

Huelva
Hospital Juan Ramon Jimenez
Ronda Exterior Zona Norte
21005 Huelva
Huelva
959201000
(Contact Person: Dr. García Martin)

Jaén
Hospital Ciudad de Ja,n Dra.
  Antonia Pizarro
Av. Ejercito Español 10
23007 Jaén
Jaén
953299000

La Coruña
Hospital Teresa Herrera
Ctra. de las Xubias
15006 La Coruña
La Coruña
981178000
(Contact Person: Dr. Leopoldo García
  Alonso)

Las Palmas de Gran Canaria
Hospital Materno Infantil
Av. Maritima del Sur s/n
35016 Las Palmas de Gran Canaria
Las Palmas de Gran Canaria
928444500
(Contact Person: Dr. Luis Peña)

Madrid
Getafe
Hospital Universitario de Getafe
Ctra. de Toledo km. 12500
28021 Getafe
Madrid
916839360
(Contact Person: Dr. Madruga)

Madrid
Hospital Doce de Octubre
Ctra. de Andalucia km 5400
28041 Madrid
Madrid
913908323
(Contact Person: Dr. Manzanares)

Madrid
Hospital Gregorio Marañon
Dr. Esquerdo 46
28007 Madrid
Madrid
915868000
(Contact Person: Dr. Hubert)

Madrid
Hospital La Paz
P§ de la Castellana 261
28046 Madrid
Madrid
913580851
(Contact Person: Dr. Antelo)

Madrid
Hospital La Princesa
Diego de León 62
28006 Madrid
Madrid
915202277
(Contact Person: Dr. Girón)

Madrid
Hospital Niño Jesús
Menendez y Pelayo 65
28009 Madrid
Madrid
915735200 ext. 276
(Contact Person: Dr. Salcedo)

Madrid
Hospital Ramon y Cajal
Ctra. de Colmenar km. 9100
28034 Madrid
Madrid
913368092/913580614
(Contact Person: Dr. Maiz)

Murcia
El Palmar
Hospital Virgen de la Arreixaca
Ctra. Madrid-Cartagena
30120 El Palmar
Murcia
968369582
(Contact Person:
 Dr. Manuel López Sanchez Solís)

Murcia
Hospital Provincial Universitario
Av. Intendente Jorge Palacios
20003 Murcia
Murcia
968256900
(Contact Person: Dr. Fernando Sanchez
 Gascon)

Málaga
Hospital Carlos Haya
Av. Arroyo de los Angeles s/n
29010 Málaga
Málaga
952390400
(Contact Person:
 Dr. Javier Pérez Frias)

Orense
Hospital Cristal Piñor
Ramon Puga 54
32005 Orense
Orense
988385500
(Contact Person: Dr. Tabares)

Oviedo
Hospital Ntra. Sra. Covadonga
Celestino Villamil s/n
33006 Oviedo

Oviedo
985108019
(Contact Person: Dr. Carlos Bousoño)

Palma de Mallorca
Hospital Son Dureta
Andrea Doria 55
07014 Palma de Mallorca
Palma de Mallorca
971750000
(Contact Person:
 Dr. Juan Figuerola Mulet)

Pamplona
Hospital Virgen del Camino
Irunlarrea 4
31008 Pamplona
Pamplona
948429400
(Contact Person: Dr. Jose Emilia Olivera)

Salamanca
Hospital Clinico
P. de San Vicente 58–182
37007 Salamanca
Salamanca
923291100
(Contact Person: Dr. Martinez)

Salamanca
Hospital Virgen de la Vega
P. de San Vicente 58–182
37007 Salamanca
Salamanca
923291200
(Contact Person: Dr. Grande)

Santander
Hospital Cantabria
Cazona s/n
39008 Santander
Santander
942202520
(Contact Person: Dr. Pedro Fernandez)

Santander
Hospital Marques Valdecilla
Av. Valdesilla 25

39008 Santander
Santander
942202520
(Contact Person: Dr. Zubano)

Sevilla
Hospital La Macarena
Av. Dr. Fedriani 3
41071 Sevilla
Sevilla
954557400
(Contact Person: Dr. Navarro)

Sevilla
Hospital Virgen del Rocio
Av. Manuel Siurot s/n
41013 Sevilla
Sevilla
954247642
(Contact Person: Dr. Dapena)

Sta. Cruz de Tenerife
Hospital Ntra. Sra. Candelaria
Ctra. Gral. del Rosario s/n
38010 Sta. Cruz de Tenerife
Sta. Cruz de Tenerife
922602000
(Contact Person: Dr. Ortigosa)

Sta. Cruz de Tenerife
Univer. Canarias
Ofra—La Laguna
38320 Sta.Cruz de Tenerife
Sta. Cruz de Tenerife
922678000
(Contact Person:
   Dr. Honorio de Armas)

Valencia
Gandia
Hospital de Francesc de Borja
Passeig de les Germanies 71
46700 Gandia
Valencia
963875936/962959200
(Contact Person:
   Dr. Manuel Oltra Benavent)

Valencia
Clinico Universitario
Av. Blasco Ibañez 17
46010 Valencia
Valencia
963862600/963862600
(Contact Person: Dr. Escribano)

Valencia
Hospital General
Av. Tres Cruces s/n
46014 Valencia
Valencia
963862900
(Contact Person: Dr. Miguel Calabuig)

Valencia
Hospital Universitario La Fé
Av. Campanar 21
46009 Valencia
Valencia
963862700
(Contact Person: Dr. Ferrer)

Valladolid
Clinico Universitario
Av. Ramon y cajal 7
47005 Valladolid
Valladolid
983420000
(Contact Person: Dr. Calvo)

Zaragoza
Clinico Universitario
Av. Gomez Laguna s/n
50009 Zaragoza
Zaragoza
976556400
(Contact Person: Dr. Lázaro)

Zaragoza
Infantil Miguel Servet
P§ Isabel la catolica s/n
50009 Zaragoza
Zaragoza
976355700
(Contact Person: Dr. Heredia)

SWEDEN

Göteborg
CF Center Pediatric Clinic
University Hospital
SU/Östra
416 85 Göteborg
46.31.3435624/46.31.3435184
(Contact Person: Anders Lindblad)

Huddinge
Pediatric Clinic University Hospital
Stockholms CF Center
B 59
141 86 Huddinge
46.8.58587359/46.8.58581410
(Contact Person: Lena Hjelte)

Lund
CF Center Medical/Lung Clinic
CF Center Medical/Lung Clinic
University Hospital
221 85 Lund
46.46.171490/46.46.146793
(Contact Person: Leif Eriksson)

Uppsala
CF Center Pediatric Clinic
University Hospital
751 85 Uppsala
46.18.665929/46.18.665853
(Contact Person: Marie Johannesson)

SWITZERLAND

Aarau
Kinderklinik Kantonsspital
5001 Aarau
41.62.8384004
(Contact Person: PD Dr. Hanspeter Gnehm/
  Dr. P. Eng)

Basel
Universitäts-Kinderspital
Römergasse 8
4005 Basel
41.61.6912626

(Contact Person:
  PD Dr. med. Jürg Hammer)

Bern
Universitäts-Kinderklinik Inselspital
3010 Bern
41.31.6329493/41.31.6329468
(Contact Person: Prof. Dr. Richard
  Kraemer/Prof. Dr. M.-H. Schöni)

Davos-Platz
Alpine Kinderklinik
Scalettastrasse 5
7270 Davos-Platz
41.81.4157070
(Contact Person: Dr. med. Bruno Knöpfli)

Gallen
Ostschweiz Kinderspital
Claudiusstrasse 6
9000 ST. Gallen
41.71.3244111
(Contact Person: Dr. med. P. Eng)

Geneve
Hôpital Cantonal Universitaire
30Bd. de la Cluse
1211 Geneve 4
41.22.3729902
(Contact Person: Dr. Dominique Belli/
  Dr. Thierry Rochat/Dr. Susanne Suter)

Lausanne
Centre Hospitalier Universitaire Vaudois
  CHUV
Service de Pédiatrie
1011 Lausanne
41.21.3145631
(Contact Person: PD Dr. Michel Roulet)

Luzern
Pädiatrische Klinik Kinderspital/
  Kantonsspital
Kinderspital/Kantonsspital
6000 Luzern 16
41.41.2053151
(Contact Person: Dr. J. Spalinger)

Zurich
Universitäts-Kinderspital
Steinwiesstrasse 75
8032 Zurich
41.1.2661111
(Contact Person: PD Dr. Christian Braegger/
  Prof. Dr. F. Sennhauser)

UNITED KINGDOM

Aberdeen
Royal Aberdeen Children's Hospital
Aberdeen AB9 2ZG
Fax: 01224 840727
(Contact Person: Dr. R. Brooker)
Children: Yes

Belfast
Belfast City Hospital
Adult CF Unit
Belfast City Hospital
Belfast BT9 7AB
028 90 329241
  Fax: 028 90263546 (326614)
(Contact Person: Dr. S. Elborn)

Belfast
Royal Belfast Hospital for Sick Children
Falls Road
Belfast, BT12 6BE
Fax: 028 90235340
(Contact Person: Dr. A Redmond)
Children: Yes

Birmingham
Birmingham Heartlands Hospital
Bordesley Green East
Birmingham, B9 5SS
0121 776 6611 X4475/
  0121 766 6611 X4478
(Contact Person: Dr. D. Honeybourne/
  Dr. D. Stableforth)
Children: Yes
Adult: Yes

Birmingham
The Children's Hospital
Ladywood Middleway

Birmingham, B16 8ET
0121 333 9999/Fax: 0121 333 8201
(Contact Person: Dr. P Weller)
Children: Yes

Bristol
Royal Hospital for Sick Children
St. Michael's Hill
Bristol, BS2 8BJ
Fax: 0117 928 5693
(Contact Person: Dr. S. Langton-Hewer)
Children: Yes

Cambridge
Addenbrooke's Hospital Hills Road
Cambridge, CB2 2QQ
01223 216020/012232 216878/
  Fax: 01223 216020
(Contact Person: Dr. R. Ross-Russell/
  Dr. R. Iles)
Children: Yes

Cambridge
Papworth Hospital
Papworth Everard
Cambridge, CB3 8RE
01480 830541/Fax: 01480 460969
(Contact Person: Dr. D. Bilton)

Cardiff
Llandough Hospital
Penarth
Cardiff, CF6 1XX
02920 716947/02920 715417/
  Fax: 02920 712284
(Contact Person: Prof. D. Shale/
  Dr. I. Campbell)

Cardiff
University Hospital of Wales
Heath Park
Cardiff, CF14 4XW
02920 743530/Fax: 02920 743587
(Contact Person: Dr. I. Doull)

Dundee
Ninewells Hospital & Medical School
Dundee, DD1 9SY

01382 632179/01382 632179/
    Fax: 01382 632597
(Contact Person: Dr. A. Mehta/
    Prof. R. Olver)

Edinburgh
Royal Hospital Sick Children
Sciennes Road
Edinburgh, EH9 1LF
0131 536 0000/Fax: 0131 536 0171
(Contact Person: Dr. T. Marshall)

Edinburgh
Western General Hospital
Crewe Road
Edinburgh, EH4 2XU
0131 537 1783/Fax: 0131 343 3989
(Contact Person: Dr. A. Innes/
    Dr. A. Greening)

Exeter
Royal Devon & Exeter Hospital
Barrack Road
Exeter, EX2 5DW
01392 402132/01392 402665/
    Fax: 01392 402152
(Contact Person: Dr. C. Sheldon/
    Dr. P. Oades/Dr. J. Tripp)
Children: Yes
Adult: Yes

Glasgow
Gartnavel General Hospital
Great Western Road 1053
Glasgow, G12 0YN
0141 211 3247/Fax: 0141 211 3464
(Contact Person: Dr. B. Stack)

Glasgow
Royal Hospital for Sick Children
Yorkhill
Glasgow, G3 8SJ
0141 201 0035/0141 201 0035/
    0141 201 0314
(Contact Person: Dr. N. Gibson/
    Dr. J. Paton/Dr. J. Evans)
Children: Yes

Gwent
Royal Gwent Hospital
Newport
Gwent, NP9 2UB
01633 234613X/01633 238965/
    Fax: 01633 234788
(Contact Person: Dr. I. Bowler/
    Dr. S. Maguire)

Leeds
Seacroft Hospital
York Road
Leeds, LS14 6UH
0113 206 2088/0113 206 3513/
    Fax: 0113 206 3738
(Contact Person: Dr. D. Peckham/
    Dr. S. Conway)
Adult: Yes

Leeds
St. James's & Seacroft University
    Hospital NHS
TrustBeckett Street
Leeds LS9 7TF
Fax: 0113 206 5405/0113 206 3540
(Contact Person: Dr. K. Brownlee/
    Dr. S. Conway)
Children: Yes

Leicester
Leicester Royal Infirmary
Infirmary Square
Leicester, LE1 5WW
Fax: 0116 258 7657
(Contact Person: Dr. C. O'Callaghan)

Liverpool
Royal Liverpool Children's Hospital
Alder HeyEaton Road
Liverpool, L12 2AP
Fax: 0151 252 5929/0151 252 5929
(Contact Person: Prof. R. Smyth/
    Dr. D. Heaf)
Children: Yes

Liverpool
The Cardiothoracic Centre Liverpool
NHS TrustThomas Drive

Liverpool, L14 3PE
0151 293 2390/Fax: 0151 228 5539
(Contact Person: Dr. M. Walshaw)

London
Barts & the Royal London Hospital
Unit Fielden House Whitechapel
London, E1 1BB
020 7377 7605/020 7377 7462/
  Fax: 020 7377 7033
(Contact Person: Dr. D. Empey/Dr. S. Carr)
Children: Yes
Adult: Yes

London
King's HealthcareKing's College Hospital
Denmark Hill
London, SE5 9RS
020 7346 3562 (3431)/020 7346 3215
(Contact Person: Dr. G. Ruiz/Prof. J. Price)

London
The Hospital for Sick Children
Great Ormond Street
London, WC1N 3JH
020 7405 9200×5453/Fax: 020 7829 8634
(Contact Person: Dr. C. Wallis/
  Dr. R. Dinwiddie)

London
The Royal Brompton Hospital
Sydney Street
London, SW3 6NP
020 7352 8121 bleep 1006/020 7351 8182
(Contact Person: Prof. M. Hodson/
  Prof. D. Geddes/Dr. A. Bush)
Children: Yes
Adult: Yes

London
University Hospital Lewisham
High Street Lewisham
London, SE13 6LH
020 8333 3136/Fax: 020 8690 1963
(Contact Person: Dr. C. Daman-Willems/
  Dr. J. Stroobant)

Manchester
Manchester Children's Hospital

HallCharlestown Road
Manchester, M9 7AA
0161 220 5093/0161 220 5093/
  Fax: 0161 795 7542
(Contact Person: Dr. L. Patel/Prof. T. David)

Manchester
Royal Manchester Children's Hospital
Pendlebury
Manchester, M27 4HA
(Contact Person: Dr. M. Super/
  Dr. G. Hambleton)
Children: Yes

Manchester
Wythenshawe Hospital
Southmoor Road
Manchester, M23 9LT
0161 291 2154/Fax: 0161 291 2080
(Contact Person: Dr. A.K. Webb)

Newcastle Upon Tyne
Royal Victoria Infirmary Queen Victoria
  Road
Newcastle Upon Tyne NE1 4LP
0191 232 5131 X25089/0191 284 3111
(Contact Person: Dr. C. O'Brien/
  Dr. D. Spencer)

Norwich
Norfolk & Norwich Hospital
Brunswick Road
Norwich, Norfolk NR1 3SR
01603 287544/Fax: 01603 287584
(Contact Person: Dr. C. Upton)

Nottingham
Nottingham City Hospital
Hucknall Road
Nottingham, NG5 1PB
0115 840 4775/0115 969 1169 X46475
(Contact Person: Prof. A. Knox/
  Dr. A. Smyth)

Oxford
Oxford Radcliffe NHS Trust.
John Radcliffe Hospital
Headington

Oxford, OX3 9DU
01865 221496/Fax: 01865 220479
(Contact Person: Dr. A. Thomson)

Stoke on Trent
North Staffs City General Hospital
Newcastle Road
Stoke on Trent ST4 6QC
01782 552572/01782 718392/
  Fax: 01782 713946
(Contact Person: Dr. W. Lenney/
  Dr. C. Campbell)
Children: Yes

Surrey
Frimley Park Hospital Portsmouth
Road Frimley
Surrey, GU16 5UJ
01276 604122/Fax: 01276 604148
(Contact Person: Dr. R. Knight)

Hampshire
Sheffield
Northern General Hospital
Herries Road
Sheffield, S5 7AU
0114 271 4770/Fax: 0114 226 6280
(Contact Person: Dr. F. Edenborough)

Hampshire
Sheffield
Sheffield Children's Hospital
Western Bank
Sheffield, S10 2TH
Fax: 0114 275 5364
(Contact Person: Prof. C. Taylor)
Children: Yes

Hampshire
Southampton
Southampton University Hospital NHS
Southampton, S016 6YD
Trust Tremona Road
023 80796801/023 80794862/
  Fax: 023 80794762
(Contact Person: Dr. M. Carroll/
  Dr. G. Connett)

INDEX

Note: Page locators followed by f and t indicates figure and table respectively.

A

Abdominal pain, 95
  in adults, 268
  from intestinal blockage, 92
Acapella, 43, 43f, 364f, 370–371, 371f
Accessory muscles of respiration, 26
Acetylcysteine (Mucomyst), 46, 327
Acid reflux, 98
Actigal (Ursodiol), 348
Actin, 33
Active cycle of breathing technique, 44,
  374
Admission, hospital, 137. *See also*
  Hospitalization
ADULT mnemonic, 256
Adults with CF, issues of, 265–284
  antibiotic-associated diarrhea, 268
  birth control, 272
  body organ systems, effect on
    bone health, 270
    gastrointestinal system, 267–270
    reproductive system, 270–273
    respiratory system, 266–267
  careers in health care, 279–281
  Clostridium difficile colitis, 268
  communication with other CF adults,
    284
  death, 283–284
  diabetes, 269
  education, 277–278
  employment, 279
  gallstones, 269
  health/disability insurance, 274–275
  intestinal blockage, 268
  liver disease, 269–270
  lung problems, 266–267
  marriage and family, 281
    infant feeding, 282
    sex life, 282
  medical care, 274
  overall health, 273–274
  pregnancy, 271–272
  psychological issues, 283
  unemployment, 276
  urinary incontinence, 273
  vaginal yeast infections, 272–273
Advair, 336
Advanced directives, 283
Aerobic exercise, 205, 206, 213. *See also*
  Exercise
Aerobic fitness, 207
Aerosol machine, 47, 48f
Aerosol therapy
  for asthma, 47, 48f
  during hospitalization, 148
  for mucus thinning, 46, 249
  for pulmonary exacerbations, 55
Air embolism, 147
Air hunger, 287
Airplane travel, 202
Airway
  fluid lining of, 3–4
  infection in CF in, 6–7
Airway cells, *Pseudomonas* attachment to,
  7
Airway clearance, 148
  Acapella in, 43, 43f, 370–371, 371f
  active cycle of breathing technique in,
    44, 374
  autogenic drainage in, 374
  exercise in, 45, 374
  flutter technique in, 42, 43f, 369–370,
    370f
  mist tents in, 46
  positive expiratory pressure mask
    technique in, 374
  postural drainage in, 363–369,
    364f–369f
  Quake in, 43, 44f, 371–372, 371f
  in teenagers, 247–249
  vest in, 372–374, 372f–373f
  while traveling, 201–202

Airway fluid, 3–4
  cilia in, 27, 27f
  research on, 302
Airway inflammation, treatment of,
    50–51
Albumin, 118
Albuterol, 47, 328
Alcohol, 260, 278
Allergy medicines, 340–341
Allergy shots, 341
Alpha-1-antitrypsin Z, 100
Altitude, effects on CF, 201–202
  higher altitude, 201
  low altitude, 202
Amantadine, 334–335
Americans with Disabilities Act (ADA) of
    1990, 279–280
Amikacin, 332
Amino acids, 227
Amniocentesis, 231
Amoxicillin, 330
Ampicillin, 330
Amylase, 85
Anaerobic exercise, 205–206, 213. *See also*
    Exercise
Anastomosis, 164
Anemia, due to iron deficiency, 119
"The anorexia of malnutrition", 105, 117
Antacid drugs, 344–345
Anthropometrics, 115
Antibiotics, 50, 328–334
  aerosol (nebulized), 55
  aminoglycosides, 332
  aztreonam, 334
  for bronchial infections, 250
  cephalosporins, 331
  colistimethate, 334
  decision to use, 56–57
  diarrhea associated with, 268
  imipenem, 334
  intravenous, 56
  linezolid, 333–334
  macrolides, 332
  meropenem, 334
  oral, 50, 55
  penicillins, 329–331
  for pulmonary exacerbations, 55–56
  quinolones, 333

resistance to, 57–59
  sulfa drugs, 331–332
  tetracyclines, 332–333
  vancomycin, 333
Antibloating medications, 347
Anticonstipation medicines, 346–347
Antifungal medicines, 335
Antihistamines, 341
Anti-inflammatory medications, 149,
    335–337
Antilymphocyte antibodies, 170t
Antilymphocyte drugs, 350
Antimetabolites, 170t, 351
Antireflux drugs, 345–346
Antirejection drugs. *See*
    Immunosuppressive medications
Antithymocyte globulin (ATG), 350
Antithymocyte globulin, 170t
Antiviral medications, 334–335
Appendicitis, 94
Appetite stimulants and supplements,
    348–349
Applesauce, 127–128
AquADEKs, 119
Aquagenic wrinkling of palms, 108
Arthritis, 107
Ascites, 100
Aspergillus fumigatus, in CF patients,
    38–39
Aspiration, 85
Asthma, 33
  bronchodilators for, 327–328
  exercise-induced, 209
  pulmonary function tests for, 75–76
  treatment of, 47–49, 48f
Ataluren, 302
Atelectasis, 65–66, 66f
  cause of, 65
  treatment of, 65–66
ATG (antithymocyte globulin), 170t, 176,
    179
Atgam, 170t
Augmentin, 330
Autogenic drainage, 44, 374
Autopsy, 292
Azathioprine (Imuran), 168, 170t,
    172–173
Azithromycin (Zithromax), 179

Azithromycin, 50
Azlocillin, 330–331
Azothioprine (Imuran), 351
Aztreonam, 334

B
Bacteria
    attachment of, to airway cells, 7
    biofilm production by, 305
    culture and sensitivity tests for, 78–81
Bacterial colonization, of lungs, 37–38
Bacterial infections
    in CF patients, 37–38
    prevention of, 50–53
        patient-to-patient transmission of
            bacteria, 51–52
        treating first *Pseudomonas* culture,
            52–53
Basic research, 296
Basiliximab, 170t
β-carotene, 120
Bench research, 296
Beta-agonists, 328
Bicycling
    clothes for, 218–219
    equipment for, 217–218
    preparing bicycle for, 218
    and safety considerations, 218
    starting to, 219
Bile, 85
Bile ducts, blockage of, 102
Biofilm, 305
Biopsy procedure, 181
Biopsy specimen, 176, 181, 183
Birth control, 272
Bisphosphonates, 107
Bleeding
    during bronchoscopy, 185
    from central line, 148
    in hemoptysis, 59–61
    liver transplantation and, 191
    vitamin K deficiency and, 59, 60
Bloating, medications for, 347
Blood clots, 174
Blood tests, during hospitalization, 149
Body box, 74
Body image, in teenagers, 259–260
Body mass index (BMI), 115

Bone and joint problems, 106–108
Bowel stimulants, 347
Brain dead, 159
Brain, role in regulation of breathing, 24–25
Breathing
    control of, 24–25
    difficult, in pneumothorax, 62
    respiratory muscles in, 25–26
Bronchi, 22, 23f
Bronchial artery embolization, for
        hemoptysis, 60–61
Bronchial cells, fluid secretion by, 3–4, 3f
Bronchiectasis, 32
Bronchioles, 22, 23f
Bronchiolitis obliterans, 31, 36, 178
Bronchitis, 36
Bronchitol, 304
Bronchodilators, 327–328
Bronchoscopy, 176, 182
    complications of, 183–186
        bleeding within bronchi, 185
        cough, 184
        nosebleed, 184
        oversedation, 184
        pneumothorax, 185
    in atelectasis, 66
    rejection, diagnosis of, 176
Bronchospasm, 33
Broviac catheters, 144–145
Budesonide (Pulmicort), 49
Burkholderia cepacia infection, 37, 38, 51,
        158
    prevention of, 51, 140

C
Calcium-dependent chloride channel,
        3–4, 3f
Caloric intake, inadequate, 117
Camps, CF, 194
Capillaries, pulmonary, 23
Carbenicillin, 330–331
Carbon dioxide, 22
    elimination of, 23, 24
    high levels of, 287–288
Cardiopulmonary bypass, 165
Carriers, 222
    of CF, 232–233, 232t
Cathelicidins, 28

Cayston, 313
Celiac disease, 95
Cellcept, 170t, 173
Central line, 144–148. *See also*
    Intravenous antibiotics
  care of, 146–147
    at home, 151
  complications of, 147–148
  equipment for, 146
  medications administration through,
    148
  placement of, 145
  for prolonged use, 144
  removal of, 145–146
  types of, 144
    Hickman and Broviac catheters,
      144–145
    Mediports, Infusaports, and
      Portacaths, 145
    PICC lines, 144
Cephalosporins, 331
Cervical mucus, 271
CF centers, 199, 203
CF gene, 2, 227–228
  clinical research and future treatments
    on, 298–299
  delta *F508* mutation in, 228, 229t
  mutations in, 7–10, 229
  research on, 297–299
CF Legal Information Hotline, 317
CFTR protein
  basic research on, 299–301
  clinical research and future treatments
    on, 301–302
  normal functioning of, 2–3, 3f, 7–8, 8f
Chemical sclerosing, 64
Chest pain, 69–70
Chest physical therapy (CPT), 40–42, 41f
  PD table for, 42
  in teenagers, 247
Chest radiographs, 150
Chest tube, 64
Chest x-rays, 77–78, 79f
Child development specialists, 142
Child-life workers, 142
Children
  parental involvement with, 136–137
  questions about hospitalization by, 136

Chloride channels, 3–4, 3f
Chloride ions, membrane transport of,
    3–5, 3f
Chloride secretion, normal, 3–4, 3f
Chloride transport, sodium transport
    and, 3–4
Chorionic villus sampling, 231
Chromosomes, 221
Chronic lung disease, 202
Cigarette smoke, avoidance of, 39,
    200–201, 230, 260, 278
Cimetidine (Tagamet), 344
Cirrhosis, 100
Clamshell approach, in lung
    transplantation, 164
Clinical research, 296
Clinics, visits to, 195
Clostridium difficile infection, 96
Cloxacillin, 330
Clubbing, 70–71, 70f, 107, 108
CMV infection, in lung transplant
    recipients, 178
COBRA (Comprehensive Omnibus Budget
    Reconciliation Act), 275, 276
Colace, 346
Colds, 34–35
Colistimethate, 334
Colistin, 334
Collapsed lung. *See* Atelectasis;
    Pneumothorax
College, going to, 199
Compacted DNA, 298
Complementary and alternative medicine
    products, 123
Complications, pulmonary, 59–71
  atelectasis, 65–66, 66f
  chest pain, 69–70
  clubbing, 70–71
  cor pulmonale, 68–69
  heart failure, 68–69
  hemoptysis, 59–61
  low oxygen level, 66–67
  pneumothorax, 61–65, 62f, 63f
  respiratory failure, 67–68
Computed tomographic (CT) scans, 78
Congenital bilateral absence of vas
    deferens (CBAVD), 234
Constipation, 93

Cor pulmonale, 68–69
Corticosteroids, 169t
Cough, 26–27
  hemoptysis and, 59
  in pulmonary exacerbations, 54
Cough medicines, 339–340
  cough suppressant, 340
  expectorants, 339–340
Cough reflex, 177
Cultures and sensitivities, 78–81
Cyclosporine, 154, 168, 169t, 350
Cyproheptadine (Periactin), 130, 341, 349
Cystic fibrosis (CF), 1, 221
  basic defect in, 1–12
  complications of, 59–71 (*See also*
    Complications)
  diagnosis of, 13–20 (*See also* Diagnosis)
  gastrointestinal conditions in,
    incidence of, 86t
  genetic diagnosis of, 233–234
  history of, 385
  incidence of, in different countries,
    225t
  medications for (*See* Medications)
  reading resources and websites on, 284,
    387–389
  secretion and absorption of salt and
    water in, problem of, 5–6
  sign or symptom of, 15t
  teenagers with, 245–246 (*See also*
    Teenagers)
Cystic fibrosis clinic, visits to, 39, 242
Cystic Fibrosis Foundation, 312–318
  on care for people with CF, 315–317
    advocacy, 317
    legal hotline, 317
    patient assistance, 317
    Patient Registry, 316
    pharmaceutical services, 317
    Quality Improvement Initiative, 316
  future directions for, 318
  history of, 312
  milestones of, 312–313
  mission of, 312
  research & drug development program
    of, 313–315
  resources on, 318
  support for, 317–318

Cystic Fibrosis Foundation Therapeutics,
  Inc. (CFFT), 313–315
Cystic Fibrosis Patient Assistance
  Foundation (CFPAF), 313, 317
Cystic fibrosis related diabetes (CFRD),
  104–105
  in teenagers, 254
Cystic Fibrosis Services Pharmacy, 312
Cystic fibrosis transmembrane
  conductance regulator (CFTR)
  gene, 87. *See also* CF gene
Cytomegalovirus (CMV), 171

D
Daily life
  college, going to, 199
  day care, 198–199
  friends, visits with, 200
  medications and treatments
    responsibility in, 196–198
  place to live, 201–203
  school, going to, 199
  smoke, avoidance of, 200–201
  sports and exercise in, 199. *See also*
    Exercise
  traveling, considerations for, 201–202
  in hospital, 137–139
Daclizumab, 170t
Data Safety Monitoring Board, 309
Dating, 262
Death and dying, 287–293
  of adults with CF, 283–284
  CF research and, 293
  low oxygen level and, 287–288
  lung transplantation and, 290–291
  morphine for sedation in, 288
  myths about, 289–290
  organ donation and, 292
  oxygen therapy in, 288, 377–379,
    378t
  patients' concerns about, 291
  and postmortem examination, 292
  reactions to, 291–292
Decongestants, 341
Defensins, 28
Dehiscence, 164
Deltasone, 169t
Denufosol, 303

Diabetes, 103–105
  in adults, 269
  in teenagers, 253–254
Diagnosis, 13–20
  gene testing in, 17–18
  impact of, on patient's family, 13
  learning of, 235–237
  nasal potential difference in, 2, 19
  newborn screening for, 17
  reasons for, 14, 15t
  sweat tests in, 1, 14–16
  in unusual cases, 19–20
Diaphragm, 25
Diarrhea, 117
Dicloxacillin, 330
Diet
  fiber in, 346
  high-calorie recipes for, 375–384
  low-fat, 117
  pancreatic enzymes in. See Pancreatic
    enzymes
  salt in, 112, 254
  suggestions for, 123–126, 124t, 125t
  supplements, 349
Dietitians, 142
Digestion, 116
  process of, 85–86
Digestive enzymes, 343–344, 346
  in mouth, 85
Digestive juices, 85
Digestive system. See Gastrointestinal
    (GI) tract
Digital clubbing, 70–71, 70f
Digitalis, 343
Distal intestinal obstruction syndrome
    (DIOS), 92–93
  in adults, 268
  in teenagers, 253
Diuretics, 342
DNA, 221, 226
DNase (Pulmozyme), 46–47, 249, 326–327
Docosahexaenoic acid (DHA), 118
Dominant trait, 222
Donor organs, shortage of, 159
Drainage, postural, 363–369, 364f–369f
Dronabinol (Marinol), 130, 349
Dual energy x-ray absorptiometry
    (DXA), 107

Duodenum, 84f
  digestion in, 85

E
Echocardiograms, 150
Edema, and hypoalbuminemia, 118
Elastase, 28, 89
Elastography, 101
Electrocardiograms (ECGs), 150
Elemental (predigested) formulas, 132,
    349
Embolization, bronchial artery, for
    hemoptysis, 60–61
Enemas, 347
Epithelial sodium channel (ENaC), 303
Epstein–Barr virus (EBV), 171
Erythromycin, 346
Erythromycin/sulfisoxazole, 331–332
Esomeprazole (Nexium), 99, 345
Esophagus, 84f, 85
Essential fatty acids, deficiency of, 118
Everolimus, 350
Exercise, 205–219
  aerobic, 205, 206
  for airway clearance, 374
  anaerobic, 205–206
  bicycling for, 217–219
  to clear mucus, 249
  effects of, 205–208
    in CF, 208–212
  guidelines for, 212–213
    general, 212
    medical advice, 212
    time allotment, 212–213
    type of activity, 213
  in heat, 206
    in CF, 210
  and heat training, 208
    in CF, 211–212
  pacing yourself in, 213–214
  repeated sessions of, 207–208
    in CF, 210–211
  running for, 214–216
  single sessions of, 205–206
    in CF, 208–209
  swimming for, 216–217
  tolerance, 207
    in CF, 210

Exercise-induced asthma (EIA), 209
Exercise tests, 77
Exercise tolerance, 207
  research in, 308
Exons, 227

F
The Family and Medical Leave Act
  (FMLA), 280
Family issues, 235–243
  clinic visits, 242
  couple relationships, 240–241
  explaining CF to others, 239
  in home care, 237–238
  in hospitalization, 242 (*See also*
    Hospitalization)
  learning of diagnosis of CF, 13,
    235–237
    emotions after, 236
    questions by parents on, 237
    response upon, 236
  sibling relationships, 240
  stress on family, 235, 241
  treatment of children with CF,
    239–240
Famotidine (Pepcid), 98, 345
Fat loss, in stool, 87
Fat-soluble vitamins, 119–122
Feeding tubes, 158
Fiber, dietary, 346
Fibrosing colonopathy, 90, 95, 129
Flow-volume curve, 72, 73f
Fluticasone (Flovent), 49
Flutter, 42, 43f, 364f, 369–370, 370f
Focal biliary cirrhosis, 100
Forced expired volume in 1 second
  (FEV$_1$), 72, 267
Forced vital capacity (FVC), 72
Formulas, infant, 123
Frequencer, 44, 247
Functional endoscopic sinus surgery
  (FESS), 30
Fundoplication, 99
Furosemide (Lasix), 342

G
Gallbladder, 99, 101–102
Gallium for *P. aeruginosa* infection, 305

Gallstones, 102, 269
Gastroesophageal reflux disease (GERD),
  97–99
Gastrografin enema, 91, 347
Gastrointestinal complications
  in adults, 267–270
  in teenagers, 253–254
Gastrointestinal (GI) tract
  anatomy of, 84, 84f
  function of, 84
  in patients with CF, problems in, 86,
    86t
    abdominal pain and diarrhea, 95–97
    esophagus and gastroesophageal
      reflux, 97–99
    gallbladder and bile ducts, 101–102
    liver, 99–101
    pancreas, 86–91
    small and large intestine, 91–95
  process of digestion in, 85–86
Gastrostomy (G-tube), 132, 133f
Gatorade, 212, 214
Gelfoam plug, 61
Genes, 221–222, 226–227
  for CF, 222, 227–228
Gene therapy, 234
Genetic diagnosis, 233–234
Genetic testing, 17–18
Gentamicin, 332
Giardiasis, 96
Gibson-Cooke method, 110
Glossary
  of drugs, 351–362
  of terms, 319–324
Gluten-sensitive enteropathy. *See* Celiac
  disease
GoLYTELY, 92, 268, 346
Grieving response, 236
Growth chart, 113–115, 114f
Growth hormone, 130–131, 348
Growth stimulants and supplements,
  348–349
GS9411, 304
GSK SB 656933, 307

H
Health care providers, 140, 143
Hearing test, 150

Heart failure, 68–69
Heart, role in oxygenation, 24
Heart medications, 341–343
Heat training, 208, 211–212
Helium dilution method, 74
Hemoptysis, 59–61
  in adults, 267
  in teenagers, 253
Hickman catheters, 144–145
High altitude, effects of, on CF, 201
High calorie recipes, 375–384
  artichoke pizzazz, 377
  cheesecake squares, 381
  cookbooks for, 384
  fettuccine alfredo, 375–376
  fruit pizza, 383
  German apple pie, 379
  heath bars, 382
  kid pleasin' chocolate mousse, 382
  lemon bars, 378
  milky way cake, 378–379
  miracle pudding, 382–383
  Orenstein family brownies, 379
  pasta pot, 375
  peanut butter banana shake, 380–381
  peanut butter round-ups, 377–378
  puppy chow, 383
  scotcheroos, 381
  shrimp spread, 377
  spinach pasta, 376
  sticky date pudding, 380
  sweet and sour strawberry dessert, 380
  vegetable pizza, 376
Histamine 2 (H_2) blockers, 98, 344–345
Hohn catheters, 144
Home care, of newly diagnosed child, 237–238
Home IV treatment, 151–152
Hospitalization
  activities in, 139
  admission for, 137
  clothing for, 139
  daily life in, 137–139
    infant and toddler, 138
    preschool, 138
    school-aged children, 138
    teenagers, 138–139
  ending of, 152
  for hemoptysis, 60
  infection control in, 140
  for initial CF education evaluation, 238
  nutrition in, 149
  preparation for, 136–137
  questions about, 136
  reasons for, 135
  and schoolwork, 139–140
  staff in, 140–143
    consultants, 142
    nurses, 141
    other health professionals, 142
    patient care assistant, 141
    physicians, 141–142
  tests in, 149–150
  treatments in, 143–149
Hypertonic saline, 47, 327
Hypertrophic pulmonary
    osteoarthropathy (HPOA), 107
Hypoalbuminemia, 118
Hypoelectrolytemia, 122–123
Hypomagnesemia, 122

I
Ibuprofen, 49–50, 252, 337
Icterus, 99
Imipenem, 334
Immunoreactive trypsinogen (IRT), 17, 89, 232
Immunosuppressive medications, 168, 171–172
  side effects of, 172–173
  types of, 169–170t
Imuran, 168, 170t, 172–173
InCourage vest system, 365f
Infants, salt loss in, 112
Infant Study of Inhaled Saline (ISIS) trial, 304
Infection control
  in hospitals, 140
  recommendations for, 51
Inflammation
  basic research on, 306–307
  clinical research and future treatments on, 307
Infusaports, 145
Insulin, 103
  function of, 103

production of, 86
resistance, 103
Intern, 141
Intrapulmonary Percussive Ventilator (IPV), 44
Intravenous antibiotics, 56, 250
    catheterization for, 143–144
    central line for, 144–148
    at home, 151–152
        care of, 151
        and checking up, 152
        ending of, 152
        reason for, 151
    length of treatment, 150
Introns, 227
Intussusception, 93, 93f
Iontophoresis, 110
Ipratropium, 47
Iron, deficiency of, 118–119
Itraconazole (Sporanox), 335
IV nutrition, 134

J
Jaundice, 99
Jejunostomy (J-tube), 132
Jogging, 207
Joint problems, 106–108

K
Kanamycin, 332
Ketchup Bottle Principle, 40

L
Lactulose (Cefulac, Chronulac), 346
Lansoprazole (Prevacid), 98–99, 345
Large intestine, 84f, 86
Laryngeal mask airway (LMA), 182, 184
Law of electrical neutrality, 4
Leukotriene inhibitors, 337
Levalbuterol (Xopenex), 47, 328
"Life support", 159
Linezolid, 333–334
Linoleic acid, 118
Lipase, mouth, 85
Liposomes, 298
Liprotamase, 308
Liver, 84f
    bile salts from, 85

disease, in adults, 269–270
medications, 348
transplantation, 101 (See also Liver transplantation)
Liver biopsy, 191
Liver transplantation, 188–192. See also Transplantation
    complications of, 190–191
        bleeding, 191
        blood clots, 191
        liver failure, 190–191
        rejection and infection, 190
    considerations for, 188
    continuing care after, 192
    contraindications to, 189
    results of, 192
    technique of, 190
    tests after, 191
    transplant list for, 189
Living donor lobar transplant, 166–167. See also Lung transplantation
LMA tube, for delivery of gas anesthesia, 184
Lobectomy, for hemoptysis, 61
Lower esophageal sphincter (LES), 85
Low-fat diet, 117
Lung Allocation Score (LAS), 161–162
Lung defenses, 26–28
    coughing, 26–27
    mucociliary escalator, 27–28, 27f
    in nose and mouth, 26
    other protection against infection, 28
Lung infections, 35–36
    basic research on, 304–305
    causes of, 37–39
    clinical research and future treatments on, 306
Lung problems, in adults, 266–267
Lungs
    function of, 22
    of people with CF, 246–247
    problems, in CF, 31–33
        asthma, 33
        cause of, 31
        cough, development of, 32–33
        infection and inflammation, 31–32, 32f
        progression of, 32–33

Lungs, treatment of
airway clearance techniques
breaking up mucus, 46–47
chest physical therapy, 40–46, 41f
exercise, 45
treating asthma, 47–48
airway inflammation in, 49–50
bacterial infection, 50–53
bronchial infection, 50
cigarette smoke, avoiding of, 39
general, 39
medical care, 39–40
pulmonary exacerbations, 54–56
viral infection, 53
Lung transplantation, 68, 156–167. *See also* Bronchoscopy; Transplantation
anastomosis in, 164
anteroinferior transthoracic incision in, 164
bleeding in, 174
blood clots in, 174
candidates for, 156
care after, 180–186
complications of, 173–180
early, 173–177
late, 177–179
psychological, social, and financial, 180
contraindications to, 156–158
absolute, 157–158
relative, 158
decision to proceed with, 187–188
dehiscence in, 164
double-lung, 164–165
immunosuppression for, 167–173, 169–170t
infection after, 176–179
living donor lobar, 166–167
narrowing of airway in, 175, 179
nerve damage in, 175
organ failure in, 173–174
rejection in, 175–176
acute, 175–176
chronic, 176, 178
results of, 186–187
sequential single-lung transplantation, 165–166
technique of, 163–167
test after, 182–186
transplant list for, 159–163
active and inactive patients on, 162–163
getting on, 160
LAS rule for, 161–162
waiting on, 162
Lung volumes, measurement of, 74–75
Lymphocyte-specific drugs, 169t

M
Maalox, 99
Macrolides, 332
Magnesium, deficiency of, 122
Malabsorption, 116–117
signs of, 116
Malaria, 11
Malnutrition, 113
causes of, 115–116
enzyme deficiency, 116–117
inadequate caloric intake, 117
increased use of calories, 117
weight loss due to, 113–115, 114f
Marijuana, 349
Masks
for infection control, 51–52
PEP, 247, 249, 374
Maximum voluntary ventilation (MVV), 207, 209
Mechanical ventilation, 36, 67
Meconium ileus, 91–92
Meconium peritonitis, 91
Media, culture, 79
Medical students, 141
Medications. *See also specific medications*
alphabetical listing of, 351–362
gastrointestinal/digestive system, 343–349
heart, 341–343
off-label usage, 325
respiratory system, 326–341
antibiotics, 328–334
antifungal medicines, 335
anti-inflammatory medications, 335–337
antiviral medications, 334–335
bronchodilators, 327–328

cough medicines, 339–340
leukotriene inhibitors, 337
mucolytics, 326–327
transplant-related, 349–351
upper airway, 340–341
Mediports, 145
Medrol, 169t
Megestrol (Megace), 130, 348
MELD (Model for End-stage Liver Disease), 189
Meropenem, 334
MESA (microsurgical epididymal sperm aspiration), 270–271
Metaproterenol, 47
Metered-dose inhaler (MDI), 328
Methicillin, 330
Methicillin-resistant *Staphylococcus aureus* (MRSA), 333
Methylprednisolone, 169t
Metoclopramide (Reglan), 345
Mezlocillin, 330–331
Microemulsion, 169t
Mineral oil, 346
Miralax, 92, 253, 346
Moli 1901, 303
Montelukast, 337
Morphine, 288
Mouth, digestion in, 85
Mucin, 303
Mucociliary escalator, 27–28, 27f
Mucolytics, 326–327
Mucous membranes, electrical charge across, 2
Mucus, 3
blood in, 59, 267
breaking up, 46–47
job of, 302
research on, 302–304
sticky, 1, 28
causes of, 7, 31
research on, 302
thinning drugs, 249
Multilobular cirrhosis, 100
Muromonab-CD3, 170t
Mutations, 227
Mycophenolate mofetil (Cellcept), 170t, 173, 351
Mylanta, 99

N
Nafcillin, 330
Nasal flaring, 26
Nasal polyp, 29–30
treatment of, 30
Nasal potential difference, 2
in diagnosis, 19
Nasogastric tube (NG tube), 132
Neomycin, 332
Neonatal cholestasis, 99
Neoral, 169t
Netilmicin, 332
Newborn screening, 17, 89
Nissen fundoplication, 99
Nizatidine (Axid), 344
Noninvasive ventilation, 68
Nose, 22
decongestants, use of, 341
electrical charges in, 4
filtering system of, 26
infections in, 34
polyps in, 29–30
Nucleotides, 226
Nutrition. *See also* Diet; Malnutrition and deficiencies in CF
albumin, 118
essential fatty acids, 118
fat-soluble vitamins, 119–122
iron, 118–119
magnesium, 122
salt, 122–123
and feeding problems in children, 124–125
growth and, monitoring of, 113–115, 114f
high-calorie recipes for, 375–384
in hospital, 149
importance of, 113
for infants, 123–124
school-aged children and, 124
teenagers and, 125
toddlers and preschool-aged children, 124
Nutritional treatment, 123
guidelines and suggestions for
for improving child's nutrition, 124t
for increasing calories in food, 125t

Nutritional treatment (*Continued*)
   hormones and appetite stimulants in, 130–131
   intravenous nutrition in, 134
   nutritional supplements in, 130, 131t
   pancreatic enzymes, use of, 126–130
   for teenagers, 126, 130
   tube feedings in, 132–134
Nutritionists. *See* Dietitians

O
Office of Disabled Students, 278
Off-label usage, 325
OKT3, 170t, 176, 179, 350
Omeprazole (Prilosec), 99, 345
Open lung biopsy, 185
Organ donations, 292
Oseltamivir, 334–335
Osteopenia, 106–107, 120
Osteoporosis, 106–107, 120
Oxacillin, 330
Oximetry, 76–77
Oxygen therapy, 337–339, 338f

P
Palivizumab (Synagis), 53, 335
Pancreas
   in CF, 6, 86–91, 86t
   structure and function of, 84f
Pancreatic enzyme replacement therapy (PERT), 88
   for pancreatic insufficiency treatment, 89
Pancreatic enzymes, 85, 87
   currently approved, 126
   enteric-coated, 127
   FDA approval for use of, 126–127
   use of
      how much to take, 128–129
      poor response to, 129–130
      procedure of, 127–128
      time of, 127
      who should take, 128
Pancreatic function testing, 88
Pancreatic insufficiency (PI), 87–88
   cause of, 87
   diagnosis of, 88–89
   prevalence of, 87
   treatment of, 89–90

Pancreatic lipase, 85
Pancreatitis, 90–91
Pansinusitis, on sinus x-rays, 29
Pantoprazole (Protonix), 99, 345
Parenteral nutrition. *See* IV nutrition
Partial thromboplastin time (PTT), 121
Patient Registry, of CF Foundation, 316
PELD (Pediatric End-stage Liver Disease), 189
Penicillins, 329–331
PEP mask, 43–44
Pepsin, 85
Peripheral IVs, 144
Phrenic nerves, 175
Physical education , 199
Physical therapists, 142
PICC lines, 144, 145
Pilocarpine, 110
Piperacillin, 330–331
PIVKA (protein induced by vitamin K absence) test, 122
Pleuritis, 69
Pleura, 164
Pleural space, 164
Pleurodesis, 165
Pneumonia, 36
Pneumothorax, 61–65, 62f, 63f, 185
   in adults, 267
   chest x-ray of, 62–63, 62f
   development of, 62, 63f
   in teenagers, 253
   treatment for, 63–65
Polyethylene glycol 3350, 92, 93, 346
Polyp medicines, 340
Polypectomy, 30
Portacaths, 145
Portal hypertension, 100, 101
Posttransplantation lymphoproliferative disease (PTLD), 172
Postural drainage, 363–369, 364f–369f
Predigested formulas, 132, 349
Prednisolone, 169t
Prednisone, 49, 168, 169t, 173, 252
Prehospitalization tour, 136
Preimplantation genetic diagnosis (PGD), 231
Prelone, 169t
Prenatal testing, 231

Preservation, 159–160
Preservation injury, 174
Prilosec (Omeprazole), 99, 345
Prograf, 168, 169t, 179
Program of Adult Care Excellence
        (PACE), 313
Proteases, 28
Proteomics, 300
Prothrombin time (PT), 121
Proton pump inhibitors (PPIs), 98–99, 345
Pseudomembranous colitis (PMC), 96
Pseudomonas aeruginosa infection,
        research on, 304–305
Puberty, delayed, 105
Pulmonary capillary, 23
Pulmonary exacerbation, 135
Pulmonary function tests (PFTs), 150
    in adults, 267
    in asthma, 75–76
    blood gas analysis in, 76
    during hospitalization, 150
    in infants and toddlers, 75
    lung volumes in, 74–75
    oximetry in, 76–77
    spirometry in, 71–74
Pulmozyme, 312

Q
Quake, 43, 44f, 364f, 371–372, 371f
Quality Improvement Initiative, by CF
        Foundation, 316
Quinolones, 333
Quorum sensing, 305

R
Radiographic enema therapy, 94
Ranitidine (Zantac), 98, 344
Rapamune, 170t
Recessive trait, 222
Rectal prolapse, 96–97, 97f
Reflux, 97–98
    treatment for, 98–99
Reproductive system
    of adults
        men, 270–271
        women, 271–272
    in CF, 105–106
    of teenagers, 254–255

Research, 296
    on airway fluid/mucus composition,
        302–304
    basic, 296
    on CF gene, 297–299
    on *CFTR* gene and protein function,
        299–302
    on chronic lung infections, 304–306
    clinical, 296
    on development of new drug
        treatment, 296–297
    ethics
        investigators' responsibilities, 309
        patients' responsibilities, 309–310
    on exercise tolerance, 308
    and future challenges, 308
    and future treatment, 296–310
    on gastrointestinal system and
        nutrition, 307–308
    on inflammation, 306–307
    organ/tissue donation for, 293, 310
    on psychology and education, 308
Research Development Program, by CF
        Foundation, 314
Residents, 141
Residential area, 202, 203
Residual volume, 74, 75
Respiratory failure, 24, 67–68
Respiratory infections, 34
    bacterial, 37–38
    bronchiolitis, 36
    bronchitis, 36
    fungal, 38–39
    pneumonia, 36
    upper respiratory tract, 34–35
        colds, 34–35
        sinusitis, 34
    viral, 38
Respiratory muscles, 25–26
Respiratory syncytial virus (RSV), 36, 335
    drugs for, 335
Respiratory system, 21
    airways in, 22–23, 23f
    alveoli in, 22, 23f
    anatomy and function of, 22–28
    bronchi in, 22–23, 23f
    bronchioles in, 22, 23f
    control of breathing in, 24–25

Respiratory system (*Continued*)
  gas transfer and delivery in, 23–24
  lower respiratory tract in CF, 31–33
    (*See also* Lungs)
  lung defenses in, 26–28
  respiratory muscles, role of, 25–26
  upper respiratory tract in CF, 29
    nasal polyps, 29–30
    sinuses, 29
Respiratory therapists, 142
Retrograde amnesia, 184
R117H gene mutation, 19
Ribavirin, 335
Rickets, 120
Rimantadine, 334–335
Running
  clothes for, 215
  equipment for, 214
  safety considerations for, 215–216
  starting of, 215

S
Salbutamol, 328
Saline, for thinning mucus, 249–250
Salt
  membrane transport of, 2–5
  in sweat, 2
Salt loss, 111–112
Sandimmune, 169t
Sequential single-lung transplantation,
    165–166
Scar tissue, 54
School, 200–201
Scuba diving, 202
Second-hand smoke, 39, 260, 278
Senna (Senekot), 347
72-hour fecal fat collection, 88
Sickle cell disease, 11
Sidestream smoke, 260
Sildenafil, 342
Simethicone (Mylicon), 347
Simulect, 170t
Sinuses, in adults with CF, 266
Sinusitis, 34
Sinus medicines, 340
Sirolimus, 170t, 179, 350
Small bowel bacterial overgrowth
    (SBBO), 94–95

Small intestine, 84f
  digestion in, 85–86
Smoke, avoidance of, 200–201
Smoking, 200–201
Social security disability insurance, 276
Social workers, 142
Sodium
  excess levels of, 5, 6f
  membrane transport of, 2–5
Sodium transport, chloride transport
    and, 3–4
Solumedrol, 169t
SourceCF multivitamin, 119
Spirometry, 71–74
Spironolactone (Aldactone), 342
Spleen, 100
Splenomegaly, 100
Sputum, 33. *See also* Mucus
Staphylococcus, 158
Stent, 179
Sternal bowing, 78
Steroids, 335–337, 349
  for fighting inflammation, 252–253
  for reducing inflammation, 49
Sticky mucus, 1, 28
  causes of, 7, 31
  research on, 302
Stomach, 84f
  digestion in, 85
Stool
  fatty, 87, 88
  meconium, 91
Structure-based drug design,
    300–301
Sudden infant death syndrome
    (SIDS), 98
Sulfa drugs, 331–332
Sulfisoxazole, 331
Summer camp, 202
Sweat gland
  in CF, 108–109, 109f
  normal, 108, 109f
Sweat, salty, 1, 6, 254
Sweat test, 1, 14–16, 109–110
  Gibson-Cooke method, 110–111
  in infants, 92
  for meconium ileus, 92
  problems with, 111

Swimming
    equipment for, 216
    learning, 217
    place for doing, 216
    safety considerations for, 217
    starting of, 217
Symbicort, 336

T
Tacrolimus, 168, 350. *See also* Prograf
Teenagers, 245–264
    attitude toward CF, 258–260
    body image of, 259–260
    career decisions by, 264
    and dating, 262
    decision to move away from home,
        263–264
    education planning of, 263
    medical issues facing, 246–255
    psychological and family issues faced
        by, 257–262
    relationships of
        with CF patients, 261
        with friends, 260–262
        with girl/boyfriends, 262
        with parents, 257–258
        with siblings, 258
    self-care by, 255–257
    sex for, 262–263
Testosterone, 131, 348
Tetracyclines, 332–333
TheraPEP devices, 44, 45f
Therapeutics Development Network
    (TDN), 296
Therapeutics Development Program
    (TDP), 313
"Therapeutic trial," 89
Thiazides, 342
Thrush, 329
Ticarcillin, 330–331
Timentin, 331
TOBI, 55, 306, 313
Tobramycin, 332
Total body plethysmograph, 74
Total lung capacity, 74
Trachea, 22, 23f, 27
Transbronchial biopsy, 183
Transesophageal echocardiography, 174

Transjugular intrahepatic portosystemic
    shunt (TIPS) procedure, 101
Transplantation, 154–193. *See also* Liver
    transplantation; Lung
    transplantation
    candidate for, 155
    care after, 180–186
    combination lung–liver, 192–193
    complications with, 167–180
    decision to go for, 187–188
    definition of, 154
    donor in, 154
    future of, 193
    history of, 154–155
    liver, 188–192
    lung, 156–167
    preservation before, 159–160
    recipient in, 154
    rejection in, 168
        pevention of, 168 (*See also*
            Immunosuppressive medications)
Transplant list
    for liver transplantation, 189
    for lung transplantation, 159–163
Transplant-related drugs, 349–351
Travel, 201–202
Trimethoprim–sulfamethoxazole
    (TMP-SMX), 331
Tube feeding, 132–134
TUMS, 99
Type 1 insulin deficiency diabetes
    mellitus (T1DM), 104–105

U
United Network for Organ Sharing
    (UNOS), 160
Uridine triphosphate, 10
Urinary stress incontinence, 273
Ursodeoxycholic acid (UDCA), 100
Ursodiol (Actigal), 348

V
Vancomycin, 333
Varicella (chickenpox) vaccine, 53
Varicella-zoster immune globulin
    (VZIG), 53
Varices, 100
Vas deferens, 106, 234, 255, 270, 282

Vest, 372–374, 372f–373f
Viagra, 342
Vibrating vest, 248–249
Viral infections, in CF patients, 38
Viruses as vectors, 298
Vitamin A, 120
Vitamin D, 120–121
Vitamin E, 121
Vitamin K, 121–122
    for hemoptysis, 60
Vitamins, 348
Volume-time curve, 72, 73f
Volvulus, 94
Voriconazole (Vfend), 335
VX-809, 302
VX-770 pills, 301–302

W
Weight loss, due to malnutrition, 113–115, 114f

Wheezing, 33
White blood cells, 28

X
Xopenex (levalbuterol), 328
X-rays
    chest, 77–78
    overinflation of lungs in, 79f
    of sinuses, 29
Xylocaine jelly, 184

Z
Zafirlukast, 337
Zantac (ranitidine), 98, 344
Zenapax, 170t
Zinc, 120
Zithromax (Azithromycin), 179
Zone of inhibition, 81
Zosyn, 331